PCEP

Perinatal Continuing Education Program

Neonatal Care

D1408673

BOOK II

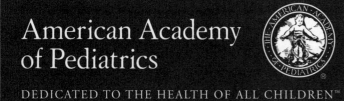

American Academy
of Pediatrics

DEDICATED TO THE HEALTH OF ALL CHILDREN™

PCEP

The original version of these self-instructional books was developed in 1978 at the University of Virginia under contract (#N09-HR-2926) from the National Heart, Lung, and Blood Institute. Subsequent versions have been developed independently by the authors.

John Kattwinkel, MD
Lynn J. Cook, RNC, MPH
Hallam Hurt, MD
George A. Nowacek, PhD
Jerry G. Short, PhD

Primary authors for the obstetrical content

Warren M. Crosby, MD
Lynn J. Cook, RNC, MPH

The neonatal resuscitation information in these books is written to be consistent with the national guidelines approved by the following groups:
  American Academy of Pediatrics
  American Heart Association
  American College of Obstetricians and Gynecologists

Several different approaches to specific perinatal problems may be acceptable. The PCEP books have been written to present specific recommendations rather than to include all currently acceptable options. The recommendations in these books should not be considered the only accepted standard of care. We encourage development of local standards in consultation with your regional perinatal center staff.

Library of Congress Control Number: 2006929344

ISBN-13: 978-1-58110-217-8
ISBN-10: 1-58110-217-8

PC0003

Continuing Education Credit

Continuing education credit is available for every perinatal health care provider who studies the Perinatal Continuing Education Program (PCEP) books. These American Medical Association (AMA) credits or contact hours/continuing education units (CEUs) are available to physicians, nurses, nurse practitioners, certified nurse midwives, respiratory therapists, and any other professional who provides care to pregnant women or newborn babies.

American Medical Association

Accreditation Statement

The University of Virginia School of Medicine is accredited by the Accreditation Council for Continuing Medical Education (ACCME) to provide continuing medical education for physicians.

The University of Virginia School of Medicine designates this educational activity for a maximum of 51 *AMA PRA Category 1 Credit(s)*™. Physicians should only claim credit commensurate with the extent of their participation in the activity.

The University of Virginia School of Medicine awards 0.1 CEU per contact hour to each nonphysician participant who successfully completes this educational activity. The CEU is a nationally recognized unit of measure for continuing education and training activities that meet specific educational planning requirements. The University of Virginia School of Medicine maintains a permanent record of participants who have been awarded CEUs.

Conflict of Interest Disclosures

As a provider accredited by the ACCME, the Office of Continuing Medical Education of the University of Virginia School of Medicine must ensure balance, independence, objectivity, and scientific rigor in all its individually sponsored or jointly sponsored educational activities. All faculty participating in a sponsored activity are expected to disclose to the activity audience any significant financial interest or other relationship (1) with the manufacturer(s) of any commercial product(s) and/or provider(s) of commercial services discussed in an educational presentation and (2) with any commercial supporters of the activity (significant financial interest or other relationship can include such things as grants or research support, employee, consultant, major stock holder, member of speakers bureau, etc). The intent of this disclosure is not to prevent a speaker with a significant financial or other relationship from making a presentation, but rather to provide listeners with information on which they can make their own judgments. It remains for the audience to determine whether the speaker's interests or relationships may influence the presentation with regard to exposition or conclusion.

The University of Virginia School of Medicine, as an ACCME provider, requires that all faculty presenters identify and disclose any off-label uses for pharmaceutical and medical device products. The University of Virginia School of Medicine recommends that each physician fully review all the available data on new products or procedures prior to instituting them with patients.

John Kattwinkel, MD, has disclosed no significant financial relationships with manufacturers of products discussed in these materials and has disclosed no off-label uses of any US Food and Drug Administration (FDA)-approved pharmaceutical products or medical devices.

Lynn J. Cook, RNC, MPH, has disclosed no significant financial relationships with manufacturers of products discussed in these materials and has disclosed no off-label uses of any FDA-approved pharmaceutical products or medical devices.

Hallam Hurt, MD, has disclosed no significant financial relationships with manufacturers of products discussed in these materials and has disclosed no off-label uses of any FDA-approved pharmaceutical products or medical devices.

George A. Nowacek, PhD, has disclosed no significant financial relationships with manufacturers of products discussed in these materials and has disclosed no off-label uses of any FDA-approved pharmaceutical products or medical devices.

Jerry G. Short, PhD, has disclosed no significant financial relationships with manufacturers of products discussed in these materials and has disclosed no off-label uses of any FDA-approved pharmaceutical products or medical devices.

Warren M. Crosby, MD, has disclosed no significant financial relationships with manufacturers of products discussed in these materials and has disclosed no off-label uses of any FDA-approved pharmaceutical products or medical devices.

AMA PRA Category 1 Credit(s)™ or Contact Hour Credit

Credit is given only for complete books, not individual educational units. Possible hours: Book I, 10.5; Book II: Maternal and Fetal Care, 15.0; Book II: Neonatal Care, 15.0; Book III, 10.5.

Required submission items

1. *Pretest and posttest answer pages* for *EACH* book studied (at the end of each book)

2. *Evaluation form* (precedes answer pages at the end of each book)

3. *Continuing education credit registration form* (ONE form per submission) (download from www.pcep.org/cec.html)

4. *Payment*, according to information given on the continuing education credit registration form (www.pcep.org/cec.html) is required.

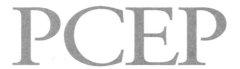

PCEP
Perinatal Continuing Education Program

BOOK I

Maternal and Fetal Evaluation and Immediate Newborn Care

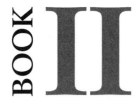

Maternal and Fetal Care

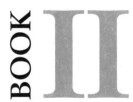

Neonatal Care

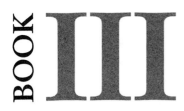

Specialized Newborn Care

Unit 1   Thermal Environment

Objectives

In this unit you will learn

A. The causes and consequences of hypothermia (low body temperature) and hyperthermia (high body temperature)

B. How to minimize heat loss in infants

C. How to control thermal environment to keep metabolic expenditure by an infant to a minimum (neutral thermal environment)

D. How to operate radiant warmers and incubators

Unit 1 Pretest

Before reading the unit, please answer the following questions. Select the *one best* answer to each question (unless otherwise instructed). Record your answers on the answer sheet that is the last page in this book *and* on the test.

1. An axillary temperature of 35.8°C (96.6°F) in a preterm infant represents

   A. Hypothermia (low body temperature)
   B. Normal body temperature
   C. Hyperthermia (high body temperature)

2. Which of the following babies does *not* need to have his/her temperature checked more often than normal routine?

   A. A term baby with hypoglycemia
   B. A 32-week baby appropriate for gestational age
   C. A 40-week baby small for gestational age
   D. A 41-week baby appropriate for gestational age

3. Which of the following methods is *most* appropriate to regulate the temperature of a term baby small for gestational age with hypoglycemia?

   A. Clothed, in a crib with blankets
   B. In an incubator, with the air temperature set at 36.0°C (96.8°F)
   C. Under a radiant warmer, with the servocontrol sensor set to keep the skin temperature of the baby's trunk at 36.5°C (97.8°F)
   D. In an incubator, with the air temperature set at 37.0°C (98.6°F)

4. Which of the following is *most* appropriate when a baby is receiving care under a radiant warmer?

   A. Set the radiant warmer to the baby's neutral thermal environment temperature and tape the servocontrol probe to the exposed side of his trunk.
   B. Set the servocontrol sensor to 36.5°C (97.8°F) and tape the probe to the exposed side of his trunk.
   C. Set the servocontrol sensor to 36.5°C (97.8°F) and tape the probe to the side of his trunk resting on the mattress.
   D. Set the servocontrol sensor to 35.5°C (97.0°F) and tape the probe to the side of his trunk resting on the mattress.

5. Which of the following methods of taking a baby's temperature is *not* recommended for frequent vital signs?

   A. Rectal
   B. Axillary
   C. Abdominal skin
   D. Any, of the above methods is appropriate for frequent vital signs

6. **True   False**   A baby whose temperature is 35.2°C (95.4°F) should have a blood glucose screening test checked.

7. **True   False**   When a baby is in the appropriate neutral thermal environment temperature range in an incubator, the baby's rectal or axillary temperature will always be normal (37.0°C or 98.6°F).

8. **True   False**   An elevated temperature is most commonly caused by an infection in a baby.

9. **True   False**   Portholes of an incubator left open can result in conductive heat loss.

10. **True   False**   A newborn who has a skin temperature of 35.0°C (95.0°F) will have a higher metabolic rate than a baby who has a skin temperature of 36.5°C (97.8°F).

11. **True   False**   Delayed drying of a baby after delivery promotes evaporative heat loss.

12. **True   False**   A baby with a slightly low body temperature requires fewer calories and less oxygen than a baby with a normal temperature.

13. **True   False**   During the first week after birth, the neutral thermal environmental range is the same for all babies of the same birth weight, regardless of gestational age.

For each question, please make sure you have marked your answer on the test and on the answer sheet (last page in book). The test is for you; the answer sheet will need to be turned in for continuing education credit.

1. What Is Temperature Control?

Temperature control means regulating a baby's body temperature with external equipment. If the thermal environment is properly controlled, a baby will not have to use extra oxygen and calories to produce heat. An otherwise healthy baby can become sick if cold-stressed.

2. How Does a Baby Produce Heat?

Babies produce heat in a different way from adults. Babies have a special substance called brown fat. They use oxygen and calories to break down this brown fat to produce heat. Preterm and small for gestational age infants have less brown fat than term infants and appropriate for gestational age infants.

Babies who are cold do not shiver to warm themselves.

Checking body temperature is the only way to know if a baby is cold.

3. How Does a Baby Lose Heat?

Babies can lose body heat *very* quickly. Body heat may be lost in any combination of 4 ways.

A. Conduction

Conductive heat loss occurs when a baby is in contact with cold objects. Examples of *preventing* conductive heat loss are
- Pre-warm receiving bed in the delivery room.
- Cover cold scale surface when weighing a baby.
- Change wet diapers and bed linens.

B. Convection

Convective heat loss occurs when cold air circulates around a baby. Examples of *preventing* convective heat loss are
- Keep delivery room warm.
- Put a hat on the baby soon after delivery.
- Keep the baby out of the draft of air conditioners.
- Keep incubator portholes closed when not working with the baby; work through portholes for procedures rather than opening the side of the incubator.
- Warm and humidify the oxygen/air mixture for babies receiving oxygen therapy.

C. Evaporation

Evaporative heat loss occurs when a liquid evaporates from a warm surface. When a baby is wet, evaporative heat loss increases significantly. Examples of *preventing* evaporative heat loss are
- Dry a baby quickly after delivery.
- Delay bathing a baby until body temperature is normal and stable for several hours.
- Change wet linen promptly.
- Warm and humidify the oxygen/air mixture for babies receiving oxygen therapy.

D. Radiation

Radiant heat loss occurs when a baby is near but not in direct contact with a cold object. The baby radiates heat to the nearest solid object. Adults experience radiant heat loss in a warm room on a cold day when they go near a closed window and feel a chill. They have not touched the window, but some of their body heat has been transmitted or radiated to the cold windowpane. In much the same way, babies in incubators lose heat to the incubator wall, which has been cooled by the room temperature. Examples of *preventing* radiant heat loss are

- Keep nursery warm, even if a baby is in an incubator.
- Keep a baby away from cold windows and walls, especially if the baby is in an open crib or a single-wall incubator.*
- Use double-walled incubators whenever possible.*

In addition to the actions listed above, some babies may benefit from special measures to prevent heat loss. For example, thermal warming packs with controlled maximum heat (commercially available) may be useful while transporting sick or small babies from a delivery room to the nursery.

 Hypothermia (low body temperature) at any time is hazardous for a baby. Becoming chilled after delivery should not be an expected occurrence.

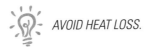 *AVOID HEAT LOSS.*

---

*Radiant heat loss is more common with single-wall incubators. Double-walled incubators are designed to reduce radiant heat loss significantly because a layer of warm air between the walls keeps the inner wall at the neutral thermal environment temperature, while the outer wall may be much colder.

Self-Test

Now answer these questions to test yourself on the information in the last section.

A1. How do babies produce heat to keep themselves warm?

_____

A2. **True False** Babies can keep themselves warm by shivering, as do adults.

A3. **True False** Babies use oxygen and calories to produce body heat.

A4. Give an example of conductive heat loss.

_____

A5. Give an example of convective heat loss.

_____

A6. Give an example of evaporative heat loss.

_____

A7. Give an example of radiant heat loss.

_____

Check your answers with the list that follows the Recommended Routines. Correct any incorrect answers and review the appropriate section in the unit.

4. How Are Temperatures Taken?

There are 3 acceptable ways to measure a baby's temperature.

A. Rectal

This is usually the first temperature taken after delivery. It gives a good estimate of deep body or core temperature, and checks patency of the anus.

Rectal measurement of a baby's temperature is seldom indicated after the initial measurement. Use of rectal thermometers may cause perforation of the colon or may result in cardiorespiratory instability due to vagal nerve stimulation.

 Measuring temperature rectally is not recommended for frequent or routine vital signs.

B. Axillary

This is the best way to take a baby's temperature for frequent vital signs. In most circumstances, an axillary temperature can be considered the same as the rectal temperature, as long as the baby's arm is kept next to his/her side while the temperature is being taken.

C. Skin

This is a convenient way to measure the temperature of a baby requiring a skin probe, such as when an incubator or radiant warmer is used in servocontrol mode. Skin temperatures are lower than axillary or rectal temperatures. Therefore, a baby's temperature should also be checked intermittently with an axillary or, in some cases, a rectal measurement.

Note: Temperature measurements taken with an ear probe are a quick way to check a baby's temperature. Tympanic measurements, however, have *not* been shown to be reliable in neonates and, therefore, are *not* recommended.

5. How Should a Baby's Temperature Be Interpreted?

A. Normal

All infants (large, small, preterm, post-term, term) have the same normal temperature.
• Axillary or rectal: 37.0°C (98.6°F)
• Skin: 36.5°C (97.8°F)

 Although a single "normal" temperature is given above, it is clear that all babies will not have this exact temperature at all times. However, this normal value should be your goal when regulating any infant's temperature.

B. Hyperthermia

An elevated or higher than normal temperature

Reasons for high body temperatures in newborns include

1. Directly Overheating a Baby

   • Under a radiant warmer with the warmer set incorrectly
   • Under certain types of phototherapy lights

2. Overheating a Baby's Environment

   • In an incubator with the temperature set incorrectly
   • In a bassinet and over-bundled in a warm room

3. Blood Infection (sepsis): In contrast to adults or older children, newborns usually do *not* have a fever when an infection is present. Some infected babies, however, will have elevated temperatures.

An overheated baby uses excessive oxygen and calories as the body's metabolism is increased. Because of a reduced ability to sweat, overheated babies may appear normal. Touching a baby's skin is not a reliable way to determine if a baby's body temperature is elevated. The only way to know if a newborn is overheated is to take the baby's temperature.

C. Hypothermia

A lower than normal temperature

Reasons for low body temperatures in newborns include

1. Blood Infection (sepsis): Hypothermia is more commonly a sign of sepsis than is hyperthermia in a newborn.

2. Heat Loss to the Environment (by conduction, convection, evaporation, and/or radiation)

A cold baby cannot shiver and may appear normal. Low body temperature cannot reliably be identified by feeling a baby's skin. The only way to know if a newborn is hypothermic is to take the baby's temperature.

 Monitor each baby's temperature. If an abnormal temperature is found, investigate the cause.

Self-Test

Now answer these questions to test yourself on the information in the last section.

B1. What are 3 acceptable ways to measure a baby's temperature?

_____

_____

_____

B2. Which method of taking a baby's temperature is not recommended for routine vital signs?

_____

B3. Which 2 methods of taking a baby's temperature will show about the same body temperature?

_____ and _____

B4. What is the abdominal skin temperature of a normal, healthy baby?

_____

B5. Which of the following is the *most* common reason for an elevated temperature in a newborn?
   A. An infection
   B. Incubator air temperature set too high
   C. Being born preterm

B6. What are 2 common reasons a baby will have a lower than normal temperature?
   A. A blood infection (sepsis)
   B. Excess caloric intake
   C. Heat loss to the environment

Check your answers with the list that follows the Recommended Routines. Correct any incorrect answers and review the appropriate section in the unit.

6. What Happens When a Baby Is Chilled or Cold-Stressed?

When babies are chilled, their metabolic rate increases. Three consequences of an increased metabolic rate are

- Hypoglycemia (low blood glucose)
- Acidosis (low blood pH)
- Hypoxia (inadequate oxygen for brain and body tissue)

A baby does not need to be severely cold-stressed to develop hypoglycemia, acidosis, and/or hypoxia. Some babies will demonstrate these findings if their temperatures drop only 1 or 2 degrees. Tiny babies are especially vulnerable to cold-stress.

A. Hypoglycemia

When an infant is chilled, the metabolic rate will increase to produce heat. This increased metabolic rate consumes glycogen stores and blood glucose faster than normal. A chilled baby may, therefore, develop hypoglycemia.

B. Acidosis

When an infant is chilled, brown fat is converted to heat and fatty acids. These fatty acids, and lactic acid from incomplete glucose breakdown, are poured into the bloodstream, resulting in lower blood pH. A chilled baby may, therefore, become acidotic. Acidosis, in turn, can cause vasoconstriction of pulmonary blood vessels, resulting in low blood oxygen levels.

C. Hypoxia

When a baby is chilled, extra oxygen is needed to produce heat. For example, when a baby's temperature drops to 35.0°C (95.0°F), twice as much oxygen is needed than at 37.0°C (98.6°F).

Chilled babies with normal lungs will increase their respiratory rates to get extra oxygen and may show signs of respiratory distress (grunting, nasal flaring, retractions, and/or tachypnea). Allowing a baby to become hypothermic, or not warming a baby who has become chilled, can make an otherwise healthy baby sick.

Chilled babies with diseased lungs may become so ill that they are not able to get enough oxygen to maintain brain and body functions. Hypothermia in a baby with respiratory disease can significantly worsen the baby's condition.

 Hypothermia can cause a healthy baby to become ill and a sick baby to deteriorate dramatically.

7. What Happens When a Baby Is Overheated?

Babies who become overheated will increase their respiratory rates, heart rates, and metabolic rates. This added stress might compromise an already sick or at-risk baby.

8. Which Babies Have Difficulty Controlling Their Own Temperatures?

Some babies are at greater risk for being cold-stressed, while others are at increased risk for being overheated. All of these babies should have their temperatures taken frequently.

A. Babies More Likely to Be Cold-Stressed

1. Preterm Babies

    Preterm babies have not had time to build up white fat for insulation or brown fat for heat production. Compared with term babies, preterm babies also have a greater surface area in relation to body weight from which to lose heat.

    They are *very* susceptible to temperature insults from the relatively cool air of delivery rooms, bathing, drafts, and inadequately warmed incubators. The smaller the baby, the greater the risk of cold-stress.

2. Small for Gestational Age (SGA) Babies

    Because they are malnourished, SGA babies do not have as much brown fat for heat production or white fat for insulation. Also, they have a relatively large surface area, for their body weight, from which to lose body heat. However, their metabolic rate may be higher than in preterm infants of comparable size. SGA babies are more likely to become either hypothermic or hyperthermic.

3. Sick Babies

    All sick babies use extra oxygen and calories just to maintain normal body functions. Their organ systems and metabolism may not be able to tolerate the additional stress of being chilled.

 While some babies are particularly vulnerable to cold-stress, any newborn—even term, healthy babies—can quickly become chilled.

It is important to protect the thermal environment of all babies.

B. Babies More Likely to Be Overheated

1. Babies in incubators

2. Babies under radiant warmers

3. Babies under phototherapy lights

Now answer these questions to test yourself on the information in the last section.

C1. What are 3 problems that may develop if a baby is chilled?

_____

_____

_____

C2. Which babies should have their temperatures taken more often?

_____

_____

_____

_____

C3. **True False**   A baby in respiratory distress can become critically ill from being chilled.

C4. **True False**   Chilled babies have increased metabolic rates.

C5. **True False**   Overheated babies have increased metabolic rates.

Check your answers with the list that follows the Recommended Routines. Correct any incorrect answers and review the appropriate section in the unit.

9. How Does Temperature Control Help to Minimize Oxygen and Caloric Requirements?

The best way to minimize oxygen and caloric requirements is to put a baby in an incubator or under a radiant warmer and supply enough heat so that heat losses and heat production are balanced at the lowest possible levels. This environment is called the neutral thermal environment (NTE). In an incubator, there is a narrow range of air temperature that provides an NTE. Under a radiant warmer, NTE is accomplished by maintaining a normal skin temperature with servocontrol.

 Neutral thermal environment (NTE) is an environment in which a baby uses the least amount of energy to maintain a normal body temperature. Different amounts of external heat are required to establish NTE for babies of different sizes and ages.

10. How Do You Determine a Baby's Neutral Thermal Environment?

A. Incubator

A baby in the appropriate NTE incubator air temperature range should maintain a skin temperature close to 36.5°C (97.8°F) and a rectal or axillary temperature close to 37.0°C (98.6°F). The details of adjusting an incubator to NTE are described in Skill Unit 2. Briefly, the procedure for determining a baby's NTE is as follows:

1. Birth to 6 Days Old

   • Estimate the baby's gestational age (Book I, Gestational Age and Size).
   • Look at Figure 1.2 on page 20 and find the appropriate temperature band on the graph for the baby's gestational age and postnatal age (days since birth).

2. Baby 7 Days or Older

   • Determine the baby's weight in kilograms.
   • Look at Figure 1.3 on page 20 and find the appropriate temperature band on the graph for the baby's current weight and postnatal age.

Example: Baby Jefferson is born at 33 weeks' gestational age and is appropriate size. What temperature should his incubator air temperature be on day 3 to provide NTE?

• Turn to the graphs on page 20. Figure 1.2 shows that the NTE temperature for a 33-week gestation baby at 3 days of age is 35.0°C (95.0°F). Set the incubator temperature to 35.0°C and monitor the baby's temperature.

At 14 days of age Baby Jefferson weighs 1.5 kg. What should the incubator air temperature be on day 14?

• Page 20, Figure 1.3 shows that the NTE temperature for a 1.5-kg baby at 14 days postnatal age is 33.5°C (92.4°F). Set the incubator temperature to 33.5°C and continue to monitor the baby's temperature.

Note: The NTE temperatures in the graphs are given as guidelines and should be considered close estimates of a baby's NTE. The NTE for an individual baby may vary a few tenths of a degree from the graph temperatures.

B. Radiant Warmer

A baby's NTE is provided by a radiant warmer when normal skin temperature is maintained using servocontrol. When skin temperature is maintained close to 36.5°C (97.8°F) (slightly lower in very big babies and slightly higher in very small babies), core or rectal temperature will be close to 37.0°C (98.6°F), and oxygen requirements will be minimal. The details of using a radiant warmer are described in Skill Unit 1. Briefly, the procedure is as follows:

1. *Keep the baby unclothed, or with only a small diaper.* This is to allow the baby's skin to absorb the radiant heat. A thin transparent plastic sheet placed over the baby (take care not to obstruct the baby's airway) may help to decrease convective and evaporative heat losses in small preterm babies.

2. *Cover the tip of the probe so it is* not *directly exposed to the radiant heat.* Usually, a commercially available reflective cover is used for this. The adhesive side holds the probe tip in place and the exposed side reflects the radiant heat so the probe measures only the baby's body temperature. Be sure the tip is completely in contact with the baby's skin.

3. *Tape the probe to the side of the baby away from the mattress.* If the baby is lying on his/her back, tape the servocontrol probe to the baby's abdomen. Tape the probe to the baby's lower back if the baby is lying on his/her stomach.

   The probe should not be placed between the baby and the mattress. That location will result in falsely high skin temperature readings and cause the baby to be *under*heated. The servocontrol mechanism will stop providing heat in response to the false temperature, until the temperature registered drops below the preset temperature. The baby's actual temperature may be significantly lower.

4. *Be sure the probe is taped to a fleshy area of the baby's trunk.* Avoid the extremities and boney prominences, such as the spine, sternum, and scapula. The probe will register falsely low temperatures when taped in these areas.

5. *Set the servocontrol mechanism to 36.5°C, "automatic" control.* This will cause the radiant warmer to turn on or off as the baby's skin temperature falls below or rises above 36.5°C (97.8°F).

C. Supplemental Oxygen

Inspired oxygen/air temperatures below a baby's NTE can cool a baby. Babies who require oxygen therapy should have the oxygen/air mixture humidified and heated to the baby's NTE temperature. This is true whether a baby is in an incubator or under a radiant warmer.

Heat from an incubator or radiant warmer will *not* adequately warm an oxygen/air mixture. A separate heated humidifier is required. The temperature setting for the heated humidifier is determined from the NTE charts, the same way that incubator temperatures are determined.

Excessively high temperatures (particularly higher than 37.0°C [98.6°F]) for oxygen/air mixture should also be avoided because they can overheat a baby.

Now answer these questions to test yourself on the information in the last section. Use the charts and flow diagram in the next section, as necessary.

D1. Providing neutral thermal environment with an incubator includes

    A. Setting the incubator air temperature to 37.0°C (98.6°F).

    B. Setting the incubator air temperature according to the baby's weight.

    C. Setting the incubator air temperature according to the baby's age and weight.

D2. The purpose of the neutral thermal environment is to

    A. Prevent overheating a baby.

    B. Individualize a baby's care.

    C. Minimize the oxygen and calories a baby needs.

    D. Increase a baby's metabolic rate.

D3. What is the neutral thermal environment incubator air temperature for a baby born at 32 weeks' gestation on the first day after birth?

    _____°C

D4. What is the neutral thermal environment incubator air temperature for a 10-day-old baby who weighs 1,300 g?

    _____°C

D5. A 1,500-g (3 lb, 5 oz) infant under a servocontrolled radiant warmer has a skin temperature of 36.4°C (97.6°F) and a rectal temperature of 37.0°C (98.6°F). Is this baby in a neutral thermal environment?

    Yes _____   No _____

Check your answers with the list that follows the Recommended Routines. Correct any incorrect answers and review the appropriate section in the unit.

11. Will Providing a Neutral Thermal Environment Always Work?

A. Incubator

The NTE incubator air temperature (see the figures on page 20) will keep a baby's temperature normal only if the baby

- Is naked in an incubator
- Does not have an infection (is not septic)
- Is appropriate size for gestational age
- Is *not* extremely small (<1,000 g or 2 lb, 3 oz)

AND sources of heat loss are controlled

- Wet diapers are removed promptly.
- Oxygen (if used) is humidified and warmed to the baby's NTE temperature.
- Incubator portholes are closed after each entry into the incubator.
- Outside walls of the incubator are not unusually cold (eg, in a cold nursery or in front of an air conditioner).

 If a baby is hypothermic in the appropriate environmental temperature, consider that there are abnormal routes of heat loss or the baby has an infection.

B. Radiant Warmers

Under a radiant warmer, a baby's skin temperature will be maintained in the normal range, even if there are extra heat losses. You should routinely check for possible sources of heat loss (cold, non-humidified oxygen, wet diapers or linens, etc) for infants under radiant warmers, even when a baby's temperature is normal. In addition, you should monitor closely for other signs of infection (Book II: Neonatal Care, Infections) because the temperature changes seen with infection will also be masked.

 When using a radiant warmer, remember to check for sources of heat loss and have a high index of suspicion for infection.

If the servocontrol probe is taped incorrectly (tip is not entirely in contact with the baby's skin) or positioned incorrectly (taped to a boney prominence or to the mattress side of the baby), the skin temperature may register "normal," but the baby's actual axillary or rectal temperature may be high or low.

 Do not rely on the skin temperature registered on a radiant warmer as the measure of a baby's temperature. Periodically use a standard thermometer to check the axillary temperature.

12. Will Managing a Baby's Temperature With Servocontrol in an Incubator Provide a Neutral Thermal Environment?

Not necessarily. Many incubators are equipped with an optional servocontrol mechanism. This mechanism can be used, with a probe taped to the baby's trunk, in much the same way that radiant warmers are used to maintain a baby's skin temperature at a set temperature. All of the possible problems with radiant warmers are also possible when servocontrol is used with an incubator.

While a baby's temperature will be normal, the baby may be using extra calories and oxygen to produce heat, with the incubator environmental temperature supplying only a small portion of the total heat the baby needs to stay warm. In addition, temperature changes associated with infection or abnormal heat loss may be masked.

To minimize these problems, it is important to use the correct technique for incubator servocontrol, which is similar to the technique used for radiant warmers. While the details of managing a baby's temperature with servocontrol in an incubator are not discussed in this unit, the main points are

1. Keep the baby unclothed, or with only a small diaper.

2. Position the probe on the side of the baby away from the mattress. If the baby is lying on his/her back, tape the servocontrol probe to the baby's abdomen. Tape the probe to the baby's lower back if the baby is lying on his/her stomach.

   The probe should not be placed between the baby and the mattress. That location will result in falsely high skin temperature readings and cause the baby to be *under*heated. The servocontrol mechanism will respond to the falsely high temperature and stop providing heat until the false temperature drops below the preset temperature. The baby's actual temperature may be significantly lower.

3. Tape the tip of the probe so it is completely in contact with the baby's skin. Be sure the entire tip is in contact with the baby's skin so the temperature registered accurately indicates the baby's skin temperature. Tape or commercially available foam pads (with adhesive back) may be used to secure the probe tip.

4. Be sure the probe is taped to a fleshy area of the baby's trunk. Avoid the extremities and boney prominences, such as the spine, sternum, and scapula. The probe will register falsely low temperatures when taped in these areas.

5. Set the servocontrol mechanism to 36.5°C, skin temperature. This will cause the incubator heater to turn on or off as the baby's skin temperature falls below or rises above 36.5°C (97.8°F). When a servocontrol probe is taped to a baby, be sure the mechanism is set to register skin temperature, *not* incubator air temperature.

13. If a Sick or Small Baby Has a Normal Body Temperature, Do You Still Have to Provide a Neutral Thermal Environment?

Yes. A baby will use minimal energy to maintain a normal temperature *only* in the NTE that is appropriate to the baby's age and weight.

A baby may have a normal rectal/axillary temperature even when not in the appropriate NTE. In this case, the baby must use considerable energy (calories and oxygen) to maintain a normal body temperature.

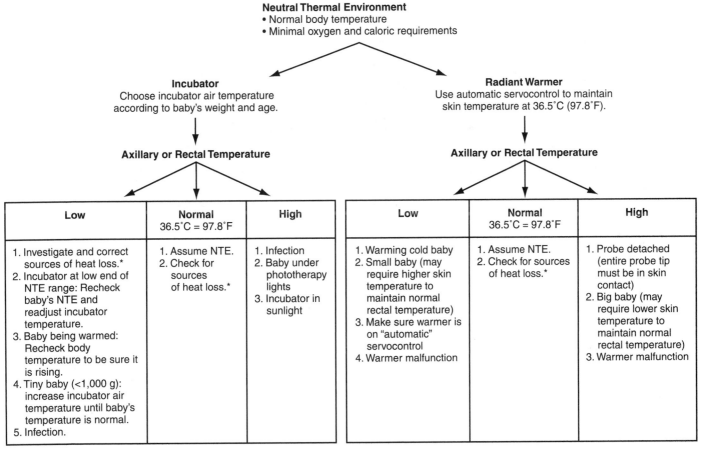

Neutral Thermal Environment
• Normal body temperature
• Minimal oxygen and caloric requirements

Incubator
Choose incubator air temperature according to baby's weight and age.

Radiant Warmer
Use automatic servocontrol to maintain skin temperature at 36.5°C (97.8°F).

Axillary or Rectal Temperature

Axillary or Rectal Temperature

Low	Normal 36.5°C = 97.8°F	High
1. Investigate and correct sources of heat loss.* 2. Incubator at low end of NTE range: Recheck baby's NTE and readjust incubator temperature. 3. Baby being warmed: Recheck body temperature to be sure it is rising. 4. Tiny baby (<1,000 g): increase incubator air temperature until baby's temperature is normal. 5. Infection.	1. Assume NTE. 2. Check for sources of heat loss.*	1. Infection 2. Baby under phototherapy lights 3. Incubator in sunlight

Low	Normal 36.5°C = 97.8°F	High
1. Warming cold baby 2. Small baby (may require higher skin temperature to maintain normal rectal temperature) 3. Make sure warmer is on "automatic" servocontrol 4. Warmer malfunction	1. Assume NTE. 2. Check for sources of heat loss.*	1. Probe detached (entire probe tip must be in skin contact) 2. Big baby (may require lower skin temperature to maintain normal rectal temperature) 3. Warmer malfunction

*Routes of heat loss commonly include incubator side opened for procedures (work through portholes), oxygen cold or non-humidified, cool nursery, wet linen, incubator near cold window, etc.

Figure 1.1. Control of Thermal Environment for Newborn Babies

Neutral Thermal Environmental Incubator Temperatures

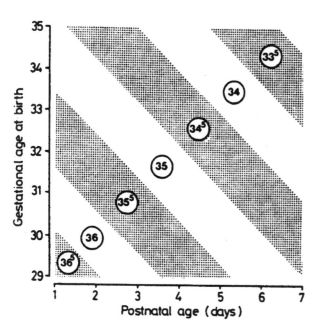

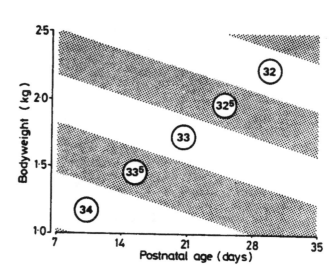

Figure 1.2. Neutral Thermal Environment (°C) During the First Week

Figure 1.3. Neutral Thermal Environment (°C) From Day 7 to 35

Incubator temperature charts are reproduced with permission from Sauer PJJ, Dane HJ, Visser HKA. *Arch Dis Child.* 1984;59:18–22.

Self-Test

Now answer these questions to test yourself on the information in the last section.

E1. A baby is in the appropriate incubator neutral thermal environment air temperature but has an axillary temperature of 35.0°C (96.0°F). What are 2 possible reasons why the baby is cold?

_____

_____

E2. **True** **False** As long as a baby is in an incubator set at the appropriate neutral thermal environment air temperature, the baby's body temperature will remain normal (37.0°C [98.6°F]).

E3. **True** **False** If a 1,800-g (4 lb) baby with respiratory distress has a normal body temperature (37.0°C [98.6°F]), he does not need to be put in a neutral thermal environment.

E4. A baby is in an incubator, with the air temperature set for the appropriate neutral thermal environment. What are 3 conditions that must be met before the baby's temperature can be expected to remain normal?

_____

_____

_____

E5. What does placing a baby in a neutral thermal environment do for the baby?

  A. Ensures that the baby will not get sick
  B. Ensures that the baby's body temperature will remain normal
  C. Ensures that the baby is using minimum energy (oxygen and calories) to maintain a normal body temperature

Check your answers with the list that follows the Recommended Routines. Correct any incorrect answers and review the appropriate section in the unit.

14. How Should a Baby's Temperature Be Regulated?

A. Clothed in a Bassinet With Nursery Temperature at 74°F to 76°F
- Full-term, well babies
- Preterm babies weighing approximately 1,600 to 1,700 g (3 lb, 8 oz–3 lb, 12 oz), who are not sick
- SGA term babies who are not sick

B. Incubator Adjusted to Appropriate NTE Air Temperature
- Preterm, appropriate for gestational age babies weighing less than 1,600 to 1,700 g (3 lb, 8 oz–4 lb)
- Sick babies who do *not* require multiple procedure

C. Radiant Warmer With Automatic Servocontrol
- Sick babies who require many procedures
- Babies whose axillary/rectal temperatures cannot be maintained at 37.0°C (98.6°F) in an incubator adjusted to NTE air temperature (abnormal routes of heat loss have been ruled out); these may include sick SGA babies, very small babies, or septic babies

D. Skin-to-Skin With Baby's Mother or Father

  1. Healthy, Term Infants

  Skin-to-skin contact between mother and baby soon after delivery will help keep a healthy, term infant warm, provided the baby is dried thoroughly and the exposed side of the infant is covered. In this situation, most women can serve as safe and effective heat sources for their infants.

  2. Small or Sick Babies, in Stable Condition

  Skin-to-skin contact between mothers or fathers and their infants has also been used for sick and preterm babies, after a baby's condition has been stabilized. For selected babies, this seems to be a safe way to provide close contact between parent and infant, while maintaining the baby's temperature. The technique carries hazards (hypothermia, disruption of therapy, etc), however, and cannot be assumed to be safe for all small or sick babies.

  Consider the risks and benefits, parental desire and preparation, and the stability of the baby's condition before undertaking skin-to-skin contact for sick or small infants. Provide ongoing monitoring of the infant's temperature and condition.

15. What Do You Do When a Baby Has a Low Body Temperature?

First, *warm the baby.* How this is done will depend on how cold the baby is.

A. Slightly Chilled Baby

A baby with a moderately low body temperature (such as 35.0°C–36.0°C or 95.0°F–96.8°F) can usually be warmed adequately in an incubator adjusted to the appropriate NTE temperature. If the baby's body temperature does not rise over 1 to 2 hours, increase the incubator temperature *slightly*, until the baby becomes warm. Warming the incubator air too quickly may induce apnea attacks, especially in preterm infants. Once the baby's temperature is normal, reestablish the NTE incubator air temperature. If a baby becomes chilled in the appropriate NTE, increase the incubator temperature, even if this means going above the NTE range. After you have begun to warm the baby, search for routes of abnormal heat loss and evaluate the baby for signs of infection (Book II: Neonatal Care, Infections), and monitor the baby for signs of cold stress: hypoglycemia, acidosis, hypoxia.

B. Severely Cold-Stressed Baby

1. In an Incubator

    • Place the baby in an incubator with the air temperature set 1°C to 1.5°C (2°F–3°F) higher than the baby's body temperature.

    • As the baby's temperature increases, increase the environmental (air) temperature to keep it 1°C to 1.5°C (2°F–3°F) above the baby's temperature.

    • When the baby's temperature reaches 37.0°C (98.6°F), set the incubator air temperature to the appropriate NTE temperature.

2. Under a Radiant Warmer

    • Attach the probe to the baby's skin and set the servocontrol to 36.5°C (97.8°F). The baby's skin temperature will rise quickly to 36.5°C, while rectal (core) temperature will rise more slowly to 37.0°C.

    • Monitor rectal temperature frequently until it is normal, then intermittent axillary temperatures may be taken.

Self-Test

Now answer these questions to test yourself on the information in the last section.

F1. A baby is born at home during the winter. Her temperature at admission to the nursery is 33°C (91.4°F). How would you warm this baby using an incubator?

_____

_____

F2. When a baby is under a radiant warmer, what temperature should be set for the servocontrol mechanism?

_____ °C or _____ °F

F3. What method for controlling the thermal environment is recommended for each of the following babies?

A. Normal, full-term, well baby: _____

B. Stable, 1,500-g preterm baby: _____

C. Sick, full-term baby *not* requiring many procedures: _____

D. Sick, preterm baby requiring many procedures: _____

E. Stable, small for gestational age, term baby: _____

F. Sick, small for gestational age, term baby: _____

F4. A baby is admitted to your nursery. You take her temperature and discover it is 35.0°C (95.0°F). How would you warm this baby?

_____

_____

F5. **True   False**   Rapid warming of incubator air temperature may lead to apnea attacks, especially in preterm infants.

Check your answers with the list that follows the Recommended Routines. Correct any incorrect answers and review the appropriate section in the unit.

Recommended Routines

All of the routines listed below are based on the principles of perinatal care presented in the unit you have just finished. They are recommended as part of routine perinatal care.

Read each routine carefully and decide whether it is standard operating procedure in your hospital. Check the appropriate blank next to each routine.

Procedure Standard in My Hospital	Needs Discussion by Our Staff	
_____	_____	1. Establish a routine of measuring body temperature frequently in all sick and at-risk babies.
_____	_____	2. Establish a policy of withholding baths from all sick babies.
_____	_____	3. Establish a policy of withholding baths from any baby until the baby's temperature has been measured and has remained normal for several hours.
_____	_____	4. Establish a policy that will ensure the continuous availability of a radiant warmer or pre-warmed incubator for any unexpected admission to the nursery.
_____	_____	5. Post the neutral thermal environment graphs and establish a policy of adjusting the environmental temperature of any occupied incubator to the appropriate neutral thermal environment temperature.
_____	_____	6. Use equipment to monitor and adjust the temperature of supplemental oxygen.

These are the answers to the self-test questions. Please check them with the answers you gave and review the information in the unit wherever necessary.

A1. They use oxygen and calories to break down brown fat.

A2. False   Babies cannot shiver to help warm themselves.

A3. True

A4. Any condition where a baby is in direct contact with a cold object (such as a cold scale, delivery room bed, etc)

A5. Any condition where cold air moves over a baby (such as cold oxygen flow, draft from an open window or air conditioner, incubator portholes left open, etc)

A6. Any condition where a liquid is allowed to evaporate from a baby's skin (such as remaining wet after delivery, giving a bath, etc)

A7. Any condition where a baby is close to a cold, solid object (such as a cold wall or closed window, cold wall of a single-wall incubator, etc)

B1. Rectal, axillary, skin

B2. Rectal

B3. Rectal and axillary

B4. 36.5°C (97.8°F)

B5. B. Incubator air temperature set too high (Note: Infection can cause a fever in a newborn, but it is uncommon.)

B6. A. A blood infection (sepsis)
    C. Heat loss to the environment

C1. Hypoglycemia, acidosis, hypoxia

C2. Babies more likely to be cold-stressed, including preterm, small for gestational age, sick babies
    Babies more likely to be overheated, including babies in incubators, under radiant warmers or phototherapy lights

C3. True

C4. True

C5. True

D1. C. Setting the incubator air temperature according to the baby's age and weight

D2. C. Minimize the oxygen and calories a baby needs.

D3. 35.5°C (96.0°F)

D4. 34.0°C (93.2°F)

D5. Yes

E1. The baby is septic and/or there are abnormal routes of heat loss.

E2. False   The body temperature may go higher or lower than 37.0°C (98.6°F) while in an appropriate neutral thermal environment temperature range. If they occur, such changes should be investigated to determine the cause for the abnormal temperature.

E3. False   The purpose of neutral thermal environment is to minimize oxygen and caloric consumption, as well as to keep a baby's temperature normal.

E4. Any 3 of the following:

Baby: • Is naked in an incubator
- Does not have an infection (is not septic)
- Is appropriate size for gestational age
- Is *not* extremely small (<1,000 g or 2 lb, 3 oz)

Sources of heat loss are controlled
- Wet diapers are removed promptly.
- Oxygen (if used) is humidified and warmed to appropriate neutral thermal environment temperature.
- Incubator portholes are closed after each entry into the incubator.
- Incubator walls are not unusually cold.

E5. C. Ensures the baby is using minimum oxygen and calories to maintain a normal body temperature.

F1. Put baby in an incubator set at 34°C to 35.5°C. Increase incubator air temperature in increments of 1°C to 1.5°C until baby's rectal/axillary temperature reaches 37.0°C (98.6°F). Set incubator air temperature to neutral thermal environment temperature after body temperature reaches 37.0°C. — OR — Put baby under a radiant warmer with skin temperature set for 36.5°C (97.8°F). Monitor rectal temperature until normal, then use axillary measurements.

F2. Exposed skin temperature of 36.5°C or 97.8°F

F3. A. Normal, full-term, well baby: clothed in crib with blanket, nursery temperature set at 74°F to 76°F

B. Stable, 1,500-g preterm baby: incubator set at the baby's neutral thermal environment temperature

C. Sick, full-term baby not requiring many procedures: incubator set at the baby's neutral thermal environment temperature

D. Sick, preterm baby requiring many procedures: radiant warmer, servocontrol set for 36.5°C skin temperature

E. Stable, small for gestational age, term baby: clothed in crib with blanket, nursery temperature set at 74°F to 76°F

F. Sick, small for gestational age, term baby: incubator with environmental temperature adjusted to keep the baby's body temperature at 37.0°C — OR — under a radiant warmer with servocontrol set for 36.5°C skin temperature

F4. Place the baby in an incubator with the air temperature set for her neutral thermal environment temperature — OR — under a radiant warmer with the skin temperature set at 36.5°C (97.8°F). Be sure to evaluate baby for possible consequences of hypothermia (hypoglycemia, acidosis, hypoxia).

F5. True

Without referring back to the information in the unit, please answer the following questions. Select the *one best* answer to each question (unless otherwise instructed). Record your answers on the answer sheet that is the last page in this book *and* on the test.

1. How should a baby's temperature be regulated when she is lying on her stomach under a radiant warmer?
    A. Set the radiant warmer to the baby's neutral thermal environment temperature and place the servocontrol probe in her rectum.
    B. Set the servocontrol sensor to regulate the baby's environmental temperature to 37.0°C (98.6°F).
    C. Set the servocontrol sensor to 36.5°C (97.8°F) and tape the probe to her back.
    D. Set the servocontrol sensor to 35.5°C (95.6°F) and tape the probe to her abdomen.

2. Which of the following babies is at *highest* risk of becoming hypothermic?
    A. 35-week, appropriate for gestational age
    B. 40-week, appropriate for gestational age
    C. 42-week, appropriate for gestational age
    D. 40-week, large for gestational age

A 2,000 g (4 lb, 61/2 oz) appropriate for gestational age baby born at 34 weeks at home arrives in your nursery at 2 hours of age, with a body temperature of 31°C (87.8°F). The neutral thermal environment temperature range for a 34-week gestational age baby on the first postnatal day is 35.0°C. Use this information to answer the questions below.

3a. Which of the following incubator temperatures would be *most* appropriate for this baby initially?
    A. 36.5°C (97.8°F)
    B. 35.0°C (95.0°F)
    C. 32.5°C (90.6°F)
    D. 31.0°C (87.8°F)

3b. By 6 hours of age, the baby's body temperature has reached 37.0°C (98.6°F). Now what is the appropriate incubator air temperature for this baby?
    A. 36.5°C (97.8°F)
    B. 35.0°C (95.0°F)
    C. 32.5°C (90.6°F)
    D. 31.0°C (87.8°F)

4. **True** **False** To put a baby in a neutral thermal environment means to make sure the incubator walls and environment are the same temperature as the baby, so heat will be neither lost nor gained.

5. A 2-day-old baby is found to have an axillary temperature of 35.0°C (95.0°F). Which of the following tests would be *least* helpful in the evaluation of this baby?
    A. Check blood oxygen level.
    B. Check for acidosis.
    C. Determine serum sodium level.
    D. Determine blood glucose level.

6. **True** **False** Rectal temperatures are the safest way to check a baby's temperature routinely.

7. **True** **False** A baby in a warm incubator in front of a cold window is at risk for radiant heat loss.

8. **True** **False** Respiratory distress may be a sign of low body temperature.

9. **True** **False** A newborn with a skin temperature of 35.0°C (95.0°F) uses more oxygen than a baby with a skin temperature of 36.5°C (97.8°F).

10. **True** **False** Putting a baby on a cold scale surface is an example of convective heat loss.

11. **True** **False** The body temperature of a baby in an incubator, with the air temperature set to the appropriate neutral thermal environment, falls to 36.0°C (96.8°F). After finding no routes of abnormal heat loss, your *first* action should be to increase the incubator temperature.

12. **True False** A healthy, term baby can become ill from being chilled.

13. **True False** A lower than normal body temperature in a newborn may be a sign of sepsis.

For each question, please make sure you have marked your answer on the test and on the answer sheet (last page in book). The test is for you; the answer sheet will need to be turned in for continuing education credit.

Skill Unit 1   Radiant Warmers

This skill unit will teach you how to operate a radiant warmer and regulate a baby's temperature using servocontrol.

Study this skill unit. Then attend a skill practice and demonstration session.

To master the skill, you will need to demonstrate correctly each of the following steps:

1. Select mode of operation.
2. Attach servocontrol probe to baby.
3. Determine temperature setting.
4. Set high and low temperature alarms.
5. Keep baby unclothed.
6. Position transparent plastic cover, if used.
7. Minimize heat loss.

Actions	**Remarks**

Deciding to Use a Radiant Warmer

1. Do you anticipate the admission of a sick or at-risk baby?

    Yes: Prepare to use the radiant warmer for this baby.

    No: Make sure the radiant warmer is clean and in operating condition.

It is generally easier to observe babies and carry out special procedures (eg, umbilical catheterization) when they are under radiant warmers than when they are in incubators.

Preparing to Use a Radiant Warmer

2. Collect the proper equipment.

   • Radiant warmer

   • Servocontrol probe

   • Cover for the tip of the servocontrol probe

3. Plug in the radiant warmer.

4. Connect the servocontrol probe to the radiant warmer.

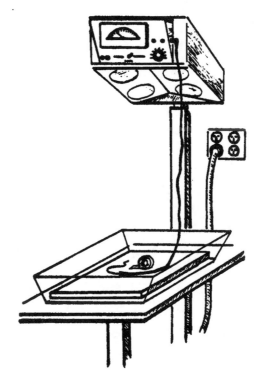

5. Place the radiant warmer on *automatic* mode.

Automatic mode means the warmer turns on and off in response to the baby's skin temperature, as it is registered by the servocontrol probe, to maintain the baby's skin temperature at the preset temperature (servocontrol).

Manual mode means that the radiant warmer will continue heating unless you turn it off. A baby can be quickly overheated.

Actions	**Remarks**

Using a Radiant Warmer

6. The infant should be unclothed to absorb the radiant heat. Leaving clothes on the baby will decrease the efficiency of heat input from the warmer.

A piece of cling film (such as Saran wrap), placed across the bed, above the baby, and attached to either side of the warmer bed or a rigid, clear plastic body tent placed over a baby, will help to decrease convective and evaporative losses, without interfering with the radiant heat needed to keep the baby warm.

If thin plastic wrap is used, be sure to keep it away from the baby's airway.

7. Decide where to place the temperature probe.

   • On the baby's abdomen (if baby is lying on back)

   • On the baby's lower back (if baby is lying on stomach)

Avoid placing the probe over boney prominences (sternum, ribs, scapula, etc) or on the baby's arms or legs. These locations will not give an accurate skin temperature but will instead register a relatively low temperature, causing the radiant warmer to put out excess heat, which may, in turn, overheat the baby

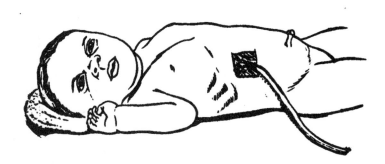

8. Securely tape the temperature probe to the baby.

Care must be taken to keep the servocontrol probe tip in constant contact with the baby's skin.

9. Cover the tip of the probe so that it is not directly exposed to the radiant heat.

To protect a baby's skin, a piece of clear adhesive dressing may be used to hold the probe tip in place on the baby's skin. A piece of opaque cloth tape or a commercially available reflective cover is then taped to the clear adhesive, over the probe tip.

10. Set the appropriate servocontrol skin temperature (36.5°C or 97.8°F).

Actions	Remarks

Using a Radiant Warmer (continued)

Check rectal temperature to make sure it is close to 37.0°C (98.6°F). If low, continue to check the baby's rectal temperature until it is normal. Then use axillary temperatures for routine monitoring.

It is important to check a baby's axillary temperature, in addition to the skin temperature registered by the servocontrol probe. A loose or incorrectly placed probe, or an incorrectly set warmer, can cause a baby to be severely overheated or underheated, even though the probe registers the desired skin temperature.

Adjust the servocontrol preset temperature higher or lower as needed to keep the axillary/rectal temperature at 37.0°C (98.6°F).

If your radiant warmer has "high" and "low" temperature alarms, set these at 0.5°C (1.0°F) above and below the preset temperature. (Many warmers have internal alarms that cannot be set manually.)

It is important to recognize a change in temperature quickly because the baby can be chilled or overheated within a short period. Know the operation and meaning of the alarms on the warmer you are using.

11. Keep the sides of the radiant warmer bed in the upright position. Minimize drafts in the room. Consider using a rigid, clear plastic "body tent" or clear plastic cling film placed across the baby and attached to either side of the warmer.

This is to minimize the baby losing heat by convection and evaporation. (See step #6.)

12. Radiant warmers can increase the baby's insensible water loss by as much as 100%. If a baby is to stay under a radiant warmer for more than several hours, it is important to increase the baby's fluid intake.

A clear plastic covering is particularly useful for decreasing insensible water losses in babies with birth weights less than 1,500 g (3 lb, 5 oz).

What Can Go Wrong?

1. Radiant warmer is placed on manual rather than automatic mode of operation.

The heating mechanism will not automatically turn off. The baby will become overheated.

2. The servocontrol probe may malfunction and the baby may be chilled or overheated when all other settings are correct.

This is rare. However, if you suspect this to be the problem, try another temperature probe. Continue frequent monitoring of the baby's temperature with a standard thermometer.

3. The baby's desired temperature is set inaccurately.

The baby will be chilled or overheated.

Actions	Remarks

What Can Go Wrong? (continued)

4. The temperature probe becomes dislodged.	The baby will become overheated. Check the baby's temperature with a second thermometer. Re-tape the probe.
5. The probe is taped over a boney prominence or on an extremity.	The temperature registered may be lower than the baby's actual skin temperature, causing the warmer to put out more heat than necessary and resulting in the baby being overheated. Be sure the probe is taped to a fleshy part of the baby's trunk.
6. The baby is lying on the probe.	While the probe should be covered to prevent *direct* exposure to the radiant heat, it should be taped to the exposed side of the baby. If the probe is between the baby and the mattress, it may register a falsely high temperature, causing the baby to be *under*heated.

Skill Unit 2   Incubators and Neutral Thermal Environment

This skill unit will teach you how to determine a baby's neutral thermal environment (NTE) and how to operate an incubator to provide a baby's NTE.

Study this skill. Then attend a skill practice and demonstration session.

To master this skill, you will need to demonstrate correctly each of the following steps:

1. Determine baby's NTE.
2. Preheat incubator to NTE.
3. Prepare water reservoir (if present and appropriate for specific incubator).
4. Transfer baby from radiant warmer to incubator.
5. Settle baby in incubator.
6. Check baby's temperature.
7. Record NTE in baby's bedside chart.

Actions	Remarks

Deciding to Use an Incubator

1. Is there a sick or at-risk baby who will stay in your nursery rather than be transferred to a regional intensive care nursery within the next few hours?

   Yes: Move this baby from a radiant warmer to an incubator as soon as any special procedures have been completed.

   No: Make sure at least one incubator is clean and in operating condition.

Remarks for 1: Keep babies who will be transferred under a radiant warmer until special procedures such as umbilical catheterization are complete or the baby is ready to be transported.

Remarks for No: It is recommended to keep a clean incubator plugged in and warm, ready to receive a baby, at all times.

Preparing to Use an Incubator

2. Prepare the bed of the incubator with clean linen.

3. Make sure the bed is properly positioned on the brackets beneath it so each end of the bed can be raised or lowered as need be.

4. Put cuffs (if used) on the portholes.

   Note: Some incubators do not have cuffs that can be attached to the portholes.

Remarks for 4: With frequent cleaning, cuffs wear out fairly rapidly. Replace them as necessary. They are useful in reducing a baby's convective heat loss because they reduce the amount of room air that can enter the incubator when the portholes are opened to provide care.

5. Check water reservoir (if present).

   • Be sure reservoir is clean.

   • Fill only with *sterile* water.

   • Cleanse the reservoir regularly while the incubator is in use.

Remarks for 5: Some very old incubators, as well as much newer incubators designed especially for extremely low birth weight babies, have a water reservoir for humidification of the incubator interior. Generally, this reservoir should be used only in new incubators designed for this, but not in much older incubators.

Beware: Water in this reservoir can easily become contaminated. When warmed by the incubator's heat, this water may provide an ideal solution for certain bacteria to grow.

Actions   **Remarks**

Setting the NTE

6. Use the NTE figures on page 20 or on page 42
    in this unit. Find the appropriate temperature
    band for the baby in your care.

    - To determine NTE for babies 0 to 6 days of
      age, estimate the baby's gestational age.

Example
Baby Thomas is 2 days old and has an estimated
gestational age of 32 weeks. Find the baby's
gestational age on the vertical scale (see arrow).

Now find the baby's postnatal age (days since birth)
on the horizontal scale (see arrow).

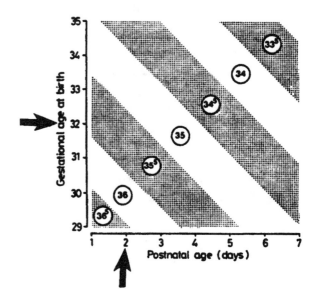

Find the area of the graph where straight lines
drawn from these 2 points cross (see arrows).

For Baby Thomas, this intersection falls in the
temperature band labeled 35.5. Baby Thomas's
NTE is 35.5°C.

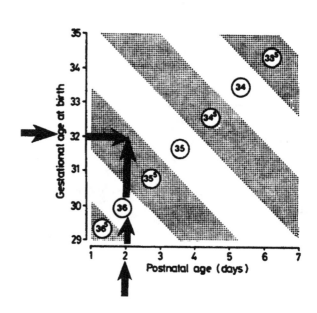

Actions   **Remarks**

Setting the NTE (continued)

- To determine NTE for babies 7 or more days of age, determine the baby's weight in kilograms.

Example
Baby Thomas is now 10 days old and weighs 1,850 g (1.85 kg). Find the baby's age on the horizontal scale (see arrow).

Now find the baby's current weight on the vertical scale (see arrow).

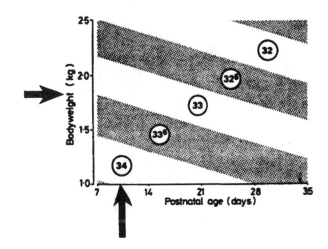

Find the area of the graph where straight lines drawn from these 2 points cross (see arrows).

Baby Thomas's NTE is now 33°C.

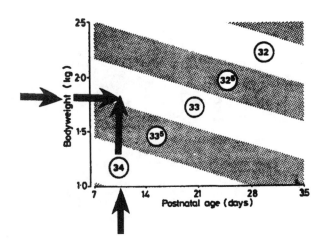

41

Neutral Thermal Temperatures

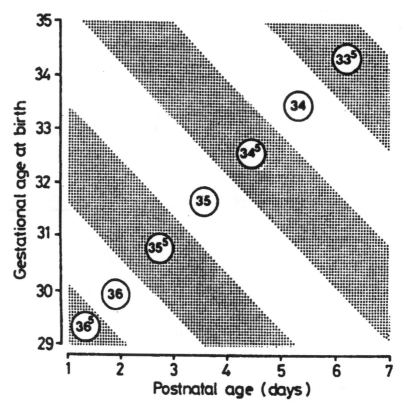

Figure 1. Neutral Thermal Environment (°C) During the First Postnatal Week (0–6 Days of Age)

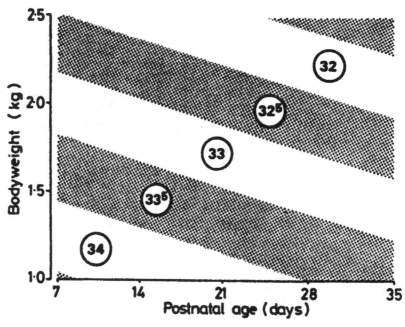

Figure 2. Neutral Thermal Environment (°C) From 7 to 35 Days of Age

Incubator temperature charts are reproduced with permission from Sauer PJJ, Dane HJ, Visser HKA. *Arch Dis Child.* 1984;59:18–22.

Actions	Remarks

Caring for a Baby in an Incubator

7. Preheat the incubator to the NTE temperature, which you have determined from the graphs.

   - Check the temperature inside the incubator.

   - Adjust the incubator temperature higher or lower as required to reach the NTE.

   - Wait 15 or 20 minutes.

   - Recheck the air temperature inside the incubator.

   - Readjust the incubator setting if necessary, wait again, and recheck the incubator temperature.

   For many incubators, the desired temperature can be set digitally. It is still important, however, to check the actual air temperature inside the incubator and readjust the temperature setting, as necessary, to achieve the desired incubator air temperature.

8. *Plan* how you will transfer the baby and any attached monitoring equipment, intravenous tubing, etc, to the incubator.

   If the baby is requiring oxygen via an oxyhood, have someone hold the tubing over the baby's nose during the entire transfer. If the baby is requiring assisted ventilation, bag-breathe for the baby during the entire transfer using the appropriate concentration of oxygen. Be prepared to resume the pre-transfer oxygen therapy *immediately,* as soon as the baby has been placed in the incubator.

   This is a *critical step* and must be done to ensure a smooth transfer with minimum stress to the baby.

   Removing an oxygen-dependent baby from oxygen for even a very brief period can make the baby's condition deteriorate severely.

9. When the incubator has reached the correct temperature, place the baby inside.

   - Open the incubator door.

   - Place the baby inside.

   - Close the incubator door as quickly as possible.

   - Work through the portholes to settle the baby.

   - Close the portholes.

   Sick and at-risk babies exposed to room temperature can be chilled very quickly. After you have settled the baby, recheck his/her temperature.

10. Check and record the incubator temperature and the baby's temperature every 30 minutes until both are stable.

11. Recheck the graphs every day and adjust the incubator setting appropriately as the baby grows.

    Record the NTE temperature in the baby's bedside chart each day.

Actions	Remarks

Caring for a Baby in an Incubator (continued)

12. Continue to keep a baby in the appropriate NTE until the baby

    • Is no longer sick

    • Weighs more than 1,600 to 1,700 g (about 3 lb, 8 oz–3 lb, 12 oz),

    • Can maintain a normal body temperature in a bassinet with shirt, diaper, and blankets

    • Continues to gain weight steadily

What Can Go Wrong?

1. NTE is set incorrectly.

   Recheck the graph for the temperature for the baby's current age and weight.

2. Some incubators are designed so that the warm air flows up the sides of the incubator. This may mean the air reaching an incubator wall thermometer is warmer than the air in the center of the incubator next to the baby.

   If this is the design of incubators in your nursery, suspend a temperature probe directly over the baby. Adjust the baby's NTE according to the temperature recorded there.

3. The baby is cold or hot in the appropriate NTE.

   • Check for routes of heat loss or gain.
     – Room temperature too cold, thus causing the baby to have excessive radiant heat loss to cold incubator walls (less likely to occur with double-walled incubators)
     – Incubator close to cold windows (heat loss) or in direct sunlight (heat gain)
     – Wet mattress or linens
     – Incubator portholes left open
     – Oxygen (if needed) not warmed to appropriate NTE (too hot or too cold)

   • Suspect sepsis.

   • Very small (<1,000 g or 2 lb, 3 oz) preterm babies *may* require special techniques to maintain their body temperatures. Care of these tiny babies is not discussed here.

   • Small for gestational age babies may become slightly overheated or underheated in an incubator adjusted according to the graphs. Raise or lower the incubator temperature as needed to keep an SGA baby's body temperature normal.

Actions	Remarks

What Can Go Wrong? (continued)

4. The incubator is set to "skin" rather than "air" temperature control.

When providing NTE as outlined in this skill unit, you are controlling the temperature of the *air* inside the incubator.

If you wish to servocontrol a baby's temperature, you need to
- Set the incubator to "skin" (not "air").

- Set the temperature of the servocontrol probe to 36.5°C (98.6°F).

- Tape the probe to the baby, as you would if using a radiant warmer.

Unit 2   Oxygen

Objectives

In this unit you will learn to

A. Identify infants who require supplemental oxygen.

B. Administer oxygen as a drug while understanding its benefits and hazards.

C. Operate the appropriate equipment for the controlled delivery of oxygen.

D. Monitor a baby's oxygenation.

Before reading the unit, please answer the following questions. Select the *one best* answer to each question (unless otherwise instructed). Record your answers on the answer sheet that is the last page in this book *and* on the test.

1. Which of the following procedures is the *best* way to measure the concentration of arterial oxygen?

    A. With an oxygen analyzer
    B. From arterial blood gas samples
    C. Check the liter-per-minute flow of oxygen
    D. From a warmed capillary blood sample

2. A baby with respiratory distress is breathing 45% oxygen and has an arterial blood oxygen concentration of 96 mm Hg. What adjustments in oxygen should be made for this baby?

    A. Change the inspired oxygen to room air.
    B. Change the inspired oxygen to 40%.
    C. Change the inspired oxygen to 50%.
    D. No changes in oxygen therapy for this infant.

3. A baby's eyes may be damaged from long periods of too much

    A. Bilirubin in the blood
    B. Carbon dioxide in the air
    C. Oxygen in the blood
    D. Oxygen in the air

4. Which of the following procedures is the *best* way to gauge the amount of oxygen an infant needs?

    A. Arterial blood gas measurements
    B. Cyanosis of the trunk and mucous membranes
    C. Degree of respiratory distress
    D. Venous blood gas measurements

5. Which of the following infants does *not* require supplemental oxygen?

    A. A preterm infant with respiratory distress and heart rate of 80
    B. A baby who appears dusky all over
    C. A baby in the delivery room with an Apgar score of 2
    D. A preterm baby with an arterial blood oxygen of 65 mm Hg

6. Which of the following is the best way to regulate the amount of oxygen an infant receives?

    A. Administer oxygen alone and regulate the liter-per-minute flow.
    B. Control the time the infant is in oxygen.
    C. Hold the oxygen source closer or farther away from the infant's face.
    D. Change the mixture of oxygen and air.

7. **True** **False** A baby with bluish-colored tongue and lips requires *immediate* oxygen therapy.

8. **True** **False** Arterial blood gas samples are not needed if continuous pulse oximetry is used.

9. **True** **False** Lung damage is a possible consequence of high inspired oxygen concentration over a prolonged period.

10. **True** **False** Capillary blood gas measurements are a reliable way to determine a baby's blood oxygen level.

11. **True** **False** Oxygen from a tank that has been in a warm room for more than 24 hours does *not* need to be heated or humidified.

12. **True** **False** A pulse oximeter uses light to estimate the degree to which hemoglobin is saturated with oxygen.

13. **True** **False** Pulse oximetry is most sensitive in detecting low blood oxygen.

For each question, please make sure you have marked your answer on the test and on the answer sheet (last page in book). The test is for you; the answer sheet will need to be turned in for continuing education credit.

Both too little and too much oxygen can be harmful.

- *Too little oxygen in the blood can cause damage to the brain and other vital organs.*
- *Too much oxygen in the blood over time can cause damage to the eyes.*
- *Too much inspired oxygen over time can cause damage to the lungs.*

1. When Does a Baby Need Supplemental Oxygen?

Babies require oxygen therapy when the concentration of oxygen in the arterial blood is low. The only sure way to determine if a baby is receiving enough or too much oxygen is to measure the amount of oxygen in the arterial blood (PaO_2 value or oxyhemoglobin saturation).

However, in emergency situations, a baby may need oxygen immediately. First, give oxygen; then obtain an arterial blood gas measurement as soon as possible. The following signs show that a baby needs oxygen:

A. Central Cyanosis
   Generally, a baby's body will look blue. This overall color change may be dramatic or it may be much less obvious. The best sign of central cyanosis is the bluish appearance of the mucous membranes (lips and around eyes).

   Central cyanosis indicates the baby needs immediate oxygen therapy. If a baby receives oxygen therapy for more than a brief period, the baby's arterial blood oxygen levels must be measured.

B. Need for Resuscitation
   When a baby's respiratory rate and heart rate are very slow or have stopped, oxygen delivery must be improved immediately to help restore the baby's vital signs. Assisted ventilation with oxygen concentrations ranging from 21% (room air) to as high as 100% will be required (Book I, Resuscitation).

C. Respiratory Distress
   Some babies have difficulty breathing and will require extra oxygen for long periods (Book II: Neonatal Care, Respiratory Distress). For these babies, it is extremely important to measure the arterial blood oxygen levels (PaO_2) frequently and to use continuous oximetry to avoid the hazards of too much or too little oxygen.

2. How Much Oxygen Do You Administer to a Baby?

A. Resuscitation
   If a baby requires resuscitation, high concentrations of oxygen (usually 100%) are generally recommended until vital signs are normal. This should take only several minutes. Your main concern at this time is getting adequate oxygen to the brain. When vital signs have returned to normal, you should attempt to lower the inspired oxygen concentration (FiO_2). Some experts recommend starting the resuscitation with a lower concentration of oxygen (eg, room air) and then increasing the concentration toward 100% as necessary.

B. Cyanosis

   1. Immediate Treatment

For cyanosis in the delivery room or in the nursery, decide on an oxygen concentration depending on the degree of cyanosis. For example, if a baby is deeply blue all over, choose 100%. If the mucous membranes are only slightly dusky, choose approximately 30%. Increasing degrees of cyanosis between these extremes will require increasing concentrations of oxygen.

Degree of Cyanosis	slightly dusky $\longrightarrow$ mucous membranes	increasing $\longrightarrow$ cyanosis	deeply blue all over
Oxygen Concentration	30% $\longrightarrow$ oxygen	increasing $\longrightarrow$ oxygen	100% oxygen

   2. Adjust According to Baby's Response

Place the baby in the chosen concentration and observe for the disappearance of central cyanosis. If the baby is still dusky or blue after a few seconds, rapidly increase the concentration until he or she becomes pink. Obtain an arterial blood gas measurement and attach a pulse oximeter as soon as possible.

C. Respiratory Distress
Babies with respiratory distress need to be given oxygen only if they are cyanotic or have a low arterial blood oxygen concentration. The amount of oxygen required depends on the degree of cyanosis and how low the PaO_2 value or oxyhemoglobin saturation is.

It is possible for a baby to be in respiratory distress, *not* be cyanotic, and still have a low PaO_2 value. These babies should have frequent arterial blood gas measurements and be given sufficient oxygen to keep the arterial oxygenation within the normal range.

Use of a pulse oximeter should *not* replace periodic arterial blood gas measurements, which measure blood pH and carbon dioxide concentration, in addition to blood oxygen concentration. A pulse oximeter is helpful in providing continuous *estimates* of arterial blood oxygen levels and should reduce the number of arterial blood measurements that are needed.

3. When Does a Baby *Not* Need Supplemental Oxygen?

A. Acrocyanosis (only hands and feet blue)
Acrocyanosis without central cyanosis is *not* an indication for oxygen to be administered. This condition may be caused by reasons other than lack of oxygen (eg, cold stress or poor peripheral blood flow).

B. Prematurity Without Respiratory Distress or Cyanosis
Preterm babies should *not* be given supplemental oxygen unless they are cyanotic or have a low arterial blood oxygen level.

4. How Should Oxygen Be Given?

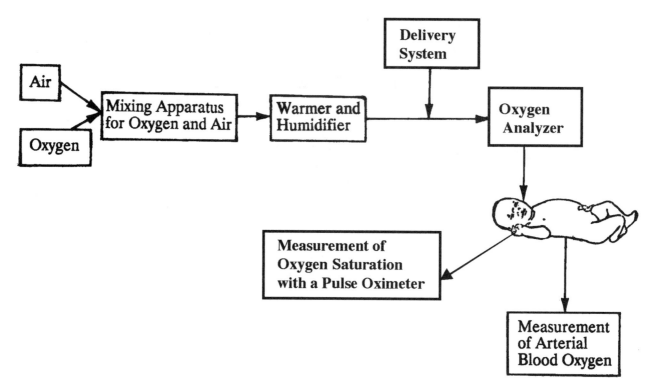

Figure 2.1. Administering and Measuring Oxygen

The concentration of oxygen in room air is 21%. To deliver supplemental oxygen (22%–100%) you should

- Mix 100% oxygen with air to provide any desired concentration of oxygen between 22% and 100%.
- Warm and humidify the oxygen/air mixture to the baby's neutral thermal environment temperature (Book II: Neonatal Care, Unit 1).
- Deliver by equipment that will prevent fluctuations in oxygen concentration.
- Measure FiO_2 precisely.
- Measure the concentration of oxygen in the baby's blood intermittently.
- Monitor oxyhemoglobin saturation continuously.

A. Mix Oxygen and Air
Oxygen from a wall outlet or tank is 100% oxygen, regardless of the liter-per-minute flow rate. The only way to get less than 100% oxygen is to mix the oxygen with air. Airflow is obtained from a wall outlet, compressed air tank, or electrical air compressor.

The flow rate of oxygen does not determine the concentration of oxygen inspired by an infant.

The amount of oxygen and the amount of compressed air mixed together determine the inspired oxygen concentration (FiO_2).

Figure 2.2 shows the *approximate* concentration of oxygen that will result from various oxygen and air liters per minute flow rates. It also shows that equal flow rates yield an oxygen concentration of approximately 61%.

An oxygen blender regulates this mixing of oxygen and compressed air automatically to provide a specified oxygen concentration. Flow meters and blenders, however, are not always precise. An oxygen analyzer should *always* be used to check the exact concentration of oxygen being delivered to a baby.

Air Liter/Minute Flow

	1	2	3	4	5	6	7	8	9	10
1			41	37	34	32	31	30	29	28
2		61	53	47	44	41	38	37	35	34
3	80	68	61	55	51	47	45	43	41	39
4	84	74	66	61	56	52	50	47	45	44
5	86	77	70	65	61	57	54	51	49	47
6	88	80	74	68	64	61	57	55	53	51
7	90	82	76	71	67	64	61	58	56	54
8	91	84	78	74	70	66	63	61	58	56
9	92	86	80	76	72	68	65	63	61	58
10	93	87	82	77	74	70	67	65	63	61

(Oxygen Liter/Minute Flow — vertical axis label)

Figure 2.2. Mixing Oxygen and Compressed Air (L/min Guide). Cells show approximate percent (%) oxygen delivered.

B. Heat and Humidify Oxygen and Air

Oxygen and air directly from wall outlets or tanks are cold and dry, even if a tank itself is warm. Oxygen and air must be warmed to avoid chilling the baby. Regulation of the temperature of the oxygen/air mixture is just as important as strict regulation of the baby's environmental temperature (neutral thermal environment). Oxygen and air must also be humidified to avoid drying the baby's mucous membranes and lung passages.

C. Prevent Fluctuations in Oxygen Concentration

Very small differences in FiO_2 can make a great difference in the amount of oxygen in the baby's blood.

The equipment used to deliver oxygen to babies who do not require assisted ventilation includes

1. Oxygen by Hood

   An oxyhood is made from clear plastic material and is placed over a baby's head. It has an inlet on one side for the oxygen/air mixture and an opening on the opposite side to fit over the baby's neck. The best way to maintain a constant FiO_2 for a baby who does not require assisted ventilation is to use an oxyhood.

2. Oxygen by Mask

    The concentration of oxygen a baby receives will vary depending on how far the mask is held from the baby's nose. There is no way to measure precisely the amount of oxygen the baby receives. Oxygen delivered by mask, however, may be adequate during the period of resuscitation. Beware: Some bag-and-mask equipment will not deliver oxygen unless the bag is being squeezed (Book I, Resuscitation).

    Delivery of oxygen directly to an incubator is *not* recommended. When oxygen is delivered in this way, the concentration cannot be precisely controlled. If a baby requires oxygen therapy beyond the period of resuscitation, an oxyhood should be used.

    Occasionally babies with chronic lung disease who require long-term oxygen therapy will be given oxygen by nasal cannula. However, this method is appropriate only for older infants, generally beyond the neonatal period, and is not discussed in this unit.

    The diagram below illustrates equipment used to deliver oxygen and monitor oxygenation in babies. (See the skill units for details.)

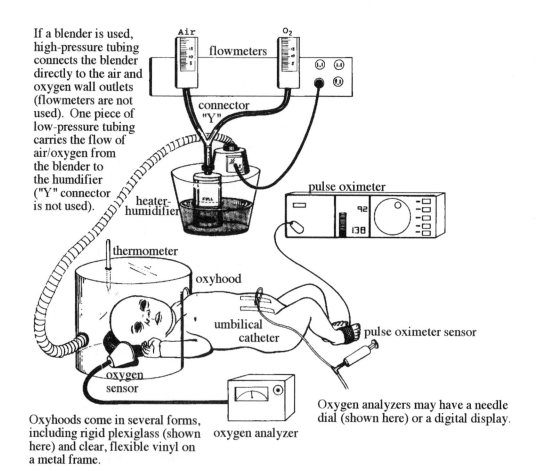

If a blender is used, high-pressure tubing connects the blender directly to the air and oxygen wall outlets (flowmeters are not used). One piece of low-pressure tubing carries the flow of air/oxygen from the blender to the humdifier ("Y" connector is not used).

Air

O_2

flowmeters

connector "Y"

heater-humidifier

pulse oximeter

thermometer

oxyhood

umbilical catheter

pulse oximeter sensor

oxygen sensor

oxygen analyzer

Oxyhoods come in several forms, including rigid plexiglass (shown here) and clear, flexible vinyl on a metal frame.

Oxygen analyzers may have a needle dial (shown here) or a digital display.

Now answer these questions to test yourself on the information in the last section.

A1. What is the only certain way to know if a baby is receiving too much or too little oxygen?

    A. Measure the arterial blood oxygen level.

    B. Observe the baby for degree of cyanosis.

A2. Name 3 situations in which supplemental oxygen may be needed.

_____

_____

_____

A3. Name 2 situations when oxygen should *not* be administered.

_____

_____

A4. What are the general principles of delivering oxygen?

_____

_____

_____

_____

_____

A5. What test must be done if a baby stays in oxygen more than a brief period?

_____

A6. If this test shows *too much* oxygen in the baby's blood, what damage could result?

_____

A7. If this test shows *too little* oxygen in the baby's blood, what damage could result?

_____

A8. When do you administer oxygen to a baby in respiratory distress?

    A. Only if the baby is cyanotic

    B. Only if the arterial blood oxygen value or oximeter reading is low

    C. If the baby is cyanotic or has a low arterial blood oxygen value or oximeter reading

Check your answers with the list that follows the Recommended Routines. Correct any incorrect answers and review the appropriate section in the unit.

5. How Is the Amount of Oxygen Measured?

Oxygen concentration should be measured in 2 ways.

1. Amount breathed by the infant (FiO_2)

2. Amount in the baby's blood, which can be measured

   - In the plasma (PaO_2)
   - On the hemoglobin in red blood cells (oxyhemoglobin saturation)

A. Inspired Oxygen

The inspired oxygen concentration is frequently abbreviated as FiO_2 (fraction of inspired oxygen). The amount of oxygen a baby breathes, the environmental or FiO_2, is measured by an oxygen analyzer. The oxygen analyzer is a sensing device that is placed near the infant's nose. Most analyzers provide a constant readout of the oxygen concentration.

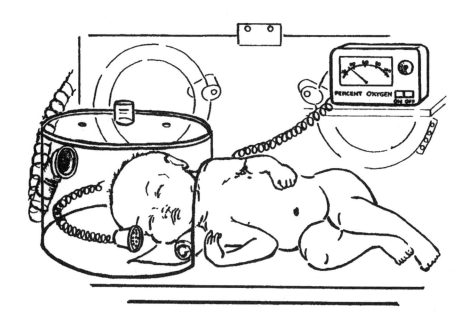

Figure 2.3. Oxyhood and Oxygen Analyzer. All aspects of a baby's care are *not* illustrated.

B. Blood Oxygen

1. Arterial Blood Oxygen

   Arterial blood oxygen levels are shown as the PaO_2 value from arterial blood gas measurements. The blood to be analyzed is usually drawn from an umbilical artery catheter. If an umbilical artery catheter has not been inserted, then an arterial blood sample may be obtained from a radial artery (see skill unit).

 Arterial blood must be used for PaO_2 determinations.

Venous and capillary blood do not give accurate estimates of oxygenation.

The desired level of PaO$_2$ in any infant (sick, well, preterm, post-term) is

45 to 75 mm Hg*

Babies with varying degrees of lung disease will require different levels of FiO$_2$ to maintain the desired arterial blood oxygen level. For example, a baby with severe respiratory distress syndrome (RDS) may require FiO$_2$ ranging up to 100% to maintain a PaO$_2$ between 45 and 75 mm Hg, while a baby with mild RDS may require only 30% FiO$_2$ to maintain a PaO$_2$ between 45 and 75 mm Hg.

2. Oxyhemoglobin Saturation

Oxygen is carried in blood by being dissolved in plasma and by attaching to hemoglobin in the red blood cells. The concentration in plasma is expressed as PaO$_2$, whereas the concentration on hemoglobin is expressed as percent saturation. When there is no oxygen bound to hemoglobin it is "0% saturated"; when the hemoglobin is carrying as much oxygen as possible, it is "100% saturated."

The desired level of oxyhemoglobin saturation in a baby is

85% to 95% saturation*

Hemoglobin changes color from blue to red as it becomes increasingly saturated with oxygen. A pulse oximeter detects the color of the blood and gives a reading expressed as percent saturation. It does this by shining a tiny light through the skin, registering the color of the light coming from the skin (which is determined by the color of blood in the capillaries), and thus estimating percent saturation, without requiring a blood sample to be drawn.

6. How Does Oxyhemoglobin Saturation Compare to PaO$_2$?

Oxygen dissolved in plasma (PaO$_2$) can range from 0 mm Hg to approximately 600 mm Hg; oxyhemoglobin saturation can range from 0% to 100%. However, when PaO$_2$ reaches approximately 60 mm Hg, the hemoglobin is almost completely saturated with oxygen, making the percent saturation nearly 100%. Therefore, if the percent saturation is more than approximately 95%, the PaO$_2$ could be either acceptable (45–75 mm Hg) or undesirably high (>75 mm Hg).

 Percent saturation as measured by a pulse oximeter is most valuable for detecting low blood oxygen.

Percent saturation is not a sensitive measure when PaO$_2$ is high.

---

*There is disagreement among experts as to the appropriate range of PaO$_2$ and oxyhemoglobin saturation. Some believe that 40 to 70 mm Hg PaO$_2$ and 88% to 92% saturation are the desired ranges.

Table 2.1. Approximate Relationship of PaO_2 and Percent Saturation

Oxyhemoglobin Saturation	PaO_2
0%–85%	0–45 mm Hg
85%–95%	45–75 mm Hg
95%–100%	75–600 mm Hg

The approximate relationship of PaO_2 and percent saturation is shown in Table 2.1 and Figure 2.4.

The shaded area of Figure 2.4 shows the approximate relationship between 85% to 95% oxyhemoglobin saturation and 45 to 75 mm Hg arterial blood oxygen level for a slightly preterm baby during the first few days following birth.

For some babies, simultaneous measurements of PaO_2 and percent saturation may give results quite different than those predicted by the graph. The precise relationship of oxygen saturation and PaO_2 is affected by several factors such as gestational age, postnatal age (age since birth), the presence of acidosis, and whether the baby has had a blood transfusion.

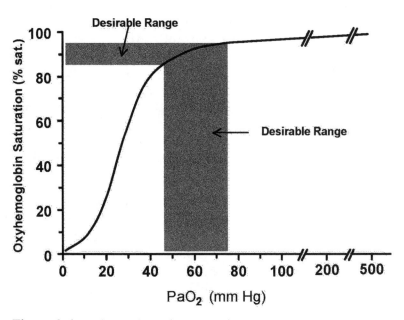

Figure 2.4. Relationship of PaO_2 and Percent Saturation

7. What Is the Best Way to Monitor a Baby's Oxygenation?

A baby's blood oxygen level will frequently fluctuate from minute to minute, particularly if the baby is distressed or undergoing any sort of procedure. A pulse oximeter can be used to monitor these changes so you will know quickly when the baby's oxygenation is persistently out of the desirable range and thus requires attention. However, because pulse oximeters only estimate the baby's oxygenation and are very inaccurate in the high range, the baby's PaO_2 should be measured intermittently with a sample of arterial blood. You should watch for the oximeter readings to stabilize to know the best time to obtain an arterial blood sample that reflects the baby's resting state (not changes that may occur with crying, stress during procedures, etc).

 The best way to monitor a baby's blood oxygen is to

- *Follow trends or changes in oxygenation with a pulse oximeter.*

AND

- *Measure PaO_2 intermittently from samples of arterial blood.*

Now answer these questions to test yourself on the information in the last section.

B1. An infant is in an FiO_2 of 50%, has a PaO_2 of 75 mm Hg, and has an oxyhemoglobin saturation of 95%. What is the inspired oxygen for this infant?

   A. 50%
   B. 75 mm Hg
   C. 95%

B2. An infant is in an FiO_2 of 35%, has a PaO_2 of 60 mm Hg, and has an oxyhemoglobin saturation of 90%. What is the oxygen concentration in the baby's blood?

   A. 35%
   B. 60 mm Hg
   C. 60 mm Hg and 90% saturation

B3. Which of the following is the best way to obtain blood for a blood oxygen measurement?

   A. From an umbilical artery catheter
   B. From an umbilical venous catheter
   C. From a heel stick

B4. The normal arterial blood oxygen level in a baby is between ____ mm Hg and ____ mm Hg.

B5. What concentration of oxygen do you administer to a deeply cyanotic baby who needs positive-pressure ventilation during resuscitation?

   A. 30%
   B. 60%
   C. 100%

B6. If oxygen needs to be administered for longer than a brief period, how much should a baby receive?

   A. Not more than 40%
   B. Enough to keep the baby pink
   C. Enough to keep the arterial blood oxygen between 45 and 75 mm Hg

B7. Pulse oximeters measure the amount of oxygen

   A. In plasma
   B. Bound to hemoglobin
   C. In inspired air

Check your answers with the list that follows the Recommended Routines. Correct any incorrect answers and review the appropriate section in the unit.

8. When Is the Concentration of Inspired Oxygen Changed?

- If the PaO_2 level is below 45 mm Hg or if the oximeter shows frequent and sustained values below 85% saturation, the FiO_2 should be increased immediately.

- If the PaO_2 level is above 75 mm Hg, or if the oximeter shows consistent values above 95%, the FiO_2 should be lowered promptly, but gradually. Use of an oximeter can help to be sure the FiO_2 is not lowered too quickly.

If the FiO_2 is lowered rapidly, the arteries to the lungs may constrict. This can seriously reduce the blood flow to the lungs and result in a much lower PaO_2 level. A consistently low PaO_2 level, regardless of the cause, may lead to brain and other tissue damage.

9. How Do You Adjust FiO_2 on the Basis of PaO_2?

If PaO_2 is low, quickly increase the FiO_2. If PaO_2 is high, decrease FiO_2 in decrements until PaO_2 is within the desired range. When PaO_2 is high it should be brought within the desired range promptly, but care should be taken to avoid dropping the FiO_2 too far or too fast. Use the guidelines in Tables 2.2 and 2.3 to adjust the FiO_2 to achieve the appropriate PaO_2 and oxygen saturation values.

Table 2.2. Recommended Responses to Arterial Blood Oxygen Values

Arterial Blood Oxygen (PaO_2) Level	Action
<45 mm Hg	Rapidly increase FiO_2 until PaO_2 is between 45–75 mm Hg. If PaO_2 fell quickly, check for change in respiratory disease (such as development of a pneumothorax) or a mechanical problem (such as displacement of an endotracheal tube).
Between 45–75 mm Hg	No change indicated.
Between 75–120 mm Hg	Decrease FiO_2 by 5%.
>120 mm Hg	Decrease FiO_2 by 10%.

Example 1: If the PaO_2 is 140 mm Hg and the FiO_2 is 70%, you should change the FiO_2 to 60% (70% − 10% = 60%).

Example 2: If the PaO_2 is 110 mm Hg and the FiO_2 is 70%, you should change the FiO_2 to 65% (70% − 5% = 65%).

10. How Can You Use a Pulse Oximeter to Adjust Inspired Oxygen?

While it is important to correct too low or too high PaO_2 values quickly to prevent tissue damage, rapid and extreme fluctuations in PaO_2 can also be hazardous. A pulse oximeter can help to guide you to change FiO_2 as quickly as possible, but without causing rapid fluctuations in PaO_2.

Table 2.3. Recommended Responses to Oximeter Readings

Pulse Oximeter Reading	Action
<85% saturation	Rapidly increase FiO_2 as much as necessary to bring the oximeter reading to 85%–95% within 1 to 2 minutes. If the PaO_2 fell suddenly, check for change in respiratory disease (such as development of a pneumothorax) or a mechanical problem (such as oxygen tubing disconnection), then obtain an arterial blood sample for PaO_2.
Between 85%–95%	No immediate action indicated. However, an arterial blood sample should be analyzed periodically for PaO_2, $PaCO_2$, and pH.
>95% saturation	Decrease FiO_2 by approximately 5% per minute until the oximeter reads 95%. Then obtain an arterial blood sample for PaO_2.

If changes in oxygenation occur during procedures such as suctioning a baby's airway or drawing a blood sample

- Stop the procedure until the oxyhemoglobin saturation returns to 85% to 95%.

and/or

- Increase the FiO_2 to maintain the oxyhemoglobin saturation between 85% to 95%. Remember to readjust the FiO_2 after completion of the procedure.

11. When Do You Obtain an Arterial Blood Gas Measurement?

If an oximeter is used, wait until the baby is relatively calm and the oximeter readings have been stable without wide fluctuations for several minutes. Then obtain an arterial blood sample as described previously. Even if the oximeter reads consistently within the normal range, if a baby has acute lung disease and is receiving supplemental oxygen, PaO_2 should be measured from an arterial blood sample several times a day.

If an oximeter is *not* used, arterial blood gas determination should be made

- Approximately every 4 hours during acute illness, if the previous PaO_2 was between 45 and 75 mm Hg and the baby's clinical condition has not changed,
- Whenever the baby's clinical condition worsens, and
- Approximately 10 to 30 minutes after each significant change in the FiO_2

12. What Are the Problems Related to Oxygen Therapy?

The chances of developing complications from too much or too little oxygen can be lessened by

- *Monitoring oxyhemoglobin saturation and*
- *Obtaining frequent arterial blood gas measurements and*
- *Making appropriate changes in FiO₂*

A. Too Little Oxygen in the Blood: Brain Damage

If a baby does not receive enough oxygen, the baby may suffer permanent brain damage. Other organs, such as the kidneys or gastrointestinal tract, may also be damaged.

B. Too Much Oxygen in the Blood: Eye Damage

Preterm infants may have serious eye damage if too much oxygen is in their blood for prolonged periods. This condition is called retinopathy of prematurity (ROP), previously termed retrolental fibroplasia.

Eye damage can occur even if the FiO_2 is relatively low. A baby with normal lungs in as little as 28% FiO_2 may have a PaO_2 as high as 150 mm Hg.

Although preterm babies with prolonged high blood oxygen concentrations are at risk for developing ROP, many other factors are also implicated in the development of ROP.

If ROP develops, the more preterm the baby the more severe the ROP is likely to be. All extremely preterm babies, regardless of the amount or duration of exposure to supplemental oxygen, and any preterm baby who received supplemental oxygen for a substantial length of time, should have an eye examination to rule out ROP (Book III, Continuing Care).

One of several factors causing ROP is high concentrations of oxygen in the blood.

C. Too Much Oxygen to the Lungs: Lung Damage

Lung damage may result from being exposed to very high FiO_2 for many days, even if blood oxygen levels are normal. Lung damage is unlikely during short-term oxygen administration.

D. Rapidly Changing Inspired Oxygen

Rapid decreases in FiO_2 can cause a sharp drop in the PaO_2 level. This may worsen a baby's condition. Higher FiO_2 may then be needed to maintain the baby's PaO_2 between 45 and 75 mm Hg.

If movement of a baby is essential (eg, to weigh a baby or obtain an x-ray), continue to give the baby oxygen by mask during the *entire* procedure.

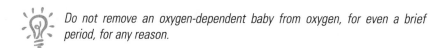

Do not remove an oxygen-dependent baby from oxygen, for even a brief period, for any reason.

13. What Are Normal Arterial Blood Gas Values and How Are Capillary and Venous Blood Gas Values Used?

A. Arterial Blood Gas Measurements

Normal Arterial Values:

pH:	7.25–7.35
$PaCO_2$:	40–50 mm Hg
PaO_2:	45–75 mm Hg

This unit focuses on how to provide oxygen therapy and how to assess and monitor a baby's oxygenation. The values for carbon dioxide and pH are given here so the different types of samples can be compared. Further discussion of the interpretation of pH and carbon dioxide concentration in assessing a baby's ventilation status, and/or need for assisted ventilation, is given in Book II: Neonatal Care, Respiratory Distress and in Book III, Review: Is the Baby Sick?

B. Capillary Blood Gas Measurements

Blood gas measurements obtained from capillary blood give close estimates of arterial blood pH and carbon dioxide concentration *if* the samples have been obtained using the proper technique. However, arterial blood oxygen concentration cannot be estimated accurately from capillary oxygen concentration. Therefore, capillary blood gas measurements should not be used to assess a baby's oxygenation.

Capillary measurements may be useful, in an emergency and when it has not been possible to obtain an arterial blood gas sample, to estimate the baby's need for assisted ventilation based on the pH and PCO_2 values. Capillary blood gas measurements, coupled with use of pulse oximetry, are also used in older babies who continue to require oxygen but do not have umbilical arterial catheters in place (Book III, Continuing Care).

Normal Capillary Values:

pH:	7.25–7.35, with proper technique
PCO_2:	40–50 mm Hg, with proper technique
PO_2:	Unreliable

Proper technique requires a well-warmed heel (to increase the blood circulation in the capillaries) and a steady blood flow after the puncture has been made. Care should be taken not to injure the baby's heel. Follow the procedure for heel sticks outlined in Blood Glucose Screening Tests (Book II: Neonatal Care, Hypoglycemia, skill).

C. Venous Blood Gas Measurements

Blood gas measurements obtained from venous blood also give close estimates of arterial blood pH and carbon dioxide concentration. The sampling technique is simpler than it is for capillary samples. Blood obtained from any venipuncture will give reliable estimates.

As with capillary blood gas measurements, venous blood gas values cannot be used to assess oxygenation, but may be useful in an emergency, and when it has not been possible to obtain an arterial sample, to estimate the baby's ventilation based on the pH and PCO_2 values.

Normal Venous Values: pH: 7.25–7.35
                          PCO_2:   40–50 mm Hg
                          PO_2:   Unreliable

Only arterial blood gas measurements give accurate information about a baby's oxygenation.

Now answer these questions to test yourself on the information in the last section.

C1. What may happen when a baby who requires additional oxygen is removed from the oxygen for a brief period?

_____

C2. **True** **False** A baby who has an arterial blood oxygen of 100 mm Hg in an inspired oxygen concentration of 22% requires continued supplemental oxygen.

C3. An infant's arterial blood oxygen is 130 mm Hg while in 45% oxygen. The concentration of inspired oxygen should

    A. Be lowered to 40%
    B. Be lowered to 35%
    C. Not be lowered at this time

C4. How long after a change in inspired oxygen concentration should a blood gas measurement be taken if an oximeter is _not_ being used?

    A. 10 to 30 minutes
    B. 60 to 90 minutes
    C. 2 to 4 hours

C5. Which 2 organs are _most_ likely to be damaged from too _little_ blood oxygen?

    A. Brain
    B. Eyes
    C. Lungs
    D. Kidneys

C6. Which organ is _most_ likely to be damaged from too _much_ blood oxygen?

    A. Brain
    B. Eyes
    C. Lungs
    D. Kidneys

C7. Which organ is _most_ likely to be damaged from supplemental inspired oxygen (even with normal blood oxygen) over a long period?

    A. Brain
    B. Eyes
    C. Lungs
    D. Kidneys

C8. A baby has an oxyhemoglobin saturation of 84% in an inspired oxygen concentration of 37%. What should you do?

    A. Increase the inspired oxygen concentration until the oxyhemoglobin saturation is between 85% to 95%.
    B. Check an arterial blood gas measurement.
    C. Both of the above.

C9. A baby is receiving 40% inspired oxygen and has an arterial blood oxygen value of 37 mm Hg. The baby appears pink. An oximeter is not available. How should her oxygen therapy be adjusted?

    A. Inspired oxygen concentration decreased to 35%, and a blood gas measurement obtained in 10 minutes.
    B. Inspired oxygen concentration increased to 60%, and a blood gas measurement obtained in 2 to 4 hours.
    C. Inspired oxygen concentration increased to 60%, and a blood gas measurement obtained in 20 minutes.
    D. Baby is pink, no change in inspired oxygen concentration is needed.

C10. An infant is in an inspired oxygen concentration of 50%, has an arterial blood oxygen of 40 mm Hg, and has an oxyhemoglobin saturation of 80%. How should you adjust the baby's inspired oxygen concentration?

    A. Increase it

    B. Decrease it

    C. No change

C11. Fill in the following chart for the normal values for arterial, venous, and capillary blood gas samples. Refer to the previous sections if necessary.

Arterial Blood	**Venous Blood**	**Capillary Blood**
PaO_2: _____	PO_2: _____	PO_2: _____
$PaCO_2$: _____	PCO_2: _____	PCO_2: _____
pH: _____	pH: _____	pH: _____

Check your answers with the list that follows the Recommended Routines. Correct any incorrect answers and review the appropriate section in the unit.

Recommended Routines

All of the routines listed below are based on the principles of perinatal care presented in the unit you have just finished. They are recommended as part of routine perinatal care.

Read each routine carefully and decide whether it is standard operating procedure in your hospital. Check the appropriate blank next to each routine.

Procedure Standard in My Hospital	Needs Discussion by Our Staff	
_____	_____	1. Periodically check oxygen delivery equipment to ensure • A precise and adjustable concentration from 22% to 100% can be achieved. • Oxygen can be humidified and warmed to a precise and adjustable temperature.
_____	_____	2. Establish a routine for monitoring the inspired oxygen concentration (FiO_2) continuously or at least every hour for every baby receiving supplemental oxygen.
_____	_____	3. If a pulse oximeter is not being used, establish a routine for obtaining an arterial blood sample • Approximately every 4 hours during acute illness, if the previous arterial blood oxygen was between 45 and 75 mm Hg and the baby's clinical condition has not changed, • Whenever the baby's clinical condition worsens, and • Approximately 10 to 30 minutes after each significant change in the FiO_2
_____	_____	4. Establish a routine for pulse oximeter use, including • Continuous oximetry monitoring for any baby receiving oxygen therapy • Adjusting FiO_2 based on oximeter readings • Obtaining arterial blood gas samples intermittently, after oximeter readings have stabilized, following a significant change in FiO_2 or worsening of the baby's clinical condition
_____	_____	5. Establish a policy that will allow sufficient oxygen to be given to keep a cyanotic baby pink until appropriate blood gas determinations are made.

6. Establish a system that ensures an ophthalmologist with experience with retinopathy of prematurity performs a dilated funduscopic examination for

- Babies born at 30 weeks' gestation or less or with birth weight less than 1,500 g

  or

- Babies with birth weight of 1,500 g to 2,000 g but with an unstable clinical course and believed to be at high risk for retinopathy of prematurity with examinations performed at

- 31 weeks' postmenstrual age for babies born at 22 to 27 weeks' gestation

  and

- 4 weeks chronologic age for babies born at 28 to 32 weeks' gestation (Book III, Continuing Care)

These are the answers to the self-test questions. Please check them with the answers you gave and review the information in the unit wherever necessary.

A1. A.   Measure the arterial blood oxygen level.
A2. Central cyanosis
     Resuscitation (21%–100%, depending on the baby's condition and response)
     Respiratory distress with low arterial oxygenation
A3. Acrocyanosis without central cyanosis
     Prematurity without respiratory distress or cyanosis
A4. Mix oxygen with air to provide desired concentration.
     Warm and humidify oxygen/air mixture to the baby's neutral thermal environment temperature.
     Prevent fluctuations in oxygen concentration (use oxyhood).
     Measure inspired concentration precisely (use oxygen analyzer).
     Measure the baby's blood oxygen concentration intermittently.
A5. Measure arterial blood oxygen level and monitor oxyhemoglobin saturation
A6. Damage to vital tissues, particularly the eyes
A7. Brain damage, as well as damage to other vital organs
A8. C.   If the baby is cyanotic or has a low arterial blood oxygen value or oximeter reading

B1. A.   50%
B2. C.   60 mm Hg and 90% saturation
B3. A.   From an umbilical artery catheter
B4. 45 mm Hg and 75 mm Hg
B5. C.   100%
B6. C.   Enough to keep the arterial blood oxygen between 45 and 75 mm Hg
B7. B.   Bound to hemoglobin

C1. If oxygen concentrations are lowered rapidly, even for a few minutes, the arteries to the lungs may constrict, reducing the oxygen flow to the body, resulting in a low arterial blood oxygen level. The arteries may stay constricted, even after the inspired oxygen concentration is increased, causing the baby to become sicker.
C2. False An arterial blood oxygen of 100 mm Hg is higher than the desired range of 45 to 75 mm Hg. Therefore, the inspired oxygen concentration should be lowered. Inspired oxygen concentration of 22% can be lowered only to 21% because that is the oxygen concentration in room air. Continued supplemental oxygen, therefore, is not required.
C3. B.   35%
C4. A.   10 to 30 minutes
C5. A.   Brain
     D.   Kidneys
C6. B.   Eyes
C7. C.   Lungs
C8. C.   First, look at the baby. If the baby's clinical appearance remains the same, then check to be sure the oximeter is functioning correctly. Check for a disconnection in the oxygen delivery system. If the baby's clinical appearance has deteriorated or if the oximeter is operating correctly, but the percent saturation remains low, immediately increase the inspired oxygen concentration.
C9. C.   The arterial blood oxygen is low, therefore the inspired oxygen concentration should be increased immediately, and another blood gas measurement obtained 10 to 30 minutes after the change in inspired oxygen concentration. Remember, a baby may appear pink and still have low blood oxygen.
C10. A.   Increase inspired oxygen concentration to keep arterial blood oxygen between 45 and 75 mm Hg and oxyhemoglobin saturation between 85% and 95%.

C11.   **Arterial Blood**   **Venous Blood**   **Capillary Blood**

   PaO_2:   45–75 mm Hg PO_2:   Unreliable PO_2:   Unreliable

   $PaCO_2$: 40–50 mm Hg PCO_2: 40–50 mm Hg PCO_2: 40–50 mm Hg*

   pH: 7.25–7.35   pH: 7.25–7.35   pH: 7.25–7.35*

*Only if proper technique is used to collect the sample. If the heel is not warmed and/or there is not a steady flow of blood during collection of the sample, the values obtained are likely to be incorrect and misleading.

Unit 2 Posttest

Without referring back to the information in the unit, please answer the following questions. Select the one best answer to each question (unless otherwise instructed). Record your answers on the answer sheet that is the last page in this book *and* on the test.

1. Which of the following statements is accurate regarding pulse oximetry?
   A. Light is used to estimate the oxyhemoglobin saturation of hemoglobin.
   B. Percent saturation of hemoglobin with oxygen is abbreviated PaO_2.
   C. Pulse oximetry is particularly sensitive in detecting high arterial oxygen concentration.
   D. Percent saturation refers to the amount of oxygen that is dissolved in the plasma of the blood.

2. A 33-week, 1-hour-old preterm baby with normal blood pressure, temperature, and heart rate is pink with mild respiratory distress and an arterial blood oxygen of 37 in 35% inspired oxygen concentration. Which of the following is the *most* appropriate action?
   A. Decrease the inspired oxygen concentration to 30% and obtain another arterial blood gas sample.
   B. Prepare for endotracheal intubation and assisted ventilation.
   C. Maintain the same inspired oxygen concentration because the baby is pink.
   D. Increase the inspired oxygen concentration to 50% and obtain another arterial blood gas sample in 20 minutes.

3. A baby is quiet and not undergoing any procedures. A pulse oximeter reads 80% with the baby in 40% inspired oxygen concentration. Which of the following should you do *first*?
   A. Obtain an arterial blood gas sample.
   B. Increase the baby's inspired oxygen concentration to approximately 60%.
   C. Obtain a chest x-ray.
   D. Listen for breath sounds.

4. Which of the following procedures is the *best* way to measure the concentration of inspired oxygen?
   A. With an oxygen analyzer
   B. Take blood gas measurements
   C. Check the liter-per-minute flow of oxygen
   D. With a pulse oximeter

5. **True   False**   For most babies, oxyhemoglobin saturation of 85% to 95% indicates an arterial oxygen concentration of 45 to 75 mm Hg.

6. **True   False**   A baby's kidneys can suffer damage from low arterial blood oxygen concentration.

7. **True   False**   In an emergency, venous blood gas measurements may be useful to assess a baby's need for assisted ventilation, but not oxygenation status.

8. **True   False**   Oxygen from a tank that has been in a warm room for 48 hours still needs to be heated and humidified.

9. **True   False**   If a baby with respiratory distress is pink in 60% oxygen, the baby can safely be removed from the oxygen briefly for simple procedures, such as weighing.

10. **True   False**   Cyanosis of the hands and feet usually indicates that the baby needs oxygen.

11. Which of the following procedures is the *best* way to gauge the amount of inspired oxygen an infant needs?
    A. Degree of cyanosis of the trunk and mucous membranes
    B. Degree of cyanosis of the hands and feet
    C. Venous blood gas measurement
    D. Arterial blood gas measurement

12. Which of the following babies should *not* have his/her inspired oxygen concentration increased?
    A. A baby in the delivery room with an Apgar score of 2
    B. A baby with blue lips and mouth
    C. A 32-week (gestational age) baby with an oxyhemoglobin saturation of 92%
    D. A 42-week (gestational age) baby with respiratory distress and a heart rate of 80

13. An infant is born with respiratory problems. It appears that he will require oxygen therapy for at least several hours. Which of the following is the *most* appropriate way to deliver this oxygen?

- **A.** With bag and mask
- **B.** Into the incubator
- **C.** With an oxygen hood
- **D.** By a funnel placed close to the face

For each question, please make sure you have marked your answer on the test and on the answer sheet (last page in book). The test is for you; the answer sheet will need to be turned in for continuing education credit.

Skill Unit 1   Administering Oxygen

Measuring Oxygen Concentration
Mixing Oxygen and Compressed Air
Heating and Humidifying an Oxygen/Air Mixture

The following 3 skill subunits will teach you how to use the equipment needed to deliver a desired amount of oxygen to a baby. You will learn how to calibrate an oxygen analyzer, heat and humidify oxygen, mix oxygen and compressed air, and measure environmental oxygen concentration.

Study these skill units; then attend a skill practice and demonstration session.

To master the skills, you will need to demonstrate correctly each of the following steps:

Calibration of analyzer

1. Connect equipment.

2. Calibrate analyzer by following the steps in the skill to adjust the sensor in 100% oxygen and check that it reads 21% oxygen in room air and/or follow the manufacturer's directions for calibrating the analyzer.

Heating, humidifying, and mixing oxygen with air

1. Set up heating/humidifying equipment.

2. Adjust temperature.

3. Connect oxygen/air source to equipment.

4. Determine liters per minute flow rates (unless a blender is being used).

5. Establish precise oxygen concentration.

6. Monitor oxyhood temperature.

The following 3 skill units will teach the techniques required for

- Measuring oxygen concentration
- Heating and humidifying an oxygen/air mixture
- Mixing oxygen and compressed air

The drawing below shows the equipment necessary for administering oxygen to a baby.

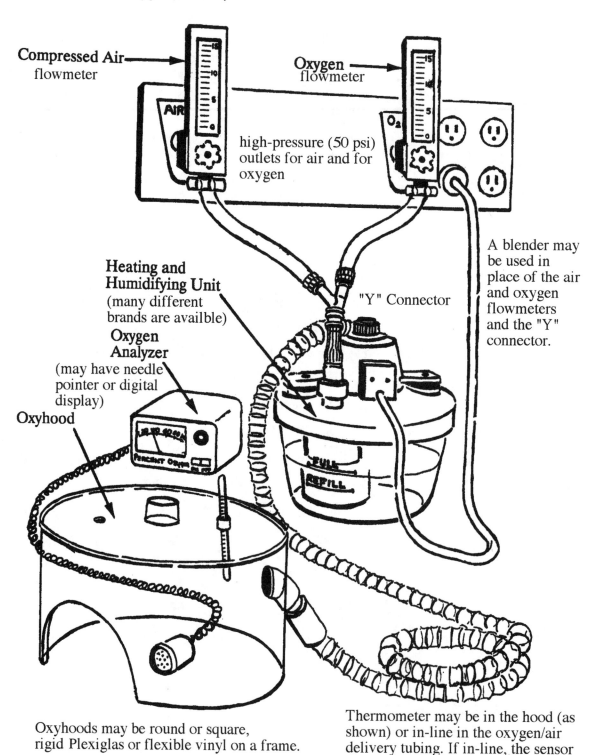

Compressed Air flowmeter

Oxygen flowmeter

high-pressure (50 psi) outlets for air and for oxygen

Heating and Humidifying Unit (many different brands are availble)

Oxygen Analyzer (may have needle pointer or digital display)

Oxyhood

"Y" Connector

A blender may be used in place of the air and oxygen flowmeters and the "Y" connector.

Oxyhoods may be round or square, rigid Plexiglas or flexible vinyl on a frame.

Thermometer may be in the hood (as shown) or in-line in the oxygen/air delivery tubing. If in-line, the sensor should be at a point close to the baby.

It is important to know the type of oxygen analyzer in use in your nursery and how to operate, calibrate, and maintain it. For example

- Some analyzers require batteries. Know when and how the batteries should be changed.

- Some require the sensor unit be changed periodically. Know when and how to do this.

- Many analyzers require periodic recalibration but the frequency of recalibration varies. Know when and how to calibrate the analyzer.

 An oxygen analyzer must be maintained and calibrated properly. It may "look as if it's working" when actually the concentration registered is not the oxygen concentration the baby is receiving. An uncalibrated analyzer is worse than no an-

Actions	**Remarks**

Deciding to Calibrate an Oxygen Analyzer

1. Will you be caring for a baby who requires oxygen therapy?	
Yes: Check the functioning of the oxygen analyzer.	Even a properly maintained oxygen analyzer will require periodic recalibration. The interval between calibrations may be 8 to 24 hours, depending on the type of analyzer. Some analyzers are designed to have the sensor changed rather than be recalibrated.
No: Make sure the analyzer is well maintained and ready for use.	

Preparing to Calibrate

2. Prepare the proper equipment.	
• Source of 100% oxygen (wall outlet or tank)	
• Flowmeter or gauge to attach to oxygen outlet or tank	If you are using an oxygen tank, be sure you have the key to open the tank.
• Oxygen analyzer	
• Appropriate tools, if any, are needed to turn the adjustment on the analyzer	
• Small plastic bag or non-sterile glove	
3. Check to see that the oxygen analyzer is in proper working condition.	Follow the operating and maintenance instructions for your nursery's analyzer.

| **Actions** | **Remarks** |

Calibrating an Oxygen Analyzer

 The method of calibration shown here may not be appropriate for all analyzers. Be sure to check the manufacturer's recommended procedure for calibrating your analyzer(s).

4. Attach a flowmeter or gauge to the oxygen source.

Do not use a heating or humidifying unit when calibrating an analyzer. It is important that the oxygen be dry during calibration. Oxygen directly from a wall outlet or tank contains no humidity.

5. Place the sensor of the oxygen analyzer into the plastic bag or non-sterile glove.

6. Turn on the oxygen source and direct the oxygen flow into the bag or glove to fill it with 100% oxygen. Squeeze the opening of the bag or glove around the oxygen tubing and sensor cord so that the bag or glove inflates slightly, but allowing enough flow to escape so that too much pressure does not build up.

7. Keep the sensor in the bag with continuous oxygen flow for at least 1 full minute.

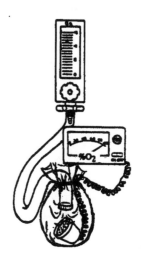

8. Adjust the calibration so that the analyzer reads *exactly* 100% oxygen.

   Note: Some analyzers are not designed to be calibrated but rather are programmed to give a signal that the whole sensor needs to be replaced.

Adjustment should be made while the sensor remains in 100% oxygen.

For analyzers with a digital display, you may need to "unlock" the higher/lower arrows before adjustments can be made. Some analyzers require a special tool to make an adjustment.

9. Turn off the oxygen flow and place the sensor in room air.

Observe if the analyzer reads 21% (room air is 21% oxygen).

10. If the analyzer does not read 21% in room air, recheck the analyzer to make sure it is in proper operating condition, then repeat steps 5 through 9.

If you have repeated steps 5 through 9 and the oxygen analyzer still does not read 100% in dry oxygen from a wall outlet or tank and 21% in room air, refer to the manufacturer's instructions. The analyzer may need to be repaired, the sensor replaced, or other measures taken.

Actions   **Remarks**

Measuring the Baby's Inspired Oxygen Concentration

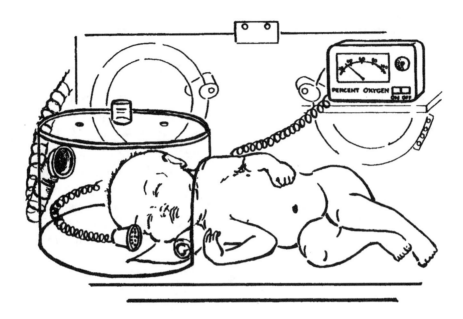

Note: The illustration is designed to show equipment needed for oxygen delivery and monitoring, not all components of a baby's care. A pulse oximeter is not shown but is commonly attached to a baby's hand or foot.

Oxyhoods come in various sizes and shapes and are made from various materials. Whatever type is used in your nursery, be sure a baby's head fits completely inside the hood. There are also several types of *oxygen analyzers*. Many have a digital display of the oxygen concentration. Thermometers are sometimes contained in a flexible wire that fits within the oxygen delivery tubing. Whatever type of *thermometer* is used, be sure it measures the temperature of the oxygen/air mixture at a point near the baby.

11.   After calibrating the oxygen analyzer, put the sensor inside the baby's oxyhood. Place the sensor near the baby's nose.

The oxygen concentration will vary slightly in different places inside the oxyhood. It is important to check the oxygen concentration near the baby's nose.

All oxygen sensors contain caustic chemicals. Normally the chemicals are sealed within the sensor, but if a sensor becomes cracked, the chemicals can leak out and burn a baby's skin. Be careful that the sensor does not come in direct contact with a baby.

12.   If possible, leave the oxygen sensor in the oxyhood for continuous monitoring of the inspired oxygen concentration. Some monitors have alarms that will signal if the oxygen concentrations fall.

If continuous monitoring is not possible, the oxygen concentration should be measured and recorded frequently (at least every hour).

Actions	Remarks

What Can Go Wrong?

Actions	Remarks
1. The analyzer shows a drop in the oxygen concentration in the oxyhood.	Check • Tubing is connected and flow rates are as previously set. • Sensor is not wet (wet sensor may give a false reading). • Analyzer calibrates properly and batteries (if needed) are fresh. • No excess water is in the tubing between the heating/humidifying device and oxyhood. • Sensor does not need to be replaced.
2. The baby is in oxygen alone (no compressed air) but the analyzer reads only 94%.	This may be OK. Because the analyzer was calibrated in 100% dry oxygen, it may only read a maximum of 94% in humidified oxygen.

Mixing Oxygen and Compressed Air

When only oxygen is delivered to a baby's oxyhood, it will result in the baby breathing 100% oxygen, regardless of the liter-per-minute flow rate.

The flow rate of oxygen (expressed in liters per minute) regulates only the speed of the oxygen flow, not the concentration. Oxygen directly from a wall outlet or tank is always 100% oxygen.

 Oxygen must be mixed with compressed air to deliver less than 100% oxygen.

The concentration of oxygen in room air is 21%. Any oxygen concentration between 22% and 99% may be achieved by mixing varying amounts of compressed air with 100% oxygen.

Actions	Remarks

Deciding to Mix Oxygen and Compressed Air

1. Do you anticipate the admission of a baby who may require oxygen therapy?

    Yes: Set up the equipment used in your nursery for mixing oxygen and compressed air.

    No: Make sure clean equipment for mixing oxygen and compressed air is available at all times.

Preparing to Mix Oxygen and Air

2. Collect the proper equipment.

   * Oxygen source
   * Compressed air source

   Oxygen and compressed air may come from wall outlets or from separate tanks. If you are using tanks, check how much gas is left in each tank. Portable air compressors may also be used to provide compressed air.

   * Heater/humidifier for oxygen/air mixture

   Many commercial units are available that will heat and humidify oxygen at the same time.

   * Oxyhood

   An oxyhood is necessary to keep a constant oxygen concentration around a baby's face.

   * Oxygen analyzer
   * Thermometer or temperature probe that can be placed in the baby's oxyhood or delivery tubing
   * *Sterile* water for the humidifier

Actions | **Remarks**

Preparing to Mix Oxygen and Air (continued)

If a blender will *not* be used, collect the following items:
- Oxygen flowmeter
- Air flowmeter
- "Y" connector
- Tubing
  - Small diameter ⟶ to connect oxygen and air sources to "Y" connector
  - Small diameter ⟶ to connect "Y" connector to heater/humidifier
  - Large diameter ⟶ to connect heater/humidifier to oxyhood

Using this equipment allows you to adjust the flow of oxygen and the flow of compressed air to achieve the desired oxygen concentration.

Regardless of the delivery system you use—with or without a blender—the concentration of oxygen should always be checked with a calibrated oxygen analyzer, near a baby's nose.

If a blender will be used, collect the following items:
- Blender (several brands are commercially available)
- Oxygen and air high-pressure tubing to connect blender to oxygen and air sources
- Tubing
  - Small diameter ⟶ to connect blender to heater/humidifier
  - Large diameter ⟶ to connect heater/humidifier to oxyhood

Blenders are easy to use because they allow you to set the desired oxygen concentration on a dial, rather than adjusting separate flow rates for oxygen and air. Blender dials, however, are frequently imprecise.

3. Connect tubing and set up heating/humidifying system.

The illustration on the second page of this skill unit shows an oxygen delivery system using the equipment listed here (without a blender). If a blender is used it replaces the oxygen and air flowmeters, tubing from the flowmeters to the "Y" connector, and the "Y" connector.

Air Liter/Minute Flow

Oxygen Liter/Minute Flow	1	2	3	4	5	6	7	8	9	10
1			41	37	34	32	31	30	29	28
2		**61**	53	47	44	41	38	37	35	34
3	80	68	**61**	55	51	47	45	43	41	39
4	84	74	66	**61**	56	52	50	47	45	44
5	86	77	70	65	**61**	57	54	51	49	47
6	88	80	74	68	64	**61**	57	55	53	51
7	90	82	76	71	67	64	**61**	58	56	54
8	91	84	78	74	70	66	63	**61**	58	56
9	92	86	80	76	72	68	65	63	**61**	58
10	93	87	82	77	74	70	67	65	63	**61**

Cells Show Approximate Percent (%) Oxygen Concentration

Actions	Remarks

Achieving Approximate Oxygen Concentration

4. Make sure an oxygen analyzer is in good working condition. Calibrate it, as necessary.	See the previous skill unit, Measuring Oxygen Concentration.
5. Decide what oxygen concentration you want to deliver (eg, 65% oxygen).	See the chart on the previous page or in the basic unit.

6. If you are not using a blender, find this oxygen concentration in the oxygen liters-per-minute flow versus air liters-per-minute flow chart of the basic unit.	In the chart you will find that a single oxygen concentration may appear at several places. For example, approximately 65% oxygen can be achieved with
	    4 L/min oxygen + 3 L/min air or
	    9 L/min oxygen + 7 L/min air

7. If you are not using a blender, select flow rates that give a combined flow of approximately 8 to 12 L/min. Use the lower end of that range for small babies, and the higher end of the range for big babies.	*High flow* rate is not necessary. High flow will increase a baby's *heat loss by convection,* even if the oxygen/air mixture is heated. *Very low flow,* however, will allow *carbon dioxide to build up* in a baby's oxyhood.
8. Open the flowmeters to the oxygen and air chosen flow rates. OR Dial the desired oxygen concentration on the blender.	

Adjusting Oxygen Concentration

9. Measure the oxygen concentration inside the oxyhood by placing the analyzer sensor near the baby's nose.	
10. Slightly increase or decrease the oxygen or airflow rate. OR Turn the dial on the blender up or down until the desired concentration is achieved. After making each adjustment wait a moment, until the analyzer needle or digital display is stable, before making another adjustment.	For example, if the flow rates selected initially give 68% oxygen, when 65% was desired, then either turn down the oxygen flow slightly or turn up the compressed air flow slightly. A properly calibrated and maintained analyzer is more accurate than a blender. Adjust the blender dial up or down until the analyzer registers the desired concentration, even if that means the percentage of oxygen shown on the blender dial is slightly above or below the concentration registered by the oxygen analyzer.
11. Recheck and record the oxygen concentration in a baby's oxyhood a few minutes after each adjustment and at least once every hour.	

Actions	**Remarks**

What Can Go Wrong?

1. The baby's $PaCO_2$ (carbon dioxide) rises.

   Check the oxygen and air combined flow rate; adjust it to greater than 8 L/min to be sure the baby is not re-breathing exhaled air. Rising $PaCO_2$ level may also mean that the baby's lung disease is getting worse and you should consider the need for assisted ventilation.

2. The oxygen concentration as measured by the analyzer is different from the concentration calculated from the chart or set on the blender dial.

   Check that tubes are connected. Remove condensed water from tubes. Check analyzer functioning and recalibrate or change sensor. If the difference persists and is not too great, consider the analyzer to be correct.

3. The baby's body temperature becomes too high or too low.

   Check that the temperature of the oxyhood is adjusted to neutral thermal environment (Book II: Neonatal Care, Thermal Environment). If the baby is cool, check that flow rate of the oxygen/air mixture is not too high. A high flow rate could cool a baby by convective heat loss.

4. The baby's blood oxygen concentration (PaO_2) or oxygen saturation (% sat.) falls quickly or the baby becomes blue.

   First, increase oxygen concentration in the oxyhood or temporarily ventilate the baby with a bag and mask and 100% oxygen until the baby is pink (and oxygen saturation is stable between 85% to 95%, if a pulse oximeter is available). Check to see that all the tubing is properly connected. Consider the possibility of a pneumothorax and obtain a portable chest x-ray. Monitor the baby's oxygenation and provide other therapy as appropriate.

Perinatal Performance Guide
Heating and Humidifying an Oxygen/Air Mixture

Actions	Remarks

Deciding to Heat and Humidify an Oxygen/Air Mixture

1. Do you anticipate the admission of a baby who may require oxygen therapy?

   Yes: Set up the equipment used in your nursery for heating and humidifying an oxygen/air mixture.

   No: Make sure clean equipment for heating and humidifying an oxygen/air mixture is available at all times.

Preparing to Heat and Humidify an Oxygen/Air Mixture

2. Collect the proper equipment.

   - Heater for oxygen/air mixture
   - Humidifier for the oxygen/air mixture

   - Thermometer or temperature probe, which can be placed in the oxyhood or in-line in the delivery system, at a point near the baby

   - *Sterile* water for irrigation

   - Tubing, oxyhood, oxygen analyzer, and other equipment needed for oxygen therapy (See previous skill units.)

   The heater must have a range of temperature settings. Although there are some humidifiers that only humidify without heating an oxygen/air mixture, these units are *not* desirable. Heated humidifiers work by heating the water used for humidification.

   Do *not* use tap water to fill the humidifier. Tap water contains numerous bacterial organisms that would multiply in the warmed water.

Heating and Humidifying an Oxygen/Air Mixture

3. Use "sterile water for irrigation" to fill the humidifying container to the "full" line.

   OR

   Connect a bag of sterile water to the heater/humidifier with intravenous (IV) tubing.

   It is important to keep the water level between the "full" and "refill" marks. A heater will not work properly unless there is sufficient water in the humidifying container. More water may need to be added periodically (frequency depends on the brand of heater/humidifier).

   Some units have a connection port for IV tubing so that sterile water fills the humidifier continuously and the system does not need to be opened to add water.

Actions   **Remarks**

Heating and Humidifying an Oxygen/Air Mixture (continued)

4. Plug in the heater.

5. Adjust the temperature setting on the heater to a medium setting.

    Some heaters may be set in degrees. If this is the case for your heater, set the temperature to a mid-point in the baby's neutral thermal environment (NTE) range (Book II: Neonatal Care, Thermal Environment).

6. Connect the heating/humidifying unit between the oxygen/air sources and the oxyhood.

7. Place the thermometer or temperature probe inside the baby's oxyhood or inside the delivery tubing, depending on the type of heater you are using. Place the thermometer or tip of the probe at a point close to the baby.

    The temperature of the oxygen/air mixture will drop several degrees as it passes through the tubing between the heating/humidifying unit and the oxyhood. It is important to measure the temperature near the baby.

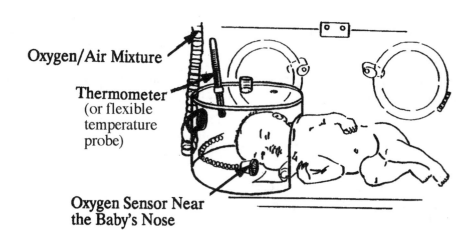

Oxygen/Air Mixture

Thermometer
(or flexible
temperature
probe)

Oxygen Sensor Near
the Baby's Nose

8. Adjust the oxygen/air mixture to the desired oxygen concentration.

    See the previous skill unit, Mixing Oxygen and Air.

    For some heaters, this may require careful, frequent monitoring and readjustment.

9. Regulate the heating adjustment until the temperature inside the oxyhood is within the baby's NTE range (Book II: Neonatal Care, Thermal Environment).

    The temperature inside the oxyhood will be determined by the temperature of the air/oxygen mixture, not by the temperature of the incubator or radiant warmer.

    Some heaters have a servocontrol mechanism. If this is the case, place the probe near the baby and set the heater temperature to a mid-point in the baby's NTE range.

Actions	Remarks

Maintaining a Heating and Humidifying System

10. Change the heating/humidifying unit and tubing periodically. This will reduce the possibility of bacteria growing within the system. The frequency of the change depends on the type of system you are using.

   To change a heating/humidifying system,

   a. Set up a clean, alternate heating/humidifying unit and tubing following steps 1 through 9.

   b. Heat the water in the clean heating/humidifying system.

   c. Quickly disconnect the old unit and connect the clean, alternate unit. Do this very quickly so the baby's oxygen is not interrupted for more than a few seconds.

   Plan ahead so the water can be heated to the appropriate temperature and the switch between "clean" and "dirty" equipment can be made quickly.

If the heater/humidifier needs to be opened to add sterile water to the water reservoir, it may need to be changed more often (usually every 24 hours) than a system that is closed with a continuous drip of sterile water to maintain the water level. Devices that contain heating wires within the delivery tubing minimize water condensation within the tubing and thus allow less chance for bacterial growth.

In-line heating wires and a closed system generally mean the system needs to be changed much less frequently (usually every 48–72 hours, or longer).

It is important to maintain the temperature of the oxygen/air mixture in the baby's oxyhood at a constant, appropriate temperature. A baby's whole body can be chilled or overheated if the temperature of the oxygen/air mixture is lower/higher than the baby's NTE (Book II: Neonatal Care, Thermal Environment, skills).

What Can Go Wrong?

1. The temperature of the oxygen/air mixture may become too cold.

   This will markedly increase the baby's oxygen and caloric requirements. Keep the temperature in the oxyhood within the baby's NTE range.

2. The temperature of the oxygen/air mixture may become too hot.

   This will severely stress the baby and increase the body temperature. Keep the temperature in the oxyhood within the baby's NTE range.

3. The humidifier may run dry.

   The unit will then not be able to either heat the air/oxygen mixture or provide humidity and the baby's mucous membranes will become dry. Check water level frequently.

4. Infection may result from inadequate cleaning of non-disposable heating/humidifying equipment.

   Change heating/humidifying equipment as recommended, according to the type of system used. Be sure all non-disposable equipment is cleaned thoroughly between uses.

Pulse Oximetry
Peripheral Arterial Blood Gas Sampling

These skill units will teach you how to monitor a baby's oxygenation using a pulse oximeter and how to obtain arterial blood samples from a peripheral artery for blood gas analysis. In Book II: Neonatal Care, Umbilical Catheters you will learn how to insert an umbilical arterial catheter and use it to obtain arterial blood gas samples.

Study these skill units, then attend a skill practice and demonstration session.

To master the skills, you will need to demonstrate correctly each of the following steps:

Pulse oximetry

1. Identify the features of an oximeter: sensor, patient cable, pulse indicator, pulse and saturation displays, alarms, etc.

2. Connect the sensor to a patient.

3. Adjust the sensor to obtain an accurate reading.

4. Set the alarms.

Peripheral arterial blood gas sampling

(Not everyone will be required to perform the skill. However, everyone should study the skill unit and learn the technique to assist with the procedure.)

1. Be aware of the risks associated with any arterial puncture.

2. Collect and prepare the appropriate equipment.

3. Locate the radial artery and cleanse the site for puncture.

4. Perform the puncture and obtain an arterial blood sample (using a model, or a baby in need of an arterial puncture).

5. Apply appropriate pressure to the puncture site for an appropriate length of time.

Note: Figures in this unit were reproduced with the permission of Nellcor Incorporated, 25495 Whitesell St, Hayward, CA 94545.

A pulse oximeter consists of 2 parts: a light that shines through the baby's skin and a light detector that measures the color of light coming through the skin. The color of the light coming through the skin is determined by the amount of oxygen carried by the hemoglobin in the red blood cells. The oximeter also detects the heart rate by sensing the pulsing of blood in the capillaries.

Some oximeters are designed to connect to a cardiac monitor so that the heart rate as determined by the pulse detector can be electronically checked against the heart rate as determined by the cardiac monitor. This comparison is made to determine the reliability of the oximeter reading.

Check the specifications of your oximeter.

• Is it supposed to be connected to a cardiac monitor?

• Is the sensor intended for use on babies? (Those made for adults generally do not work well when used on babies.)

Actions	Remarks
Deciding to Use a Pulse Oximeter	
1. Will you be caring for a baby who requires oxygen therapy? Yes: Plug in the oximeter, connect it to a cardiac monitor (if indicated), and attach the sensor cord to the monitor. No: Be sure the monitor and sensors are well maintained and ready for use.	An oximeter can be extremely valuable when caring for any baby who requires oxygen therapy. Although arterial blood gas determinations are still necessary, use of an oximeter will decrease the number of blood gases needed. Pulse oximetry also allows you to recognize very quickly the need for change in the inspired oxygen concentration a baby is receiving.
Preparing to Monitor a Baby	
2. Examine the sensor. 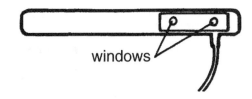	Look at the sensor head. There are 2 dot-like "windows"—one is a light emitter, the other a light detector. For the sensor to work properly, the detector must be able to "see" light coming from the emitter.

windows

Actions	Remarks

Preparing to Monitor a Baby (continued)

3. Select an appropriate site for monitoring by considering

• Size of patient	Select a thin portion of the body where the emitter light can shine through the tissue and be detected on the other side. A finger or a toe usually works best, but in a small baby, a foot or hand generally works.
• State of perfusion	The sensor must be able to detect a pulse of blood within the tissue. If your patient is very sick and has poor peripheral perfusion, select a site with relatively good perfusion. Locations closer to the heart, such as a thumb or hand, may work better than a foot or toe.
4. Wrap the sensor around the selected site, so the sensors are in contact with the baby's skin.	The 2 windows—light emitter and light detector—should be directly opposite each other.
Hold the sensor in place with Velcro or tape. (See manufacturer's recommendations.)	The wrap should be neither loose nor tight.

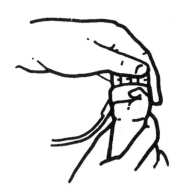 or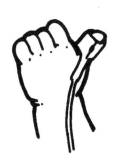

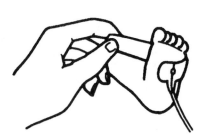 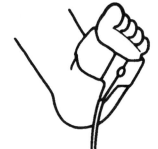 or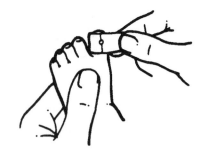

Actions	Remarks

Monitoring a Baby With Oximetry

5. Turn on the monitor.

The monitor will "search" for a pulse. If a pulse is detected, the monitor will indicate so with a flashing light-dot, a vertically stacked series of horizontal light-bars, and/or a tone that is activated with each heartbeat.

6. Adjust the sensor, if necessary, until the baby's pulse is displayed and is coincident with the heartbeat signal displayed on the cardiac monitor.

Although a baby can be monitored with a pulse oximeter alone, simultaneous use of a cardiac monitor will help in determining the reliability of the oximeter readings. Also, any baby sick enough to require oximetry probably should also have continuous electronic cardiorespiratory monitoring (Book I, Is the Baby Sick?).

7. When the heart rate displayed on the cardiac monitor and on the oximeter agree (within approximately 5 beats per minute), note the percent saturation displayed by the oximeter.

Be careful. Occasionally an oximeter will display a percent saturation reading even though the pulse is not being detected reliably. In such cases, the percent saturation reading is inaccurate.

Oxygen saturation displayed by a pulse oximeter is accurate only when the oximeter is correctly detecting the pulse.

8. If the baby is under a bright light, shield the sensor by covering it lightly with opaque material.

The detector in the sensor is supposed to "see" only light from the emitter. If the baby is under phototherapy or bright procedure light and the sensor is not shielded, the sensor may not work or a false reading may be obtained.

9. When the oximeter reading is relatively stable, obtain an arterial blood sample for determination of PaO_2. Note the oximeter reading at the time the sample is drawn.

Oximetry is valuable for following trends and changes in a baby's oxygenation, but does not replace the need for precise measurement of arterial PaO_2 (as well as $PaCO_2$ and pH).

10. Set the low and high alarms.

   Low: 85% sat

   High: 95% sat

Actions	Remarks

What Can Go Wrong?

1. The oximeter continues to "search" but cannot find a pulse, or there is a pulse displayed, but no percent saturation displayed.

Try readjusting the sensor or applying it to a new site that has better perfusion. Slight readjustments in the position of the light emitter and/or light detector can make the difference between a non-functional and a functional sensor. Be sure, too, that the "windows" are clean. Tiny bits of debris can interfere with the sensor. The sensor may not be plugged in securely to the monitor, or the sensor may be damaged.

2. The heart rate and percent saturation readings fluctuate rapidly.

This is usually motion artifact caused by an active baby, although some of the fluctuations may be real.

3. The percent saturation readings are misinterpreted to be the PaO_2, as determined from an arterial blood sample.

Remember that PaO_2 measures the oxygen dissolved in plasma, which is reported as "mm Hg." An oximeter measures oxygen bound to hemoglobin, which is reported as "% sat." Although the 2 values should correlate (see the basic unit), the exact numbers will not be the same.

4. The oximeter reading seems to be inaccurate.

Check to be sure that the pulse oximeter pulse rate is the same as the heart rate as determined by a cardiac monitor. If they are different the sensor may need to be adjusted. Also, check to be sure the sensor is shielded from bright light.

Peripheral Arterial Blood Gas Sampling

Actions	Remarks

Deciding to Obtain a Peripheral Blood Gas Sample

1. Obtain a peripheral arterial blood gas (ABG) sample if the baby needs a blood gas determination and does not have an umbilical arterial catheter (UAC) in place.	This may be done • When it is anticipated that a baby will require supplemental oxygen for only a few hours • To check a baby's ventilation and oxygenation status before undertaking an umbilical catheterization procedure • When UAC insertion has been unsuccessful, or it was necessary to remove the catheter
Use a UAC (Book II: Neonatal Care, Umbilical Catheters) whenever possible to obtain frequent blood gas samples.	There are several reasons ABG samples taken from a UAC are preferred to peripheral ABG samples. • A sample obtained with a needle may cause the baby to cry vigorously and therefore give a falsely low PaO_2 value and/or a falsely high or low $PaCO_2$ value. • Peripheral ABG samples may be difficult to obtain. • A peripheral puncture is more stressful for the baby than is sampling done from an umbilical catheter. • Certain complications may develop as a result of a needle puncture. • Venous blood, and not arterial blood, may be obtained with a peripheral sample.
2. Be aware of the risks and complications that are associated with peripheral arterial punctures.	Proper technique will minimize the occurrence of these complications and allow the same puncture site to be used repeatedly.
Possible complications include • *Hematoma* (a swollen, "black and blue" mark caused by bleeding from the vessel into the surrounding tissue)	A hematoma may result from • Repeated punctures and excessive probing with the needle to find the artery • Inadequate pressure applied to the artery after the procedure is completed

Actions	Remarks

Deciding to Obtain a Peripheral Blood Gas Sample (continued)

	A hematoma may cause • Tissue or nerve damage due to pressure • Difficulty in obtaining additional arterial samples from that site by obscuring the artery
• *Nerve damage*	Nerves often run parallel to arteries and may be damaged if punctured repeatedly. Pressure from a hematoma may also cause nerve damage.
• *Thrombus formation* (blood clot attached to the wall of a blood vessel)	A thrombus may develop after numerous punctures into the same spot in an artery. This can cause partial or complete blockage of the blood flow.
• *Embolus* (blood clot, air bubble, or other plug that is carried by the bloodstream)	An embolus can lodge in a blood vessel, obstruct the blood flow in that vessel and, thereby, cut off the blood supply to the tissues the artery perfuses. Both thrombi and emboli can cause severe tissue damage.
• *Arterial spasm*	Any artery that has been punctured may "clamp down" or constrict completely. This may or may not have serious consequences, depending on the amount of collateral circulation (blood flow to the same tissues but through different vessels) and the length of time the artery is in spasm.
• *Infection*	This may be a superficial soft tissue infection, such as might occur as a result of any needle puncture. If the bone is penetrated, osteomyelitis (bone infection) can occur. Although this is rare, osteomyelitis can be extremely difficult to treat and may cause severe, permanent damage.
3. Be aware of the advantages and special hazards associated with the puncture site chosen. These are listed and illustrated on the following pages.	Arterial blood gas determinations are often extremely important for determining therapy. Always try to obtain a sample from the lowest-risk site first. If this is unsuccessful, however, it may be necessary to obtain an ABG sample from a site associated with more risk.

Actions	Remarks

Deciding to Obtain a Peripheral Blood Gas Sample (continued)

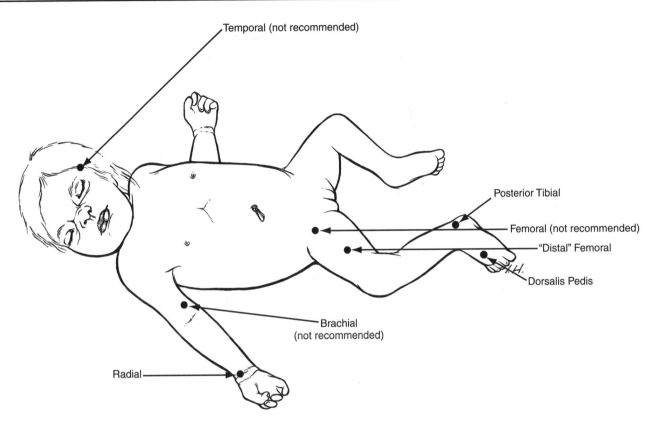

Temporal (not recommended)

Posterior Tibial

Femoral (not recommended)

"Distal" Femoral

Dorsalis Pedis

Brachial
(not recommended)

Radial

Radial Artery

Advantages
- No large veins nearby: therefore, almost 100% assurance that any blood obtained is arterial.
- Good collateral circulation via ulnar artery.
- Position of artery is stable, making it relatively easy to penetrate the artery.

Hazards
- Those for all arterial punctures

The radial artery is the recommended site for peripheral ABG sampling in newborns.

Brachial Artery

Advantages
- Collateral circulation via 3 small arteries

Hazards
- Those for all arterial punctures
- Deeper artery, not easily stabilized, tends to roll when puncture attempted
- High likelihood of obtaining venous blood
- Possibility of median nerve damage

Because collateral circulation is not ensured, brachial artery puncture should be avoided.

Actions	**Remarks**

Deciding to Obtain a Peripheral Blood Gas Sample (continued)

Distal Femoral Artery

Advantages

- Large vessel, penetrated fairly easily if leg held in proper position

Hazards

- Those for all arterial punctures
- High likelihood of obtaining venous blood from femoral vein
- Limited collateral circulation, making arterial spasm, thrombus, or embolus formation particularly hazardous

Dorsalis Pedis Artery

Advantages

- Good collateral circulation

Hazards

- Those for all arterial punctures
- Small artery, therefore difficult to puncture

Posterior Tibial Artery

Advantages

- Good collateral circulation
- No large veins nearby, therefore relative assurance that any blood obtained is arterial
- Position of artery is stable, making it relatively easy to penetrate artery

Hazards

- Those for all arterial punctures
- Possibility of posterior tibial nerve damage

Temporal Artery

Advantages

- Easily palpated, stable artery

Hazards

- Those for all arterial punctures
- Thrombus or embolus could cut off blood supply to an area(s) of the brain

"Distal femoral" is in the mid-thigh region, where the muscles make a "V" when the baby is supine with his/her leg is held in a "frog-like" position.

Temporal arteries should be AVOIDED as sampling sites in newborns.

Actions	**Remarks**

Deciding to Obtain a Peripheral Blood Gas Sample (continued)

Femoral Artery at Groin

Advantages
- Large artery in stable position, therefore penetrated relatively easily

This site (femoral artery at the groin) should be AVOIDED for arterial punctures in newborns.

Hazards
- Those for all arterial punctures
- No collateral circulation because femoral artery divides below the groin, therefore arterial spasm, thrombus, or embolus occurring at the groin can damage entire leg
- Traumatic damage and/or infection of the hip joint
- High likelihood of obtaining venous blood from femoral vein, which runs parallel with the artery

If complications occur, the consequences are often extremely serious.

Preparing for a Radial Artery Puncture

Note: The radial artery is the most commonly used site for peripheral ABG sampling. With care, this site may be used repeatedly with little chance of adverse consequences. The steps below are, therefore, restricted to the technique for radial artery puncture.

4. Collect the following equipment:

In addition to the equipment listed, a second person is usually needed to draw blood into the syringe once the artery has been punctured.

- Pre-heparinized syringe

- Alcohol swab

- Sterile gauze pad

- #25 g butterfly needle with 12-inch tubing

Pre-heparinized syringes are commercially available and contain powdered heparin. Syringes containing 50 units of heparin are preferable to those containing 100 units.

Many hospitals have replaced butterfly needles with small catheters that are introduced into the blood vessel over introducing needles. Other hospitals have only safety catheters where the needle snaps into a protecting sheath after the catheter enters the vessel. The details of these devices are not described in this program.

Note: If your hospital does not have pre-heparinized syringes, you may "heparinize" a syringe by drawing liquid heparin (1,000 units/mL concentration) into a 1.0-mL syringe the full length of the barrel and then ejecting all of the heparin out of the syringe again. Only the heparin left in the hub of the syringe should be allowed to remain. Too much heparin in the syringe may dilute the sample and cause falsely low blood gas values.

Actions   **Remarks**

Performing a Radial Artery Puncture

5. Hold the baby's wrist in extension.

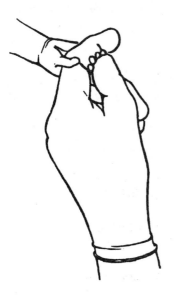

The wrist should be neither flexed nor hyperextended. The artery is most easily penetrated when the wrist is held in a neutral position. A second person holds the baby and withdraws blood into the syringe when the puncture is successful. It is generally less awkward, however, if the person performing the puncture also holds the baby's hand.

6. Using your index finger, palpate the baby's wrist for the radial pulse.

The best place to feel the radial pulse is on the thumb side of the baby's wrist, just above the first wrist crease.

7. Clean the baby's wrist with the alcohol swab.

8. Open the sterile gauze pad.

9. Remove the needle or rubber cap from the heparinized syringe, and save it for later capping of the syringe.

10. Place the heparinized 1.0-mL syringe (without cap or needle attached) on the sterile gauze pad.

11. Take the sheath off the butterfly needle and the cap off the tubing.

The tubing should be uncapped so blood can flow into the tubing as soon as the artery is punctured.

12. Grasp both "wings" of the butterfly needle and quickly insert it into the spot where the artery was palpated. (See illustration on next page.)

A 45° angle with the tip of the needle entering the skin at the first wrist crease should be used.

Actions   **Remarks**

Performing a Radial Artery Puncture (continued)

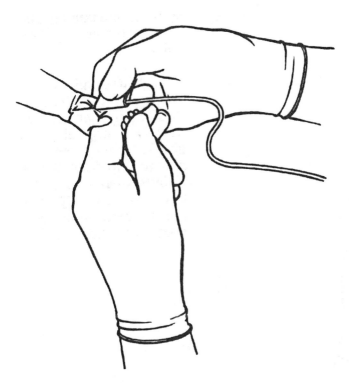

13. If blood is not immediately seen in the butterfly tubing, withdraw the needle slowly. Stop withdrawing the instant blood is seen in the tubing.

You may have gone through both sides of the artery and need to withdraw the needle until it is within the vessel.

14. If no blood enters the tubing, continue to withdraw the needle until it almost exits from the skin.

15. Palpate the artery again and reinsert the needle in another quick thrust.

Try not to make tiny jabbing advances of the needle. These are rarely successful and tend to cause more tissue damage than do decisive, "clean" insertions of the needle.

16. If you have made several unsuccessful attempts at puncturing the artery, withdraw the needle completely and start the procedure over again with a fresh butterfly needle.

The butterfly needle you were using may have become plugged with tissue during the puncture attempt(s).

17. As soon as blood is seen in the butterfly tubing, the second person should attach the heparinized syringe to the tubing.

Blood should be seen pulsating and/or flowing very rapidly within the tubing. This is evidence of a good arterial sample.

Actions	**Remarks**

Performing a Radial Artery Puncture (continued)

18. The second person then *gently* pulls back on the syringe while the first person holds the butterfly needle steady in the artery.

If the blood stops flowing, it may be necessary for the first person to reposition the needle slightly.

19. Withdraw blood into the tubing and syringe until the necessary volume has been obtained.

As with any laboratory test for a baby, obtain only the minimum amount of blood required for the test. There is 0.3 mL volume in 12 inches of butterfly needle tubing. Many blood gas machines require 0.3 mL or less for analysis.

20. The second person then places the gauze pad on the baby's wrist and presses firmly as soon as the first person withdraws the butterfly needle.

21. Aspirate any blood remaining within the butterfly tubing into the syringe.

22. Disconnect and discard the butterfly needle and tubing from the syringe.

23. All air bubbles should now be removed from the syringe, so that only blood remains within the syringe.

If air bubbles are allowed to remain within the syringe, the bubbles might affect the oxygen and carbon dioxide levels in the blood. The PaO_2 result would be falsely high and the $PaCO_2$ result would be falsely low.

24. Cap the syringe with a rubber stopper or clean needle and needle cover.

25. If there will be a delay of more than 10 to 15 minutes between the times the sample is collected and analyzed, the syringe should be placed in ice.

Metabolism of the blood cells continues within the syringe. If there is a delay between the time the sample is collected and analyzed, metabolism could result in a falsely low PaO_2 value. When the sample is chilled by being placed in ice, the metabolic rate is brought almost to a standstill and will not affect the results.

26. The second person should continue to hold the puncture site for a minimum of 3 minutes.

    Pressure is generally required for a minimum of 3 minutes but may be needed for 5 minutes or longer in very sick babies.

The pressure should be firm and constant but not so hard as to occlude the blood flow to the baby's hand. The baby's hand should remain pink and not turn white, or purple. Firm, steady pressure will prevent the baby from losing any unnecessary blood and will also prevent the formation of a hematoma.

Actions	**Remarks**

What Can Go Wrong?

1. You may not obtain any blood.	Consider the following actions: • Try a new needle because the first one may have become clogged with body tissue. • Take a short break from the procedure, then start from Step 1, perhaps using the baby's other wrist. Do *not* persist in numerous fruitless attempts because they will only traumatize the wrist and stress the baby. • Ask someone else to attempt the procedure. This procedure is akin to peripheral IV insertion in that even very skilled individuals have "bad days."
2. You may obtain venous blood rather than arterial blood.	In well-oxygenated babies with normal blood pressure, arterial blood will • Be a brighter, more vivid red color than venous blood • Flow more rapidly than venous blood • Sometimes be seen to pulsate within the butterfly tubing In sick babies with low arterial oxygen concentration and/or low blood pressure, it may be impossible to detect any differences between the appearance of venous and arterial blood. The best way to be sure you have obtained arterial blood is to select a puncture site where there is little chance of penetrating a vein. A venous blood gas can be helpful to estimate pH, PCO_2, and HCO_3 but is of no value in estimating the state of oxygenation.
3. Hemorrhage from the site may occur.	Someone should apply continuous pressure to the puncture site for a minimum of 3 minutes, or as long as required for the bleeding to stop. Do *not* apply a pressure bandage because this may be too tight and severely restrict the circulation, or too loose and allow the baby to bleed into the bandage. Do *not* leave the baby unattended until you are certain the bleeding has stopped. Pressure may be required for 5 minutes or longer in very sick babies who have a tendency for prolonged clotting time. Observe the site after pressure is released to be certain bleeding does not restart.

Actions	**Remarks**

What Can Go Wrong? (continued)

4. The baby's hand may turn white during or immediately following the procedure.	This indicates that the artery has gone into spasm, cutting off all blood flow to the hand.
	*Immediately wrap the **opposite** arm and hand in a warm compress.* This is done to dilate the blood vessels in that hand and hopefully to cause a sympathetic response with dilation of the vessels in the affected hand.
	*Do **not** wrap the **affected** hand.* If the affected arm and hand were wrapped, the warmth of the compress would increase the metabolic demands of the tissues, thereby increasing the need for blood flow in an area where the circulation is already compromised.
5. A hematoma may develop.	This is due to bleeding under the skin and results from repeated punctures and excessive probing with the needle or from inadequate pressure applied to the puncture site. Again, apply pressure to the wrist as soon as the needle is withdrawn and maintain firm, steady pressure until the bleeding has stopped completely. If a hematoma develops, it will make it much more difficult to obtain additional blood samples from that site.
6. The puncture site may become infected.	Use careful aseptic technique. Use a new butterfly needle every time you completely withdraw the needle from the skin and make another insertion.

Unit 3   Respiratory Distress

Unit 3 Pretest

Before reading the unit, please answer the following questions. Select the *one best* answer to each question (unless otherwise instructed). Record your answers on the answer sheet that is the last page in this book *and* on the test.

1. To determine if a baby is cyanotic, which of the following is the *best* part of the baby's body to examine?
   A. Nail beds
   B. Feet
   C. Lips
   D. Nose

2. An infant's respiratory rate is 70 respirations per minute. This breathing pattern is called
   A. Normal
   B. Tachypnea
   C. Apnea
   D. Flaring

3. What causes respiratory distress syndrome (RDS) in the newborn?
   A. Congenital malformation of the upper airway
   B. Polycythemia (thick blood)
   C. Pneumothorax
   D. Immaturity of the lungs

4. Which of the following infants is *not* at increased risk for respiratory distress?
   A. Baby born in a taxicab during the winter
   B. A term baby whose nails are meconium stained
   C. A 38-week appropriate for gestational age baby whose mother's membranes had been ruptured for 6 hours before delivery
   D. A baby with a 5-minute Apgar score of 2

5. A baby has respiratory distress. You note asymmetrical movement of the chest, with breath sounds louder on the left side. Which of the following actions is *most* appropriate for this baby?
   A. Obtain an electrocardiogram.
   B. Obtain a chest x-ray.
   C. Position baby with right side down.
   D. Insert an oral airway.

6. If a preterm baby stops breathing for 10 seconds, this is considered
   A. Normal, unless accompanied by bradycardia or cyanosis
   B. Always abnormal and requiring immediate treatment

7. Which of these may be a cause of apnea (choose the letter that identifies the correct answers)?
   1. Imbalance in blood chemistry such as low blood glucose, calcium, or sodium
   2. Infections
   3. Low blood volume
   4. Temperature change such as when a cold baby is being warmed
      A. 2, 3
      B. 3, 4
      C. 1, 2, 4
      D. 1, 2, 3, 4

8. A baby with respiratory distress has an apnea spell. What should you think about this?
   A. Apnea is normal in babies with respiratory distress.
   B. Apnea shows the baby is getting worse quickly.

9. What percentage of babies weighing less than 1,000 g (2 lb, 3 oz) will have at least one apnea spell?
   A. <20%
   B. 50%
   C. 75%
   D. >90%

10. When a baby is being bag-breathed for an apnea spell, it is important to _____ the rate of assisted breathing before stopping assistance.
    A. Decrease
    B. Increase
    C. No change

11. **True** **False** Three hours after birth, an infant shows mild grunting and nasal flaring. This is probably normal.

12. **True** **False** Babies frequently cannot breathe through their mouths by themselves.

13. **True** **False** A baby in respiratory distress who is grunting probably has stiff lungs.

14. Which of the following babies is at *highest* risk for developing a pneumothorax?
    A. Term baby with congenital heart disease
    B. Term baby whose mother had hydramnios
    C. Preterm baby with respiratory distress syndrome
    D. Preterm baby requiring an exchange transfusion

15. A baby with a pneumothorax is *least* likely to develop
    A. High blood pressure
    B. Sudden cyanosis
    C. Abdominal distension
    D. Shift in location of heart sounds

16. The possible consequences of a pneumothorax include all of the following, *except*
    A. Hypoxia
    B. Intraventricular hemorrhage
    C. Anemia
    D. Acidosis

17. Approximately _____ of healthy, term newborn babies will develop a pneumothorax.
    A. 0.1%
    B. 1%
    C. 5%
    D. 10%

18. **True** **False** A pneumothorax should be considered any time there is a sudden deterioration in a baby's condition, even if the baby is recovering from an illness.

For each question, please make sure you have marked your answer on the test and on the answer sheet (last page in book). The test is for you; the answer sheet will need to be turned in for continuing education credit.

Part 1: Respiratory Distress

Objectives

In Part 1 of this unit you will learn to

A. Identify infants at risk for respiratory distress.

B. Identify infants with respiratory distress.

C. Understand the causes of neonatal respiratory distress.

D. Understand the principles of therapy for infants with respiratory distress.

E. Take appropriate emergency actions for infants with respiratory distress.

1. What Are the Signs of Neonatal Respiratory Distress?

There are 5 signs of respiratory distress in the newborn. They are

- Tachypnea (rapid breathing)
- Intercostal retractions
- Nasal flaring
- Grunting
- Cyanosis

A. Tachypnea

Normal newborn respiratory rate may be erratic with brief periods of very rapid respirations, mixed with periods of no breathing for a few seconds. For this reason, when vital signs are taken on a newborn, respirations should be counted for a full minute.

Sustained respirations greater than 60 per minute are abnormal. This is called tachypnea.

B. Intercostal Retractions

These may be seen each time an infant inhales. The skin between the ribs is pulled in as the baby tries to expand lungs that may be stiffer than normal.

C. Nasal Flaring

The nostrils widen with each inspiration as the baby attempts to move more air into the lungs.

D. Grunting

This is one of the most important signs of respiratory distress in the newborn. It is heard during the expiratory phase of the breathing cycle in an infant with decreased pulmonary compliance (stiff lungs). In an attempt to hold open the alveoli (air sacs in the lungs), an infant will exhale against a partially closed glottis (upper airway). The resulting noise may be heard as a grunt or even a whine or cry repeated with each expiration. Occasionally, the grunt may be heard only with a stethoscope on the chest.

E. Cyanosis

Central cyanosis indicates an abnormally low blood oxygen level. Absence of cyanosis, however, is *not* a reliable indicator of normal oxygenation.

It is not uncommon for a baby to show tachypnea, grunting, flaring, and/or retractions, but without cyanosis, and still have low arterial blood oxygen concentration. In addition, an extremely anemic baby may *not* show cyanosis despite having a low blood oxygen level.

 A pink baby may still have a low PaO$_2$ level.

Normal newborns may have a ruddy skin color, which is sometimes mistaken for cyanosis. In addition, acrocyanosis (blue hands and feet) may be seen normally in a newborn and is not, by itself, an indicator of respiratory distress or low blood oxygen. Central cyanosis involves a more generalized blueness or duskiness, and can best be determined by observing mucous membranes, such as the lips.

Mucous membranes should be used to determine the presence or absence of cyanosis.

If cyanosis is suspected, check blood oxygen level with an arterial blood gas and/or pulse oximetry.

2. When Is It Normal and When Is It Abnormal for an Infant to Show Signs of Respiratory Distress?

During the first hour after delivery, mild tachypnea, retractions, flaring, and/or grunting may occasionally be seen in a normal infant who will not later exhibit respiratory distress. This is because the infant is absorbing lung fluid and the circulation is readjusting to the extrauterine environment.

Central cyanosis is *never* normal and always requires prompt investigation and treatment. Likewise, severe or worsening tachypnea, retractions, flaring, and/or grunting within the first hour after birth also requires investigation.

Signs of respiratory distress are present

- *Whenever tachypnea, retractions, flaring, or grunting persist beyond 1 hour after birth*

  and/or

- *Any time severe or worsening tachypnea, retractions, flaring, or grunting develop*

  and/or

- *Any time cyanosis is present*

Now answer these questions to test yourself on the information in the last section.

A1. What are the 5 signs of respiratory distress?

_____

_____

_____

_____

_____

A2. What part of a baby's body should you examine to determine if the baby is cyanotic?

_____

A3. An infant, 30 minutes after birth, is pink but shows mild grunting and nasal flaring. You check the baby's vital signs and they are normal. What would you do next?

    A. Observe the baby for the next 30 minutes.

    B. Act now to treat the respiratory distress.

A4. An infant, 2 hours after birth, shows mild grunting and nasal flaring. Is this normal or a sign of respiratory distress?

_____

A5. At 3 hours after birth, a 1,900-g (4 lb, 3 oz) baby develops mild grunting, intercostal retractions, and nasal flaring and has a respiratory rate of 80, but is pink all over. It is 4:00 am. What should you do?

Yes	No	
___	___	Assist the baby's breathing with bag and mask ventilation.
___	___	Take the baby's vital signs.
___	___	Attach a cardiac monitor to the baby.
___	___	Feed the baby to prevent hypoglycemia.
___	___	Attach a pulse oximeter to the baby.

Check your answers with the list that follows the Recommended Routines. Correct any incorrect answers and review the appropriate section in the unit.

3. What Are the Causes of Neonatal Respiratory Distress?

There are many causes of neonatal respiratory distress. They may be divided into

- *Obstructive problems* (a mechanical obstruction preventing air from getting into the lungs or preventing lung expansion)
- *Primary disorders of the lung*
- *Miscellaneous group of non-pulmonary problems*

A. Obstructive Problems

    1. Anything that obstructs the airway, from the nose to the air sacs in the lungs, will result in respiratory distress.

        Infants breathe through their noses and seldom through their mouths. In general, babies are able to breathe through their mouths only when they are crying. When at rest, babies may suffocate if their nasal airway becomes obstructed.

- *Mucus* in the nasal passageways is a common cause of respiratory distress.
- A *misplaced phototherapy mask* may also obstruct the nose.
- Other less common causes include congenital abnormalities of the airway such as *choanal atresia* (congenital obstruction of the nasal passageways) or *Robin Syndrome* (congenitally small mandible, which causes the tongue to obstruct the pharynx).

    2. Conditions that restrict lung expansion within the chest cavity will result in respiratory distress.

- The most common of these is a *pneumothorax*. This is a rupture in the lung tissue, which allows air to leak from the lungs and become trapped in the space between the lungs and the rib cage, thus forming a large "bubble" that inhibits the lungs from expanding with inhalation.
- A rare cause is *diaphragmatic hernia*. This is a congenital defect in the diaphragm that allows the abdominal contents to enter the chest cavity, thus compressing the lungs and greatly restricting their ability to expand normally with inhalation.

B. Primary Lung Problems

    1. The most common of these is respiratory distress syndrome (RDS). This is caused by an immaturity of the lungs. The mature lung produces substances called "surfactants" that coat the alveoli and allow them to remain open during exhalation. Without surfactants, the alveoli collapse during exhalation and are difficult to open with the next breath. As a result, the lungs are stiff and difficult to inflate.

 Respiratory distress in the neonate has many causes, only one of which is respiratory distress syndrome (RDS).

RDS is caused by lack of lung surfactants.

2. Other primary lung problems include

- *Aspiration syndrome:* This occurs when a fetus aspirates contaminated amniotic fluid into the lungs. This is particularly severe when the amniotic fluid contains meconium that is inhaled. A newborn may aspirate fluid at delivery or later with feedings in the nursery or mother's room.

- *Bacterial or viral pneumonia:* The baby's lungs may become infected before birth (the mother may or may not show signs of infection).

- *Transient respiratory distress of the newborn* or transient tachypnea of the newborn: Some babies, particularly those born by cesarean section, may have delayed absorption of lung fluid after birth. These babies may have mild to moderate signs of respiratory distress.

C. Non-Pulmonary Problems

Respiratory distress may also result from anything that causes

1. Abnormally high or low blood flow to the lungs

Decreased blood flow to the lungs may result from *hypotension* (which may be due to blood loss or sepsis), *congenital heart disease,* or *severe hypoxia and acidosis* (which may cause the blood vessels supplying the lungs to constrict).

2. Increased demand for oxygen

Cold stress increases the body's demand for oxygen. For acutely ill babies, *excessive handling* and *oral feedings* may also increase oxygen demands.

3. Abnormally high or low number of red blood cells

Anemia may result from blood loss or hemolytic disease. Regardless of the cause of anemia, there are a decreased number of red blood cells to carry oxygen to the muscles and organs.

Polycythemia (an excess of red blood cells) may cause the blood to become too thick to move easily through the lungs and may result in respiratory distress.

 Many times correction of non-pulmonary, underlying problems can significantly diminish or completely eliminate a baby's respiratory distress.

Now answer these questions to test yourself on the information in the last section.

B1. **True** **False** Babies usually breathe through their noses. They usually cannot breathe through their mouths.

B2. What causes respiratory distress syndrome (RDS)?

    A. A blockage in the airway between the nose and lungs
    B. Immaturity of the baby's lungs and the resulting lack of surfactants needed to keep the alveoli open
    C. Inhalation of amniotic fluid into the lungs
    D. Low blood volume
    E. Thick blood

B3. What causes respiratory distress? Choose as many as needed.

    A. A blockage in the airway between the nose and lungs
    B. Immaturity of the baby's lungs and the resulting lack of surfactants needed to keep the alveoli open
    C. Inhalation of amniotic fluid into the lungs
    D. Low blood volume
    E. Thick blood

B4. List 2 obstructive causes of respiratory distress.

_____

_____

B5. Besides respiratory distress syndrome, list 2 primary lung problems that cause respiratory distress.

_____

_____

B6. List 3 non-pulmonary problems that may cause respiratory distress.

_____

_____

_____

Check your answers with the list that follows the Recommended Routines. Correct any incorrect answers and review the appropriate section in the unit.

4. Which Infants Are Prone to Developing Respiratory Distress?

Observe the following babies closely and frequently for signs of respiratory distress:

A. Preterm Infants

Lungs may be immature with insufficient surfactants, so that a baby may develop respiratory distress syndrome. Preterm babies are also at higher risk for developing an infection, which may take the form of bacterial or viral pneumonia.

B. Infants Following Difficult Births

Blood flow to the lungs may be decreased due to pulmonary vasoconstriction, a baby may have aspirated meconium, or a pneumothorax may have resulted from resuscitative efforts.

C. Infants of Women With Diabetes Mellitus

Regardless of gestational age, infants born to diabetic women are delayed in their ability to produce surfactants and, therefore, are more likely to develop respiratory distress syndrome.

D. Infants Born by Cesarean Section

Infants born by cesarean delivery are more likely to have delayed absorption of lung fluid (transient respiratory distress of the newborn) than infants delivered vaginally.

E. Infants With Maternal Risk Factor(s) for Infection

Infants born to women with fever, rupture of membranes for 18 hours or longer, or foul smelling/cloudy amniotic fluid are at particular risk for developing bacterial pneumonia. Maternal history of group B beta hemolytic streptococci (GBS) cervical or rectal colonization or bacteriuria during this pregnancy, or previous GBS-infected baby, increases the risk for neonatal GBS infection.

See Book II: Maternal and Fetal Care, Perinatal Infections and Book II: Neonatal Care, Infections for more information about surveillance, as well as intrapartum and neonatal management, of these risk factors.

F. Infants With Meconium-Stained Skin

Meconium aspiration may have occurred.

G. Infants Born to Women With Hydramnios

Hydramnios (excess amniotic fluid) may result from any of several causes. One cause is when fetuses are unable or are too weak to swallow amniotic fluid. These babies may have esophageal atresia and tracheoesophageal fistula or central nervous system depression.

Hydrops fetalis (generalized fetal edema) is also associated with hydramnios. These babies may have respiratory distress from pulmonary edema.

H. Infants With Other Problems

The increased oxygen needs of severely cold-stressed infants may lead to respiratory distress. If perinatal blood loss has occurred, respiratory distress can result from decreased blood flow to the lungs to pick up oxygen and/or from insufficient red blood cells to carry an adequate amount of oxygen from the lungs to perfuse the rest of the baby's body and organs. Thus cold stress, hypovolemia, hypotension, and/or anemia and their associated complications may result in respiratory distress. (See 3C on page 114.)

5. What Should Be Done to Evaluate an Infant Who Shows Signs of Respiratory Distress?

Any infant with tachypnea, intercostal retractions, nasal flaring, or grunting persisting beyond the first hour after birth, or with cyanosis at any time, should be given oxygen and other emergency treatment, as indicated by physical examination findings.

Based on the physical findings, consider transillumination and/or chest x-ray, pulse oximetry and arterial blood gas, screening tests, and evaluation for sepsis.

A. Physical Examination (See Table 3.1.)

Table 3.1. Physical Findings Associated With Respiratory Distress

Observation	Action	Comments
1. **Tachypnea** (respiratory rate faster than 60 breaths/min)	• Check vital signs. • Obtain chest x-ray. • Review perinatal history.	The **most common sign of respiratory distress.** Use a process of elimination to rule out possible causes.
2. **No air flow into lungs**	• Suction mucus. • Attempt to pass nasogastric tube, insert oral airway (choanal atresia). • If Robin syndrome, position prone: Insert 12F catheter as a nasopharyngeal tube to prevent occlusion by the tongue.	Consider the possibility of obstruction due to **mucus, choanal atresia,** or **Robin syndrome.**
3. **Meconium staining**	• Suction the airway as soon as the baby is born. • Consider suctioning below the vocal cords if the baby is depressed at birth.	If amniotic fluid is meconium stained, **meconium** may be in the baby's airway (Book I, Resuscitation).
4. **Decreased breath sounds on one side, asymmetrical chest movement,** and/or **sudden onset of cyanosis**	• Obtain transillumination and/or chest x-ray.	Baby may have developed a **pneumothorax.**
5. **Grunting** is predominant sign	• Obtain chest x-ray.	This indicates the baby has stiff lungs (**poor lung compliance**).
6. **Cyanosis** of mucous membranes	• Give oxygen. • Obtain chest x-ray.	Assume that any infant with blue mucous membranes has **low blood oxygen.**
7. **Sunken abdomen**	• Pass nasogastric tube to withdraw swallowed air and decompress stomach. • Position at 45° head-up angle. • If in severe respiratory distress, intubate trachea and bag breathe.	Babies with **diaphragmatic hernias** have sunken abdomens because the intestines are in the chest. Avoid distending the gastrointestinal tract with air.
8. **Pale baby, weak pulses,** and/or **poor peripheral perfusion**	• Obtain blood pressure, hematocrit, and white blood cell count with differential.	Babies with low blood pressure related to **blood loss** or related to **sepsis** may exhibit signs of respiratory distress (Book II: Neonatal Care, Blood Pressure, Infections).
9. **Excessive** and/or particularly thick **mucus**	• Suction mucus. • Pass nasogastric tube. • Obtain chest x-ray. • Position baby at 45° head-up angle.	Babies with **esophageal atresia** may aspirate secretions. X-ray will show nasogastric tube coiled in blind esophageal pouch.

B. Transillumination and Chest X-ray

Transillumination is the technique of holding a bright light against the body to detect a collection of air. The chest may be transilluminated to detect a pneumothorax.

A positive transillumination may be sufficient evidence to insert a needle or tube into the chest to relieve a pneumothorax if other indications, such as vital signs or arterial blood gases, are rapidly deteriorating. If the baby's condition allows intervention to be delayed for a brief time, you may want to obtain a chest x-ray to confirm the presence and location of a pneumothorax before insertion of a needle or tube.

A follow-up chest x-ray should be taken to assess position of the chest tube and/or evacuation of the pneumothorax, as well as to detect other disorders such as pneumonia or respiratory distress syndrome.

C. Pulse Oximetry and Arterial Blood Gas

For a newborn who requires increased inspired oxygen for longer than a brief period or who has persistent respiratory distress

- Monitor oxygen saturation with a pulse oximeter.
- Determine arterial blood oxygen, pH, carbon dioxide, and bicarbonate.

Oxygenation (PaO_2) and acid-base status (pH, $PaCO_2$, and bicarbonate) may be measured from blood drawn from an artery. Oxygenation may also be estimated by a transcutaneous oximeter while acid-base status is measured from a blood sample.

It is inadequate to measure only oxygenation without determining acid-base status.

A baby may be severely acidotic and/or have a high CO_2 level requiring immediate treatment and still have normal oxygenation.

D. Screening Tests
- Hematocrit
- Blood glucose screen
- White blood cell count and differential

E. Evaluation for Sepsis and/or Pneumonia

Some babies with respiratory distress may have bacterial pneumonia, which is indistinguishable, by chest x-ray, from respiratory distress syndrome (RDS). Many experts advise obtaining a blood culture and starting antibiotic therapy in any newborn with respiratory distress (Book II: Neonatal Care, Infections). If the blood culture result is reported as negative in 2 to 3 days, the antibiotic therapy may then be discontinued.

6. What General Support Measures Are Indicated for Any Infant With Respiratory Distress?

General principles of therapy for any infant with respiratory distress include

• Improve oxygen delivery to lungs.

• Improve blood flow to lungs.

• Minimize consumption of oxygen.

A. Improve Oxygen Delivery to the Lungs

This is most easily accomplished by increasing the oxygen concentration in the infant's environment (Book II: Neonatal Care, Oxygen). Extreme care must be taken to avoid delivering excess or insufficient oxygen.

 Too little oxygen in the blood can cause brain damage. Too much oxygen over time can cause damage to other systems, particularly the eyes and lungs.

Appropriate oxygenation can be determined by measurement of arterial blood gases or proper use of a pulse oximeter. Environmental oxygen should be regulated to maintain arterial blood oxygen levels 45 to 75 mm Hg or 85% to 95% saturation.

Some babies with respiratory distress require ventilatory assistance beyond increased environmental oxygen. These babies

• Generally require more than 45% to 50% inspired oxygen to maintain an arterial blood oxygen (PaO_2) between 45 to 75 mm Hg, and/or
• Have severe, recurring apnea, and/or
• Have evidence of respiratory failure or an arterial carbon dioxide concentration ($PaCO_2$) greater than approximately 55 to 60 mm Hg

These babies may require either continuous positive airway pressure or intermittent positive-pressure ventilation, depending on the cause and severity of the respiratory distress. For babies with respiratory distress syndrome, administration of surfactant may also be appropriate. These procedures and treatments require special equipment and expertise, and are discussed in other units.

B. Improve Pulmonary Blood Flow

Adequate pulmonary blood flow depends on

• Maintenance of arterial blood oxygen in 45 to 75 mm Hg range or oxygen saturation between 85% to 95%

• Correction of acidosis

• Assurance of an adequate circulating blood volume

• Assurance of an adequate number of red blood cells

Hypoxia and acidosis each constrict pulmonary blood vessels and thus decrease pulmonary blood flow, with a resultant further decrease in arterial blood oxygen levels.

The most common causes of *metabolic acidosis* include
- Insufficient arterial oxygen
- Poor tissue perfusion from low circulating blood volume or from myocardial failure and low blood pressure
- Cold stress
- Infection

 Severe metabolic acidosis (pH less than 7.2 with serum bicarbonate less than 15–16 mEq/L) indicates severe illness. The cause must be determined and treated.

While the cause is being determined, metabolic acidosis may be treated by intravenous administration of dilute sodium bicarbonate. The dose is 1 to 2 mEq/kg (depending on the severity of acidosis) in a 0.5 mEq/mL concentration. This should be given *slowly,* at a rate no faster than 1 mL/minute.

Severe *respiratory acidosis* (pH less than 7.2, $PaCO_2$ equal to or greater than approximately 55 to 60 mm Hg) indicates respiratory failure. Sodium bicarbonate should *not* be used in this situation. In most cases, the treatment for respiratory acidosis is assisted ventilation.

 As a general rule, sodium bicarbonate should not be given unless
- *Serum bicarbonate level is less than 15 to 16 mEq/L.*
- *$PaCO_2$ level is less than 40 to 45 mm Hg.*
- *There is adequate spontaneous or assisted ventilation.*
- *Cause of acidosis is being assessed and treated.*

A *low blood pressure* may require treatment with a blood volume expander. A newborn in respiratory distress with a *low hematocrit*, less than 35%, may require a blood transfusion (Book II: Neonatal Care, Blood Pressure).

Babies with *very high hematocrit* values can develop respiratory distress from viscous blood that becomes compacted in small pulmonary capillaries, with subsequent reduction in blood flow through the capillaries. Be sure blood is drawn from a vein for hematocrit determination, because heel stick hematocrits are frequently falsely high.

If a venous or arterial hematocrit is greater than 65% to 70% and the baby has otherwise unexplained respiratory distress, a type of exchange transfusion can be done to lower the hematocrit. A dilutional partial exchange transfusion is accomplished by removing some of the baby's blood and replacing it with normal saline. See Book III, Unit 4 and consult with your regional center staff if a reduction exchange is considered.

C. Decrease Oxygen Requirement

You can do several things to minimize a baby's oxygen consumption. These measures include

- Providing an appropriate neutral thermal environment

- Warming and humidifying inspired oxygen/air mixture

- Withholding oral feedings (adequate hydration and some caloric requirements can be met with intravenous fluids)

- Handling a baby as little as possible

  - Do not bathe the baby.

  - Do not perform an extensive physical examination.

  - Perform only essential procedures, with minimal, gentle handling.

These principles apply to the care of babies with acute respiratory distress during the first several days after birth. If a baby requires oxygen for a prolonged period, care practices may change somewhat, depending on the baby's gestational age, postnatal age, and condition.

Self-Test

Now answer these questions to test yourself on the information in the last section.

C1. List at least 3 groups of infants who are at risk for developing respiratory distress.

_____

_____

_____

C2. What should be done, in addition to a physical examination, for a baby showing signs of respiratory distress?

_____

_____

_____

C3. If grunting is the primary physical symptom, you would suspect the baby has _____ lungs. You would obtain a _____ to help evaluate the cause.

C4. If a catheter cannot be passed through the nose of a baby with respiratory distress, you would suspect the baby has _____. You would immediately insert _____ in the baby's mouth.

C5. If a baby with respiratory distress suddenly turns blue, you would suspect the baby has _____. You would perform a _____ and obtain a _____ to confirm the diagnosis.

C6. If a baby in respiratory distress soon after birth has a hematocrit of 30%, the baby probably experienced _____. You should prepare to give _____.

C7. If arterial PaO_2 is low, increase the baby's _____ to avoid damage to the baby's

_____.

C8. If arterial PaO_2 is very high, you should _____ the amount of inspired oxygen to avoid damage to organs such as the _____ and/or _____.

C9. If arterial $PaCO_2$ is high and pH is low, you should
   A. Ventilate the baby.
   B. Give sodium bicarbonate.

C10. If arterial $PaCO_2$ is normal and pH is low, you should
   A. Ventilate the baby.
   B. Give sodium bicarbonate.

Check your answers with the list that follows the Recommended Routines. Correct any incorrect answers and review the appropriate section in the unit.

Part 2: Apnea

Objectives

In Part 2 of this unit you will learn

A. The definition of apnea

B. Which babies are likely to develop apnea

C. The causes of apnea

D. What to do for an apneic baby

1. What Is Apnea?

Apnea means cessation of breathing for longer than a 15-second period or for a shorter time if there is bradycardia or cyanosis. Many normal newborns will have brief breathing pauses or "periodic breathing," but these pauses are not apnea episodes.

2. Which Babies Are at Risk for Apnea?

A. Preterm Babies

Thirty percent of all preterm babies weighing less than 1,800 g (4 lb) will have at least one apneic spell. The chances of apnea occurring increase as birth weight decreases. Essentially all babies with birth weights less than 1,000 g (2 lb, 3 oz) will have at least one apneic spell.

 A preterm baby who is stable and doing well can suddenly have a severe apneic spell.

B. Babies With Respiratory Distress

Any newborn, regardless of birth weight, may develop apnea as a complication of respiratory disease.

 When a baby with respiratory disease has an apneic spell, assume the baby's condition is deteriorating rapidly.

Active intervention is indicated (eg, increased oxygen, intubation, assisted ventilation, correction of acidosis, and/or other measures, as needed).

C. Babies With Metabolic Disorders

Low blood glucose, calcium, or sodium can all result in apnea. Babies who are acidotic (low blood pH from too much acid in their blood) may become apneic.

D. Babies With Infections

Apnea may be the first sign of sepsis or meningitis.

E. Cold-Stressed Babies Who Are Being Warmed

Cold babies are likely to have apneic spells as they are being warmed.

F. Babies With Central Nervous System Disorders

Babies with seizures may occasionally stop breathing during a seizure. Babies with central nervous system hemorrhage or rapidly progressing hydrocephalus may also develop apnea.

G. Babies With Low Blood Volume or Low Hematocrit

Babies with low blood volume or anemia may develop apnea as the first sign of their condition.

H. Babies Who Experience Perinatal Compromise

Babies may develop many of the problems mentioned previously (metabolic disorders, central nervous system damage, etc) after a period of hypoxia and/or acidosis. Apnea spells may also result.

I. Babies Whose Mothers Received Certain Medications

Depressant drugs, such as narcotics, given to a woman during labor will cross the placenta and may cause apnea in the baby.

3. How Should Apnea Be Anticipated and Detected?

All of the babies mentioned previously are at risk for developing apnea. They should have heart rate and respirations monitored electronically. See Book I, Unit 4 skill.

A. Heart Rate Monitor

Set the alarm to sound when the heart rate falls below 100 beats per minute.

B. Respiratory Monitor

Set the alarm to sound when there is a 15- to 20-second period without respiratory efforts.

Self-Test

Now answer these questions to test yourself on the information in the last section.

D1. **True** **False** Apnea means any stoppage of breathing in a newborn, no matter how long the stoppage may be.

D2. A baby stops breathing for 10 seconds and has blue lips. Is this baby having an apnea spell?

_____ Yes _____ No

D3. List at least 5 problems that put a baby at risk for apnea.

_____

_____

_____

_____

_____

D4. All babies at risk for apnea should be electronically _____ .

Check your answers with the list that follows the Recommended Routines. Correct any incorrect answers and review the appropriate section in the unit.

4. What Should You Do When a Baby Has an Apneic Spell?

A. Glance at the Cardiorespiratory Monitor

A quick glance at the monitor screen will let you know if the electrocardiogram and respiratory signals are clear.

Many monitors will also show what preceded the apneic spell (eg, whether bradycardia or absence of chest movement came first).

B. Look at the Baby

1. If the baby is blue and/or apneic

   First, stimulate the baby to resume breathing. In many cases this involves merely stimulating the skin by rubbing the baby's extremities or back. Babies will often quickly resume breathing after light stroking. Sometimes, more vigorous rubbing of the skin may be needed.

   If mild or moderate stimulation does not result in resumed respirations, do not persist in these efforts. Use a bag and mask to bag-breathe for the baby until the heart rate is normal and spontaneous respirations resume.

   You may need to decrease the rate of bag-breathing and at the same time stimulate the baby before spontaneous breathing resumes. This is because assisted ventilation may have removed some of the stimulus to breathe.

   Use supplemental oxygen if cyanosis persists after assisted or spontaneous ventilation is established.

2. If the baby is pink, has a normal heart rate, and is breathing

   In this case, the episode may represent a

   • True apneic spell with spontaneous resumption of breathing by the baby

   or

   • Malfunction of the monitor (Check placement of the leads on the baby, monitor settings, and functioning.)

C. Record Your Observations and Actions

5. What Should You Think of When a Baby Has an Apneic Spell?

As noted previously, apnea may be caused by many different disorders, or may have no identifiable cause. However, all of the treatable causes must be considered before attributing the apneic spell to "apnea of prematurity."

The following actions are not indicated with every apneic spell. However, with the first spell, or if the spells become more frequent or severe, all actions should be considered.

• If the baby has respiratory disease, it may be rapidly worsening. Obtain an arterial blood gas and increase respiratory support for the baby. Obtain a chest x-ray.

• Check blood glucose.

- Check if the baby aspirated milk or formula while feeding.
  - Could the baby have aspirated while nipple feeding?
  - Does the baby have a nasogastric or orogastric tube that may have slipped out of the stomach and allowed milk or formula to go into the lungs?
  - Did the baby vomit and aspirate vomitus?

- Measure blood pressure.

- Check body and environmental temperature (including oxygen/air temperature if the baby is receiving supplemental oxygen).

- Check hematocrit.

- Consider the possibility of sepsis or meningitis and review recent feeding history, baby's vital signs, tone, and activity. Consider obtaining white blood count and differential, blood and cerebrospinal fluid cultures, and starting antibiotics.

- If a cause still has not been found, check serum calcium, sodium, and pH.

- Consider the possibility of a patent ductus arteriosus, particularly if the baby is significantly preterm. Listen for a heart murmur and check for bounding pulses.

- Consider the possibility that the apneic spell was a type of seizure activity. Review the history for evidence of perinatal compromise and evaluate the baby's neurologic status.

6. What Should Be Done if the Apnea Is Recurrent and/or Severe?

Most preterm babies with apnea require no more intervention than occasional stimulation.

If the spells occur frequently (more than a few each day), other therapies such as continuous positive airway pressure, drugs (theophylline or caffeine), or mechanical ventilation may be required. These babies generally require long-term intensive care, and such treatments are not discussed in this unit.

7. When Can Apnea Monitoring Be Discontinued?

Most experts agree that the chances of recurrent apnea are very small if all of the following are true:

- Acute illness has resolved
- Baby weighs more than 1,800 g (4 lb) and has reached a gestational age of 35 weeks or older
- Baby has been apnea-free for 7 to 8 consecutive days

Note: These guidelines are intended to apply only to babies during the first few weeks after birth and should not be used for babies who stop breathing at several months of age (acute life-threatening event, formerly termed "near-miss sudden infant death syndrome").

See Book III, Specialized Newborn Care, Continuing Care for more information regarding apnea monitoring and treatment in stable, growing preterm babies.

Self-Test

Now answer these questions to test yourself on the information in the last section.

E1. **True False** Whenever a preterm baby has an apneic spell it is reasonable to assume it is due to "apnea of prematurity."

E2. If an apneic baby does not breathe spontaneously after mild to moderate tactile stimulation, what should you do *next*?

_____

E3. List at least 6 screening procedures that should be considered for a baby who has suffered an apneic spell.

1. _____

2. _____

3. _____

4. _____

5. _____

6. _____

E4. When can apnea monitoring be discontinued?

1. _____

2. _____

3. _____

Check your answers with the list that follows the Recommended Routines. Correct any incorrect answers and review the appropriate section in the unit.

Part 3: Pneumothorax

Objectives

In Part 3 of this unit you will learn

A. The definition of a pneumothorax

B. Which babies are at risk for developing a pneumothorax

C. How to detect a pneumothorax

D. The consequences of a pneumothorax

E. How to treat a pneumothorax

1. What Is a Pneumothorax?

A pneumothorax is a collection of air (pneumo) within the chest cavity (thorax). It results from a tiny rupture in the lung tissue that allows air to leak outside the lung. This air forms a pocket between the lung tissue and the chest wall, compressing the lung. For this reason, a pneumothorax is sometimes referred to as "collapsed lung." More than one pneumothorax, or ruptures in both lungs, are called pneumothoraces.

The air pocket may become so large that it also causes a shift in the normal position of the heart. A pneumothorax in the baby's left chest cavity shifts the heart toward the right, while a pneumothorax in the right chest causes the heart to shift toward the baby's left side. The pneumothorax and shifted heart position can be seen by chest x-ray.

2. Which Babies Are At Risk for a Pneumothorax?

Approximately 1% of all well, term newborn babies develop a spontaneous pneumothorax. Most of these babies show no signs, and the pneumothorax resolves without treatment.

Much more frequently, babies with lung disease develop pneumothoraces as a complication of their lung disease. The risk increases with increasing severity of lung disease. A pneumothorax is most likely to occur in

A. Babies Receiving Positive-Pressure Ventilation

  If a baby is receiving continuous positive airway pressure (CPAP), the higher the CPAP pressure, the greater the risk of a pneumothorax. Likewise, if a baby is receiving assisted ventilation with a mechanical respirator or by bag-breathing, the higher the pressure, the greater the risk of a pneumothorax. These higher-than-normal pressures required to achieve adequate oxygenation increase the risk of a pneumothorax. Techniques for CPAP and assisted ventilation are discussed in separate units in Book III, Specialized Newborn Care.

B. Babies With Poor Lung Compliance

  Whether they require CPAP or assisted ventilation, babies with poor lung compliance (stiff lungs) are at higher risk for developing a pneumothorax. For example, a baby with respiratory distress syndrome requiring oxygen therapy via an oxyhood, CPAP, or assisted ventilation may develop a pneumothorax.

C. Babies Who Have Aspiration Syndrome

  Aspiration of a foreign substance such as meconium, blood, or amniotic fluid places the baby at risk for development of a pneumothorax because the aspirated material creates a ball-valve effect in the small branches of the airway. When the baby inhales, the airways expand slightly and the air and oxygen flow past these bits of foreign material and into the alveoli. However, during exhalation the airways collapse around the foreign matter. This means that the trapped gas keeps the alveoli abnormally inflated during exhalation.

This process can continue until the alveoli are so over-inflated that a rupture in the lung tissue occurs.

D. Babies Who Required Resuscitation

High ventilation pressures may be required during resuscitation of a sick baby. While it is always important to resuscitate a baby as quickly and effectively as possible, some babies will develop a pneumothorax as a result of the bag-and-mask or bag-and-endotracheal tube ventilation that was required.

3. What Are the Signs of a Pneumothorax?

In addition to the risk factors, there are certain signs and arterial blood gas values that are important indicators that a baby has developed a pneumothorax. A baby may have one or several of the following findings:

A. Clinical Findings

- Sudden onset of cyanosis.

- Increase or decrease in respiratory effort or rate.

- Breath sounds that are louder over one lung. However, because breath sounds radiate easily across the small chest of a newborn, a difference in breath sounds may be impossible to detect, even with a large pneumothorax.

- Shift in the location where the baby's heartbeat is best heard.

- One side of the chest becomes higher than the other. The pneumothorax may cause hyperexpansion of the affected side of the chest.

- Development of abdominal distension. The pneumothorax pushes the diaphragm down, compressing the abdominal organs and making the belly appear distended.

- Development of low blood pressure, when the blood pressure had been normal. Pressure from the pneumothorax on the major veins inhibits blood return to the heart, causing a decrease in circulating blood volume, which then results in lower blood pressure.

- Deterioration in appearance, with mottling of the skin and sluggish peripheral blood flow (when the skin is pressed, the blanched area is slow to turn pink again).

B. Oxygen Saturation and Arterial Blood Gas Changes

When a pneumothorax occurs, oxygen saturation drops acutely and arterial blood gas values change as the lung is unable to expand fully. Pressure from the pneumothorax compresses the alveoli in large areas of the lung and interferes with the normal exchange of oxygen and carbon dioxide.

If oxygen saturation and clinical changes are detected early enough, they may be seen before dramatic changes in arterial blood gas values occur. Typical changes in arterial blood gas values include

- Decrease in arterial oxygen (PaO_2) concentration

- Increase in arterial carbon dioxide ($PaCO_2$) concentration

- Decrease in blood pH

4. What Should You Do When You Suspect a Baby Has Developed a Pneumothorax?

Several things will need to be done rapidly, depending on how sick the baby appears. Your first action should always be to maintain the baby's oxygenation. Then proceed to detect and treat the pneumothorax.

1. Quickly increase the baby's inspired oxygen concentration until the baby is pink. If not already in place, attach a pulse oximeter to the baby to monitor oxygenation. Adjust the baby's inspired oxygen concentration to maintain normal saturation (85%–95%).

2. If an umbilical arterial catheter is in place, obtain an arterial blood gas sample. Do *not* wait for the results before taking further action. Proceed with techniques to detect a pneumothorax.

3. Transilluminate the baby's chest. Based on the results of the transillumination, and the baby's clinical condition, you may need to insert a needle into the baby's chest and aspirate the pneumothorax as an emergency measure.

4. Obtain a portable chest x-ray as soon as possible. Following detection of a pneumothorax, several follow-up x-rays may also be needed to evaluate treatment (needle aspiration and/or chest tube insertion).

5. If an arterial blood gas sample could not be obtained earlier, obtain one now. Provide oxygen therapy and respiratory support as indicated by the arterial blood gas (ABG) results. You will probably need to obtain several ABGs as the baby's condition changes and treatment is provided. Even if a pulse oximeter is being used, ABGs are necessary to monitor the baby's PaO_2, $PaCO_2$, pH, and serum bicarbonate and to adjust therapy accordingly.

5. How Is a Pneumothorax Detected?

A. Transillumination

A baby's chest may be illuminated with a bright light to detect a pneumothorax. Light penetrates air better than tissue. Therefore, the area of the pneumothorax "lights up," creating a "positive" transillumination.

A large pneumothorax can be detected easily and quickly with transillumination, but a small pneumothorax may not be seen clearly. A small pneumothorax may still be present even though a transillumination is "negative."

Immediate treatment should be undertaken for a baby with a clearly positive transillumination whose condition is deteriorating. Do not wait for a chest x-ray.

B. Chest X-ray

When the baby's condition is stable, or there is any question about the transillumination, obtain a chest x-ray. The details of transillumination and x-ray interpretation for a pneumothorax are presented in the skill units.

6. What Are the Consequences of a Pneumothorax?

A. Hypoxia and Acidosis

Pressure on the heart and lungs from the pneumothorax pocket of air may restrict adequate air movement to the lungs or blood flow from the heart.

B. Intraventricular Hemorrhage (IVH)

- Decreased venous return to the heart from cerebral veins occurs as a result of compression by the pneumothorax on the heart and major blood vessels.

- Hypercarbia (high blood CO_2) and peripheral arterial constriction usually accompany the development of a pneumothorax, thus causing an acute increase in blood flow to the brain.

Decreased venous drainage from the brain together with increased blood flow to the brain are thought to be responsible for the increased occurrence of intraventricular hemorrhage in babies with pneumothoraces. Because cerebral blood vessels of preterm babies are particularly fragile, preterm infants are at highest risk for intraventricular hemorrhage.

7. When Do Pneumothoraces Occur?

A. Healthy Babies

In healthy newborns, pneumothoraces may develop at delivery. This is due to the high inspiratory pressures the baby creates with the first few breaths. As noted previously, pneumothoraces in otherwise healthy infants are rarely symptomatic and should not be treated unless a baby develops significant respiratory distress.

B. Sick Babies

In sick babies, pneumothoraces may occur at the time of resuscitation or at any time during their illness. High CPAP and assisted ventilation pressures increase the risk. A pneumothorax should be considered any time there is a sudden deterioration in the baby's condition, even if the baby is recovering from an illness.

C. Babies With a Pneumothorax

Development of one pneumothorax increases the chance of developing additional pneumothoraces, either on the same side as the original pneumothorax or on the opposite side.

A blocked chest tube may also lead to redevelopment of a pneumothorax in the already affected side.

8. How Is a Pneumothorax Treated?

If a pneumothorax is small and the baby is not in respiratory distress, no treatment is required. In these cases, the pneumothorax will gradually resolve spontaneously, over several hours.

If a baby is symptomatic, however, needle aspiration and/or chest tube placement may be used to relieve a pneumothorax.

A. Needle Aspiration

If a baby's condition is deteriorating rapidly, a needle or percutaneous catheter is placed through the chest wall and into the collection of air. A stopcock and syringe are attached to the needle or catheter and the air is aspirated. Needle aspiration is a temporary measure, performed in an emergency. It is usually followed by placement of a chest tube.

B. Chest Tube Placement

A chest tube may be inserted initially, if the baby's condition is relatively stable, or may be inserted after needle aspiration of the pneumothorax. After insertion, a chest tube is attached to low, continuous suction using a 3-chamber or preset valve system until the rupture in the lung heals and the air leak stops.

The step-by-step details of these 2 procedures are described in the skill units.

Now answer these questions to test yourself on the information in the last section.

F1. A pneumothorax is _____ .

F2. Which babies are at highest risk for a pneumothorax?

_____

_____

_____

_____

F3. True False Bag-breathing during resuscitation should be strictly limited to prevent the development of a pneumothorax.

F4. List at least 4 signs that a baby with a pneumothorax may develop.

_____

_____

_____

_____

F5. When a baby has a pneumothorax, you would expect the PaO_2 concentration to _____,

the $PaCO_2$ to _____, and the blood pH to _____.

F6. True False All term babies with a spontaneous pneumothorax should have a chest tube placed to relieve the pneumothorax.

F7. A pneumothorax

   A. Can be a life-threatening condition
   B. Is a minor complication of positive-pressure ventilation
   C. Occurs only in term newborns
   D. Occurs only in babies on ventilators
   E. Will always cause intraventricular hemorrhage

F8. What are 2 techniques used to treat a pneumothorax?

_____

_____

F9. True False If a pneumothorax is present, a transillumination will always be positive.

F10. True False A chest x-ray should always be obtained before treatment of a pneumothorax.

Check your answers with the list that follows the Recommended Routines. Correct any incorrect answers and review the appropriate section in the unit.

Recommended Routines

All of the routines listed below are based on the principles of perinatal care presented in the unit you have just finished. They are recommended as part of routine perinatal care.

Read each routine carefully and decide whether it is standard operating procedure in your hospital. Check the appropriate blank next to each routine.

Procedure Standard in My Hospital	Needs Discussion by Our Staff	
_____	_____	1. Establish a routine of using a pulse oximeter to monitor oxygenation of any baby with respiratory distress, starting from the time the distress is first noted.
_____	_____	2. Establish a routine for obtaining the following for any baby with respiratory distress, within 30 minutes of the onset of distress:
_____	_____	• Vital signs (temperature, pulse, respirations, and blood pressure)
_____	_____	• Physical examination
_____	_____	• Portable chest x-ray
_____	_____	• Arterial blood gas
_____	_____	• Hematocrit from venous or arterial (not capillary) blood
_____	_____	• Blood glucose screening test or laboratory test
_____	_____	• Blood culture and/or white blood cell count with differential
_____	_____	3. Establish a policy to allow sufficient oxygen to be given to keep a cyanotic baby pink until appropriate blood gas determinations are made.
_____	_____	4. Establish a policy of withholding baths and oral feedings from any acutely ill baby who has respiratory distress or receives supplemental oxygen.
_____	_____	5. Provide continuous electronic cardiorespiratory monitoring for all babies at risk for apnea.
_____	_____	6. Be prepared to provide immediate transillumination for any baby in your nursery.
_____	_____	7. Establish a system for obtaining a chest x-ray and an arterial blood gas within 30 minutes of the time a pneumothorax is suspected.
_____	_____	8. Be prepared to provide immediate needle aspiration of a pneumothorax.
_____	_____	9. Establish a policy that will ensure the presence of a sterile chest tube insertion tray in the nursery at all times.

These are the answers to the self-test questions. Please check them with the answers you gave and review the information in the unit wherever necessary.

A1. Tachypnea
   Intercostal retractions
   Nasal flaring
   Grunting
   Cyanosis

A2. Mucous membranes (eg, lips)

A3. A. Observe the baby for the next 30 minutes

A4. Tachypnea, retractions, nasal flaring, or grunting after the first hour of life indicates respiratory distress.

A5. This baby is now sick. You would

Yes	No	
___	_x_	Assist the baby's breathing with bag-and-mask ventilation.
_x_	___	Take the baby's vital signs.
_x_	___	Attach a cardiac monitor to the baby.
___	_x_	Feed the baby to prevent hypoglycemia.
_x_	___	Attach a pulse oximeter to the baby.

B1. True

B2. B. Immaturity of the baby's lungs and the resulting lack of surfactants needed to keep the alveoli (air sacs) open

B3. A, B, C, D, and E all cause respiratory distress.

B4. Any 2 of the following:
   • Mucus
   • Mechanical obstruction, such as a misplaced phototherapy mask
   • Choanal atresia
   • Pneumothorax
   • Diaphragmatic hernia
   • Robin syndrome

B5. Any 2 of the following:
   • Aspiration syndrome
   • Pneumonia
   • Transient respiratory distress

B6. Any 3 of the following:
   • Hypotension
   • Congenital heart disease
   • Cold stress
   • Anemia
   • Polycythemia
   • Hypoxia and acidosis

C1. Any 3 of the following:
   • Preterm infants
   • Infants with difficult deliveries
   • Infants born to women with diabetes mellitus
   • Infants born by cesarean section
   • Infants born to women with fever, prolonged rupture of membranes, foul-smelling amniotic fluid, and/or risk factors for GBS infection

- Meconium-stained babies
- Babies born to women with hydramnios
- Babies with other problems, such as cold-stress, hypotension, anemia, polycythemia, etc

C2.
- Monitor with pulse oximetry
- Obtain
  Arterial blood gas
  Chest x-ray
  Hematocrit
  Blood glucose screen
  White blood cell count and differential
- Consider blood culture and antibiotics.

C3. Stiff, chest x-ray
C4. Choanal atresia, an oral airway
C5. A pneumothorax, transillumination, chest x-ray
C6. Perinatal blood loss, a blood transfusion
C7. Inspired oxygen concentration, brain
C8. Decrease, eyes and/or lungs
C9. A. Ventilate the baby.
C10. B. Give sodium bicarbonate.

D1. False   Breathing pauses are normal in newborns. Apnea is when breathing stops for longer than 15 seconds or for a shorter period if accompanied by cyanosis or bradycardia.
D2. Yes
D3. Any 5 of the following:
1. Preterm
2. Rapidly worsening respiratory disease
3. Metabolic disorder such as low blood glucose, calcium, sodium, or acidosis
4. Sepsis or meningitis
5. Rewarming of cold-stressed baby
6. Central nervous system disorder
7. Low blood volume or low hematocrit
8. History of severe hypoxia and/or acidosis
9. Maternal depressant drugs during labor
D4. Monitored, with heart rate and respiratory monitor.

E1. False   There are many causes of apnea. Each should be considered before deciding it is due to apnea of prematurity.
E2. Bag-breathe for the baby; give oxygen if cyanosis is present and persists after ventilation is established.
E3. Any 6 of the following:
1. Arterial blood gas
2. Chest x-ray
3. Blood glucose
4. Blood pressure
5. Baby's temperature, environmental temperature, and oxygen/air temperature (if supplemental oxygen is being used)
6. Hematocrit
7. Evaluate for sepsis and meningitis
8. Evaluate for a patent ductus arteriosus
9. Evaluate for seizures; assess neurologic status
10. Serum sodium, calcium, and pH
11. Evaluate oral feeding

E4.   1. Acute illness has resolved.
      2. Baby weighs 1,800 g (4 lb) or more and has reached a gestational age of 35 weeks or older.
      3. Baby has been apnea-free for 7 to 8 consecutive days.

F1.   A collection of air within the chest cavity, between the lung and the chest wall, that results from a rupture in the lung tissue, allowing air to leak outside the lung

F2.   Babies receiving positive-pressure ventilation
      Babies with poor lung compliance (stiff lungs), as seen with respiratory distress syndrome
      Babies with aspiration syndrome
      Babies requiring resuscitation

F3.   False   High pressures may be needed to ventilate a baby adequately. The pressure needed should be given and not limited, but unnecessarily high pressures should be avoided. You should be aware that a possible complication of assisted ventilation is a pneumothorax, but that possibility should not restrict resuscitation efforts.

F4.   A baby with a pneumothorax may develop any of the following signs:
      • Sudden onset of cyanosis
      • Increase or decrease in respiratory effort or rate
      • Breath sounds louder over one lung
      • Shift in location of heart sounds
      • Unequal chest expansion
      • Abdominal distension
      • Low blood pressure, especially when it had been normal
      • Deterioration in appearance with poor peripheral perfusion

F5. PaO_2 concentration to *decrease*
      $PaCO_2$ concentration to *increase*
      blood pH to *decrease*

F6.   False   Otherwise healthy babies who are in no respiratory distress do not need treatment for a spontaneous pneumothorax. Treatment is needed only if a pneumothorax becomes symptomatic.

F7.   A. Can be a life-threatening condition

F8.   Needle aspiration
      Chest tube placement

F9.   False   A small pneumothorax may not give a positive transillumination. Also, as you will learn in the skill unit, a clear transillumination may be difficult to obtain in obese babies.

F10. False   You should not wait for a chest x-ray if the transillumination is clearly positive and the baby's condition is worsening rapidly.

Unit 3 Posttest

Without referring back to the information in the unit, please answer the following questions. Select the **one best** answer to each question (unless otherwise instructed). Record your answers on the answer sheet that is the last page in this book *and* on the test.

1. What are the 5 signs of neonatal respiratory distress?

   _____

   _____

   _____

   _____

   _____

2. To determine if a baby is cyanotic, which of the following is the *best* part of the baby's body to examine?

   A. Feet
   B. Mouth
   C. Hands
   D. Ears

3. An infant, 30 minutes after birth, shows mild grunting and nasal flaring but is not cyanotic. You check the baby's vital signs and they are normal. What would you do *next*?

   A. Attach a pulse oximeter to the baby.
   B. Assist the baby's breathing with bag and mask.
   C. Administer 60% oxygen.
   D. Intubate immediately.

4. Which of the following may cause respiratory distress in the newborn?

   A. Congenital heart disease
   B. Hypothermia
   C. Anemia
   D. All of the above

5. Which infants are at increased risk for developing respiratory distress? (Choose the letter that identifies the correct answers.)

   1. Preterm infants
   2. Infants who have been resuscitated
   3. Infants with meconium staining
   4. Infants with low blood pressure
      A. 1, 3
      B. 1, 2
      C. 1, 2, 3
      D. 1, 2, 3, 4

6. **True   False**   Thirty minutes after birth, an infant shows mild grunting and nasal flaring but is not cyanotic. This is probably normal.

7. **True   False**   Babies breathe mainly through their mouths.

8. You observe that a baby is in respiratory distress in the delivery room. You attempt to pass a nasogastric tube but it will not advance farther than 1 inch. What is the *first* thing that should be done for this baby?

   A. Obtain a chest x-ray.
   B. Insert a needle into his chest cavity.
   C. Insert an oral airway.
   D. Administer sodium bicarbonate.

9. A preterm baby with respiratory distress is grunting and has nasal flaring. Her arterial hematocrit 2 hours after birth is 25%. Which of the following is *most* important to do for this baby?

    A. Give her a blood transfusion.

    B. Administer sodium bicarbonate (1–2 mEq/kg).

    C. Insert a nasogastric tube.

    D. Withdraw 10 mL/kg of blood and replace it with 10 mL/kg of normal saline.

10. Which of the following babies has had an apneic spell?

    A. A baby who stops breathing for more than 20 seconds

    B. A baby who grunts and breathes irregularly

    C. A baby who turns blue while breathing

    D. A baby who grunts and has a heart rate of 120 beats per minute

11. Which babies should be monitored for apnea? (Choose the letter that identifies the correct answers.)

    1. Term baby with an infection

    2. Baby weighing less than 1,800 g (4 lb) with no respiratory problems

    3. Baby with hypoglycemia

        A. 1, 2

        B. 1, 3

        C. 2, 3

        D. 1, 2, 3

12. A preterm baby with respiratory distress has an apnea attack. Her heart rate is 90. What is the *first* action that should be taken for this baby?

    A. Provide assisted ventilation with bag and mask.

    B. Rub the baby's arms and legs.

    C. Administer epinephrine.

    D. Administer theophylline.

13. A baby is at risk for apnea. Which of the following is the *most* appropriate procedure for this baby?

    A. Place the baby in low-flow oxygen.

    B. Obtain an electrocardiogram.

    C. Attach a cardiorespiratory monitor.

    D. Place the baby in Trendelenburg position.

14. Which of the following babies is at *highest* risk for developing a pneumothorax?

    A. Post-term baby with polycythemia

    B. Term baby with hypoglycemia

    C. Post-term baby who aspirated maternal blood at delivery

    D. Term baby with choanal atresia

15. Refer to the following normal arterial blood gas values when answering the next question.

$$PaO_2: \quad 45\text{–}75 \text{ mm Hg}$$

$$PaCO_2: \quad 40\text{–}50 \text{ mm Hg}$$

$$pH: \quad 7.25\text{–}7.35$$

Which of the following blood gas results would you be *most* likely to find in a baby with a pneumothorax?

    A. $PaO_2 = 96$, $PaCO_2 = 37$, pH = 7.36

    B. $PaO_2 = 38$, $PaCO_2 = 29$, pH = 7.18

    C. $PaO_2 = 75$, $PaCO_2 = 30$, pH = 7.30

    D. $PaO_2 = 42$, $PaCO_2 = 66$, pH = 7.19

16. Which of the following signs is *most* likely to occur in a baby with a pneumothorax?

   A. Sudden cyanosis
   B. Vomiting
   C. Hypothermia
   D. Cardiac arrhythmia

17. A baby in respiratory distress has a pneumothorax. You have increased the inspired oxygen concentration, but the baby remains cyanotic. What should you do *next*?

   A. Monitor with a pulse oximeter and obtain another chest x-ray.
   B. Perform needle aspiration or insert a chest tube and obtain another chest x-ray.
   C. Place the baby in reverse Trendelenburg position (head up, feet down).
   D. Aspirate the baby's stomach contents.

18. True   False   Healthy newborns sometimes develop pneumothoraces but may not develop signs of respiratory distress.

For each question, please make sure you have marked your answer on the test and on the answer sheet (last page in book). The test is for you; the answer sheet will need to be turned in for continuing education credit.

Skill Unit 1   Detecting a Pneumothorax

These skill units will teach you how to detect a pneumothorax. Two techniques will be covered: transillumination and chest x-ray. Not everyone will be required to learn how to transilluminate a baby's chest with a fiberoptic light or to interpret chest x-rays. However, everyone should read this unit and attend a skill session to learn equipment, sequence of steps, and correct positioning of a baby to assist with these skills.

Note: The illustrations for these separate skill units are not meant to be linked to each other, although the baby appears similar throughout. The transillumination and chest tube insertion skills show left pneumothoraces, while a right pneumothorax is illustrated in the needle aspiration skill, and x-rays of both left and right pneumothoraces are shown.

Study these skill units; then attend a skill practice and demonstration session. To master the skills you will need to demonstrate correctly each of the following skill steps:

Transillumination
1. Position the "baby."
2. Set transillumination light to proper setting(s).
3. Darken room.
4. Maintain the "baby's" therapy: oxygen delivery, thermal environment, intravenous (IV) infusions, etc.
5. Position tip of fiberoptic light on "baby's" chest.
   • Mid-axillary area
   • Mid-clavicular area

Chest X-ray: Anterior-posterior view
1. Place the "baby" in a supine position
   • In an incubator
   • Under a radiant warmer
2. Maintain the "baby's" therapy: oxygen delivery, thermal environment, IV infusions, etc.
3. Reposition tubes and/or wires, as necessary and appropriate.
4. Shield the "baby's" genitalia and caution others within range of x-ray beam to move or put on a lead apron.
5. Restrain the "baby," if necessary.

Chest X-ray: Lateral view
1. Place the "baby" in a lateral decubitus position (with "correct" side up)
   • In an incubator
   • Under a radiant warmer

147

2. Maintain the "baby's" therapy: oxygen delivery, thermal environment, IV infusions, etc.

3. Reposition tubes and/or wires, as necessary and appropriate.

4. Shield the "baby's" genitalia and caution others within range of x-ray beam to move or put on a lead apron.

5. Restrain the "baby," if necessary.

6. Hold x-ray plate in proper position.

Note: While useful results depend on carrying out these skills correctly, interpretation of findings is not included in these checklists. Physicians, and selected nurses, may be asked to participate in a workshop for interpretation of transillumination and chest x-ray findings.

Perinatal Performance Guide
Transillumination

A chest x-ray is obtained any time a pneumothorax is suspected. The benefit of transillumination is that it can be done easily at the bedside, and more quickly than an x-ray can be obtained. This allows immediate treatment of a large, life-threatening pneumothorax without waiting for x-ray evaluation.

Actions	Remarks

Anticipating the Need for Transillumination

1. Is there a clinical indication that the baby might have developed a pneumothorax?
    - Sudden cyanosis
    - Increase in respiratory rate
    - Unequal breath sounds
    - Unequal chest size
    - Development of abdominal distension
    - Shift in location of heart sounds
    - Low blood pressure (especially if it had been normal)
    - Mottled skin with poor peripheral blood flow

    Yes:
    - Obtain an arterial blood gas measurement immediately.
    - Prepare to transilluminate the baby's chest.
    - Connect an oximeter to the baby, if not already being monitored.

    Remarks: When a pneumothorax first develops, a baby may show only one of these signs. Often the most important initial sign is the sudden deterioration in a baby's condition. As the pneumothorax worsens, more changes may become evident.

    Be sure to increase the baby's inspired oxygen concentration and provide other supportive therapy as necessary.

    If a baby does not have an umbilical arterial catheter and a peripheral arterial blood gas cannot be obtained quickly, or if the baby's condition is deteriorating rapidly, it will be necessary to confirm and treat the pneumothorax immediately, before obtaining an arterial blood gas.

2. Do the blood gas or oximeter values suggest the occurrence of a pneumothorax?
    - Decrease in PaO_2 or % saturation
    - Increase in $PaCO_2$
    - Acidosis

    Yes: Transilluminate the baby's chest.

    Remarks: These changes are typical during development of a pneumothorax. However, sometimes the PaO_2 does not decrease and, at first, the $PaCO_2$ level may increase only slightly.

    Changes in blood gas values or O_2 saturation may also reflect worsening lung disease. Blood gas values must be interpreted together with the baby's clinical appearance.

    Whenever there is sudden clinical deterioration, a pneumothorax should be suspected, and transillumination performed and/or a chest x-ray obtained.

Actions	**Remarks**

Transilluminating a Baby's Chest

3. Obtain the transillumination light. Plug it in at the baby's bedside.	A transillumination light is a high-intensity fiberoptic light that shines through the end of a flexible metal tube.
4. Position the baby supine.	
5. Turn out the nursery lights and darken the room as much as possible.	
6. Position the tip of the light firmly against the baby's chest at the mid-axillary area between the fourth and sixth interspaces.	The surface of the fiberoptic light should be held flat against the baby's chest, pressed firmly but gently against the chest wall.
7. Turn on the fiberoptic light to its highest intensity setting.	
Shine the light first on one side of the baby's chest and then the other.	Look for a difference in the amount of transillumination between the side with the suspected pneumothorax and the opposite side.

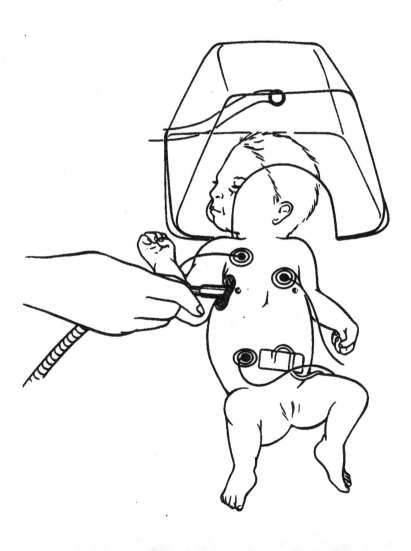

Actions   **Remarks**

Transilluminating a Baby's Chest (continued)

8. Observe the area of the baby's chest that lights up. A large pneumothorax will show up as a bright area that extends throughout the air that is trapped outside of the lung, but within the chest cavity. This is shown in the illustration (shown at right) as a shaded area on the baby's chest.

9. Move the transilluminating light to anterior parts of the chest and to the opposite side to look for positive transillumination there as well. When there is no pneumothorax the light will form a narrow symmetrical halo around the light source (shown below).

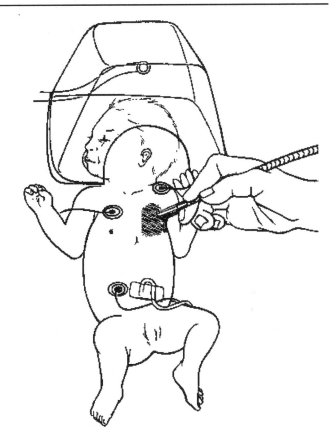

Transillumination Positive

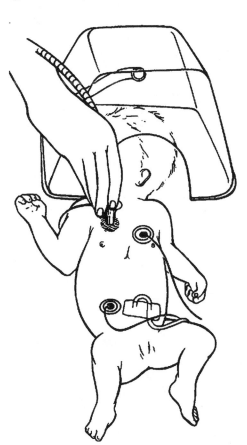

Transillumination Negative

10. Repeat steps 8 and 9 to double-check your findings.

Compare both sides. Although it is possible to have bilateral pneumothoraces, this is quite rare. Usually, a large pneumothorax will appear as a lighting up of the affected side (shown above).

Transillumination of the unaffected side would show only a narrow halo around the light (shown at left).

Actions	Remarks

Interpreting the Transillumination Findings

11. Normal (negative transillumination)

- The area that lights up will be a symmetrical ring or halo around the tip of the fiberoptic light and generally will not extend more than 1 cm from the light source.

- The size of the translucent area will be equal for both sides of the baby's chest.

Thin preterm babies will normally transilluminate more than full-term babies, even when there is no pneumothorax.

A clear transillumination may be difficult to obtain in babies born at term and in obese babies.

12. Abnormal (positive transillumination)

- The translucent glow will be larger on one side of the chest than on the other.

- The translucent area on the side with the pneumothorax will often have an irregular pattern.

The air collection of the pneumothorax lights up. Rarely, there will be a bilateral pneumothorax, in which case both sides of the chest will transilluminate positively.

13. Suspicious

- It is difficult to be sure if the area of translucent glow on one side of the chest is larger than that on the other side.

A large pneumothorax will almost always show a positive transillumination. A small but clinically significant pneumothorax may not show a definite positive transillumination.

Using the Transillumination Information

14. Negative transillumination

- If the baby's clinical appearance and/or blood gas values still suggest a pneumothorax, obtain a chest x-ray.

Continue to provide oxygen therapy, assisted ventilation, and other supportive therapy as necessary.

15. Positive transillumination

- If the baby's condition is deteriorating, relieve the pneumothorax immediately with needle aspiration or chest tube insertion.

- If the baby's condition is stable, you may wish to obtain a chest x-ray before chest tube insertion.

This is a life-threatening situation. If the baby's vital signs are deteriorating, or if adequate oxygenation cannot be achieved, immediate decompression of the pneumothorax is required. Do not wait for a chest x-ray.

16. Suspicious

- A suspicious transillumination should always be evaluated with a chest x-ray.

If the baby's condition deteriorates, transilluminate the chest again. Also, be sure to investigate other causes of a marked deterioration in the baby's condition (eg, a dislodged or occluded endotracheal tube).

Actions	**Remarks**

What Can Go Wrong?

1. The fiberoptic light may not be bright enough.	Be sure that the light is always set on the highest intensity setting.
2. The room may not be dark enough.	It may not be possible to see the full area of translucent glow.
3. You may not hold the tip of the light firmly enough against the baby's chest wall.	This will prevent complete transillumination, and a pneumothorax may be missed.
4. You may not hold the tip of the fiberoptic light flat against the baby's chest.	When you transilluminate a baby's chest, shift the angle of the light slightly until the largest area of translucent glow is seen.
5. You may hold the light under a skin fold and get excessive false transillumination.	Be certain to place the tip of fiberoptic light flat against the baby's chest.
Note: Significant edema can also cause a false transillumination.	
6. You may insert a chest tube unnecessarily.	It is always best to confirm a positive transillumination with a chest x-ray, unless the baby's condition is rapidly deteriorating.

Perinatal Performance Guide
Chest X-Ray Evaluation

Complete chest x-ray evaluation of a newborn will *not* be covered in this skill unit. A few key points that are important to the x-ray evaluation and identification of a pneumothorax are presented. In almost all circumstances, an anterior-posterior view of the chest is adequate. Lateral views are helpful occasionally; these are discussed where appropriate. Determination of chest tube placement by x-ray is also covered.

Actions	Remarks

Preparing a Baby for Chest X-ray

1. Position the baby supine. The baby's shoulders, back, and hips should be flat, without rotation either to the left or to the right.	Rotation will cause the body structures to appear distorted in size and malpositioned. Accurate evaluation cannot be made from an x-ray taken when the baby is rotated.
2. Be sure the baby's oxygen therapy, thermal environment, intravenous infusions, etc, are maintained without interruption during the x-ray procedure.	If the baby is in an incubator, the x-ray can easily be taken through the top of the incubator. This will not interfere at all with the evaluation of the chest x-ray. The small hole that is in the center of the top of most incubators will appear on the x-ray as a symmetrical lucent circle. Because it is perfectly round it is easily identified as an artifact and should not be confused with an abnormal finding.
3. If possible, remove any tubes or wires that drape across the baby's chest.	Cardiac monitor leads attached to the anterior or posterior surface of a baby's chest may need to be removed during an x-ray and replaced as soon as the procedure is completed. Monitor leads attached to the sides of a baby's chest do not need to be removed during an x-ray.
4. Shield the baby's genitalia from exposure to the x-rays. This can be done by placing a lead glove or other piece of x-ray opaque material across the baby's pelvis.	This will also help to immobilize the baby's legs and keep the hips flat during the x-ray.
5. Take the x-ray when the baby is quiet. Do not take a chest x-ray when a baby is crying vigorously.	Ideally the x-ray should be during inspiration but this is difficult to do with a baby's rapid respiratory rate. Also, because of a baby's small breaths, little difference is seen between inspiratory and expiratory films. However, an x-ray taken during forceful crying may appear as if the lungs are completely collapsed and will not allow accurate interpretation.

Positioning a Baby for a Chest X-ray

The illustration below shows the correct position of a baby for an anterior-posterior chest x-ray. Note that the baby's shoulders, back, and hips are flat against the x-ray plate; the genitalia are shielded with x-ray opaque material; and the oxygen therapy is maintained, as are all other components of the baby's care (not shown). The x-ray beam is shown as a circle but is actually a rectangular pattern and should cover both sides of the chest to include the lung periphery.

Although not shown, a baby may remain inside an incubator for this procedure, with the x-ray taken through the top of the incubator.

Once properly positioned, some very sick babies may not need to be restrained during an x-ray. If the baby is at all active, you should wear lead gloves to hold the baby or use restraints to immobilize the baby's extremities. If needed, use restraints only during the very brief period when the x-ray is taken.

If the x-ray beam is vertical (as shown here), there will be no detectable radiation beyond 6 ft. If the x-ray beam is horizontal (as shown later) a lead apron is necessary to shield staff and other patients.

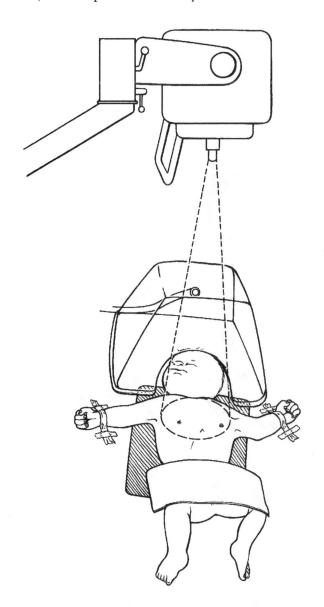

Actions	Remarks

Evaluating a Chest X-ray for a Pneumothorax

6. Assess the chest x-ray for rotation. Do this by comparing the length of the anterior ribs on the left and right sides.	When the film is not rotated, the ribs will appear of equal length.
7. Assess the x-ray for any asymmetry between the right and left sides.	Asymmetrical findings generally indicate an abnormality and should be further evaluated.
8. Look for typical asymmetric findings seen with a pneumothorax.	
• **Compression of the affected lung:** Edge of the lung should be clearly visible.	If the lungs are stiff, complete collapse will not be seen and may limit the degree of heart shift.
• **Shift of midline structures:** This can occur in varying degrees.	Sometimes there is a drastic shift in the heart location while at other times there is only a lucent curve above the heart as the pneumothorax crosses the midline.
• **Downward displacement of the diaphragm** on the affected side.	This causes a clinical appearance of abdominal distension. Even without a pneumothorax, the left diaphragm is usually slightly lower than the right.

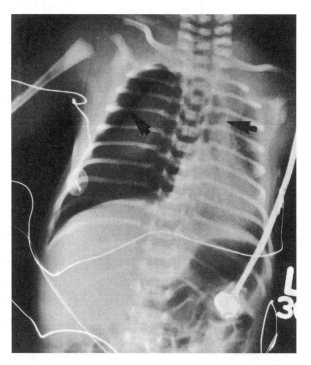

Figure 3.1. Chest X-ray—Pneumothorax. Note lung edge, flat diaphragm, and shift of midline structures in right pneumothorax.

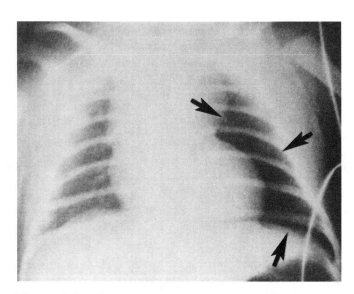

Figure 3.2. Chest X-ray—Anterior Pneumothorax. Note hyperlucency without a visible lung edge in left anterior pneumothorax.

Actions	**Remarks**

Clarifying Questionable Findings

- Hyperlucent area ringing the superior, lateral, and/or inferior edges of the lung.

  The area corresponds with the location of the pneumothorax air collection.

- *One lung field that is more lucent than the other.* (Figure 3.2)

  Sometimes the air collection is completely anterior, overlying the whole lung, and does not show a ring at the edge of the lung. Lateral x-ray may be needed to confirm a pneumothorax.

9. If you are not sure if a pneumothorax is present on the anterior-posterior chest x-ray, obtain a lateral view.

10. Put the baby in a lateral decubitus position. The lung suspected of having the pneumothorax should be up, and the unaffected side should be down.

    The baby's shoulders, back, and hips should be at right angles to the bed. The trapped air will "rise," shifting from the anterior chest to the lateral chest and outlining the lung.

11. Extend the superior arm over the baby's head.

12. Place the x-ray plate flat across the baby's back, also at right angles to the bed.

    The x-ray beam will be positioned horizontally across the baby's bed.

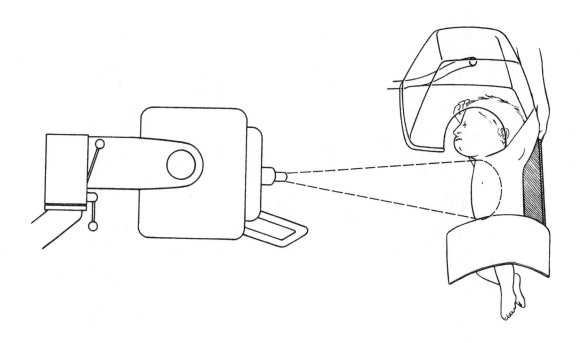

Actions	**Remarks**

Determining Chest Tube Placement

13. Obtain a follow-up chest x-ray any time a chest tube is inserted. This is done to determine if the

    • Chest tube is positioned properly

    • Pneumothorax has been completely evacuated

14. Assess the position of the chest tube. It should be directed toward the baby's head and then curved toward the midline.

    Remark: The tip may touch but should not press against the mediastinal structures.

15. Assess the position of the holes in the chest tube. These will appear as small concave areas on the edge of the tube.

    Remark: Because the holes are not outlined in radiopaque material, it may not be possible to assess the position of all of them. However, if the tube position is adjusted, be sure that all of the holes stay within the baby's chest cavity.

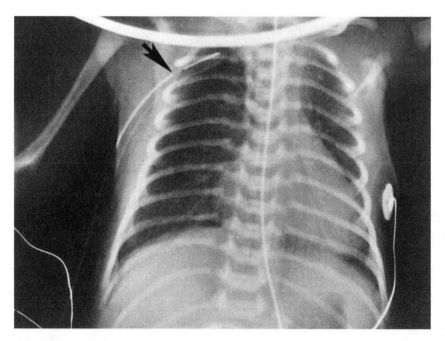

Figure 3.3. Incorrect Placement of Chest Tube. Note that the tube has been placed very high, and a hole (arrow) is outside the chest cavity.

Actions   **Remarks**

Determining Chest Tube Placement (continued)

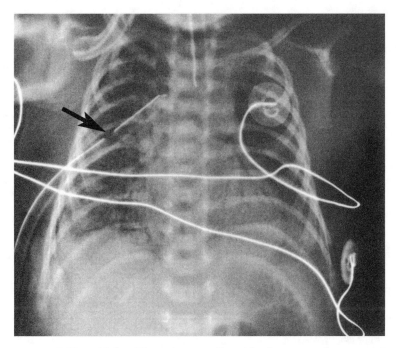

Figure 3.4. Correct Placement of Chest Tube. There is a small residual pneumothorax at the superior aspect of the lung. The arrow points to one of the holes in the chest tube.

16. Determine if the pneumothorax has been evacuated. If the pneumothorax is still present, several things should be considered.

• The chest tube is **positioned incorrectly.**

  – **Placed posteriorly:** The pneumothorax may be anterior to the lung while the chest tube has been placed behind the lung.

  – **Inserted too far:** On the x-ray, measure the length that the tube needs to be withdrawn. Withdraw the chest tube that amount by using the black marks printed on the catheter as reference points.

  – **Not inserted far enough:** The chest tube must be withdrawn and a new one inserted under sterile conditions.

On an anterior-posterior x-ray, it is not possible to tell whether the chest tube is in front of or behind the lung. To differentiate this you would need to obtain a cross-table view with the baby supine. The x-ray plate is held vertically against the baby's opposite chest wall, and the x-ray taken horizontally across the baby's chest.

Actions	**Remarks**

Determining Chest Tube Placement (continued)

– The chest tube **suction apparatus is not functioning correctly.**	Recheck the system. See also the following skill units.
– The chest tube and system are working but the **x-ray was taken before all of the air could be withdrawn.**	If you believe this to be the case and the baby's clinical condition has improved, obtain a second follow-up chest x-ray in 30 minutes.
– Tube positioned correctly but **not all of the air is accessible to the chest tube.**	Change the baby's position to redistribute the air pockets, allowing complete evacuation.
– **One chest tube is not adequate.**	It is very rare, but a second chest tube may be needed. Before a second chest tube is inserted, thoroughly evaluate the position and functioning of the first chest tube.

Note: A small residual pneumothorax may not need treatment if the baby's vital signs are stable and oxygenation is adequate.

What Can Go Wrong?

1. You misdiagnose a small pneumothorax.	Ask a second person to help you read the chest x-ray and/or obtain another x-ray 30 minutes later. If a pneumothorax is present, it will probably be larger and may have shifted location, making it easier to detect.
2. One pneumothorax is diagnosed and treated but the baby's condition again deteriorates suddenly. Transilluminate the baby's chest again and/or obtain another chest x-ray.	A pneumothorax may have developed in the other lung or the chest tube may not be working, allowing the original pneumothorax to recur. Be sure to assess other factors that could have caused a rapid deterioration, such as inadequate ventilation, dislodged endotracheal tube, etc.

These skill units will teach you how to aspirate a pneumothorax in an emergency and how to place and secure a chest tube. You will also learn how to maintain a chest tube and how to manage chest tube suction. Not everyone will be required to learn how to relieve a pneumothorax. However, everyone should read this unit and attend a skill practice session to learn the equipment and sequence of steps so they can assist with needle aspiration and chest tube insertion. Everyone will be required to know how to maintain a chest tube safely.

Study these skill units then attend a skill practice and demonstration session. To master the skills you will need to demonstrate correctly each of the following steps:

Needle aspiration

1. Collect the equipment and, wherever possible, connect the pieces together.

2. Position "baby."

3. Restrain "baby," if necessary.

4. Locate the third intercostal space at the mid-clavicular line.

5. Cleanse this area.

Chest tube insertion: set up suction

1. Collect the equipment.

2. Assemble the pieces together.
    • Add water to the suction control and the water seal chambers or set up the preset valve system.
    • Connect tubing to the universal adapter and to the suction source.

Chest tube insertion: prepare "baby"

1. Collect the equipment and prepare the "sterile" tray.

2. Position "baby."

3. Continue therapy and maintain support systems: oxygen delivery, thermal environment, intravenous (IV) infusions, etc.

4. Monitor "baby" with a cardiac monitor and an oximeter.

5. Reposition tubes and/or wires, as necessary and appropriate.

6. Locate the fourth intercostal space and sixth rib at the mid-axillary area.

7. Cleanse this area.

* * *

8. Tape the chest tube in place.

9. Turn on and adjust the suction.

10. Tape all tubing connections.

11. Identify whether air is being evacuated from "baby's" chest.

12. Demonstrate how to check for leaks in the system.

Note: While successful relief of a pneumothorax depends on carrying out these skills correctly, actual insertion of a needle or chest tube is not included in these checklists. Physicians, and selected nurses, may be asked to participate in a demonstration and practice workshop for needle aspiration and chest tube insertion on models.

Actions	Remarks

Deciding When to Use Needle Aspiration

1. Is the baby's clinical condition deteriorating rapidly?

   Yes: Use needle aspiration to relieve the pneumothorax.

   No: Insert a chest tube to relieve the pneumothorax, or wait for spontaneous resolution if baby is not symptomatic.

Needle aspiration is used as an emergency procedure prior to placement of a chest tube.

Preparing the Baby and Equipment

2. Collect the following equipment:

   - 21- or 23-gauge butterfly needle
     or
     19- or 21-gauge percutaneous catheter
   - Short IV connecting tubing (T-connector) for use with a percutaneous catheter
   - 3-way stopcock
   - 10-mL or 12-mL syringe
   - Povidone-iodine or equivalent antiseptic solution
   - Alcohol swabs
   - Sterile water swabs

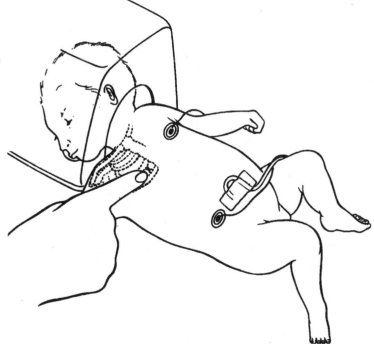

3. Position the baby supine.

4. If necessary, restrain the baby or have someone hold the baby still.

5. Determine the location of the third intercostal space at the mid-clavicular line.

   Be certain to avoid insertion at or near the nipple area.

6. Prep this area with antiseptic solution then wipe thoroughly with alcohol swabs.

Allow the povidone-iodine or chlorhexidine to dry, then remove it *completely* from the baby's skin by wiping with alcohol or sterile water swabs. If left in place, either of these antiseptics can cause marked skin irritation.

Actions   **Remarks**

Preparing the Baby and Equipment (continued)

7. Attach the butterfly needle to the 3-way stopcock and the syringe.

8. Turn the stopcock so it is open between the butterfly needle and syringe (shown below).

Note: A percutaneous catheter (not shown) may also be used. With this, the short IV connecting tubing (T-connector) and stopcock should be connected but cannot be attached to the catheter until after it is inserted and the needle introducer removed.

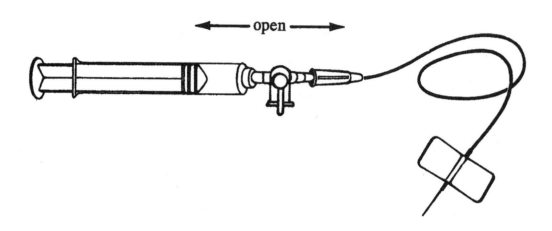

←— open —→

Evacuating the Air

9. Take the wings of the butterfly needle or the percutaneous catheter between your thumb and forefinger.

10. Hold the needle or catheter perpendicular to the chest wall and insert it into the third intercostal space, just above the fourth rib.

The intercostal blood vessels run just below each rib. You avoid hitting these by inserting the needle just above the rib.

11. *If a butterfly needle is used,* as soon as the needle enters the skin, a second person should begin to "pull back" on the syringe plunger.

Stop inserting the needle as soon as you get an air return. Hold it in this place.

The air should come back easily with gentle pulling. Do not pull forcibly on the syringe plunger.

If a percutaneous catheter is used, stop inserting the catheter as soon as a "pop" is felt, indicating the pleural space has been entered. Hold the catheter in place. A second person should remove the needle introducer and attach the IV connecting tubing (T-connector) and stopcock, then begin to aspirate air by gently pulling back on the syringe plunger. Air withdrawal should come easily. Do not pull back forcibly.

Hold the needle or catheter still. Do not allow it to advance any farther into the chest cavity.

Actions

Remarks

Evacuating the Air (continued)

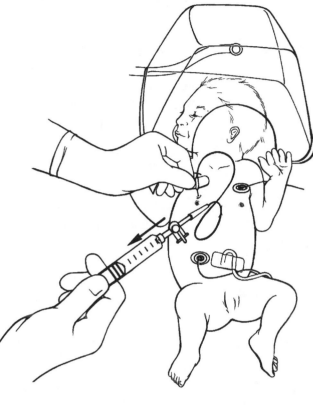

12. Continue to hold the butterfly needle (shown) or percutaneous catheter (not shown) in place while the second person gently pulls back on the syringe plunger to aspirate the air collection.

    You should begin to see a decrease in the baby's respiratory distress as the air is withdrawn.

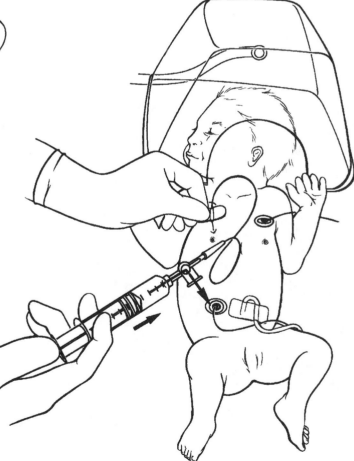

13. After the syringe has filled with air from the pneumothorax, close the stopcock to the needle or catheter and open it between the side port and the syringe.

14. Empty the syringe of air by pushing the air out through the side port. (Note direction of arrows in the illustrations.)

Actions	Remarks

Evacuating the Air (continued)

15. Continue to repeat this process until you can no longer aspirate air easily from the chest cavity.

16. As soon as you can no longer aspirate air easily from the chest cavity, withdraw the butterfly needle or percutaneous catheter.

    This is done so that the re-expanded lung is not punctured by the needle. If using a catheter, some clinicians will decide to tape the catheter in place until an x-ray has been obtained and read.

17. A dressing is not needed over this site. The baby's skin and tissues will close tightly over the puncture point preventing any air from entering from the outside.

18. Reassess the baby's condition, and consider inserting a chest tube.

    In many, but not all, cases a chest tube will need to be inserted following needle aspiration of a pneumothorax.

Perinatal Performance Guide
Chest Tube Insertion

Actions	Remarks

Preparing the Equipment

1. Collect the following equipment:
    - 1% xylocaine
    - Small syringe with 26-gauge needle
    - Mask
    - Sterile gloves
    - Povidone-iodine or equivalent solution
    - Alcohol swabs
    - Sterile water swabs
    - Sterile 2 × 2's
    - Sterile drapes
    - #15 knife blade
    - Knife handle
    - Small curved hemostat
    - Kelly clamp
    - 10 F and 12 F chest tubes with trocar
    - 3-0 suture on curved needle
    - Needle holder
    - 1/2-inch adhesive tape
    - Clear adhesive dressing
    - Cotton-tipped swabs
    - Universal adapter (to fit between chest tube and suction tube)
    - 3-bottle suction apparatus
    - Suction source

    Most of these items can be kept prepared on a sterile tray in the nursery.

2. Set up the suction apparatus. This should be a 3-bottle water seal system or a system that works with preset valves.

    *Disposable units that incorporate all of the principles of the 3-bottle system are commonly available.**

3. Fill the section marked "suction control chamber" to between the 5- and 10-mL mark.

    Usually much lower suction levels are required for babies than are commonly used for adults. In almost all circumstances, chest tubes are placed in babies to evacuate air, not blood or fluid (which would require higher suction pressures).

---

*A Pleur-evac set-up is shown on the next page. Other 3-bottle commercially available products have chambers with similar function but may be labeled differently. Some of these products may regulate pressures with preset valves, rather than water seals.

Actions   **Remarks**

Preparing the Equipment (continued)

4. Fill the section marked "water seal chamber" to
    the fill line.

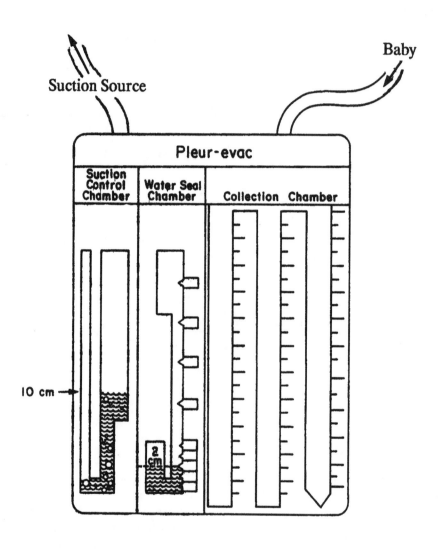

5. Connect the suction tubing to the suction
    source.

    Do not, however, turn on the suction yet.
    (The illustration may be misleading because
    bubbles will not appear in the suction control
    chamber until the suction is turned on.)

6. Using aseptic technique, connect the universal
    adapter to the patient's drainage tube.

    Keep the patient end of the universal adapter
    covered with sterile gauze. Put this end near the
    baby so it can be connected to the chest tube as
    soon as it is inserted.

Actions	**Remarks**

Preparing the Baby

7. Position the baby so that the side with the pneumothorax is at a 60° upright angle.

Place a blanket roll behind the baby's back.

During the procedure, a second person will need to hold the baby's uppermost arm over his or her head.

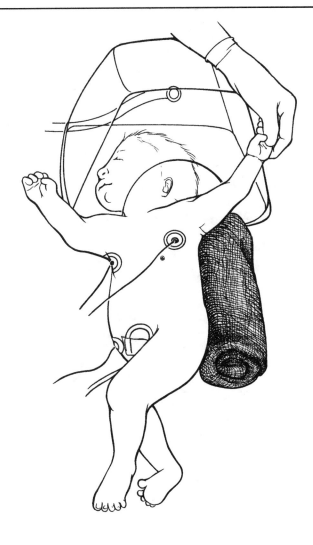

8. Maintain the baby's medical support. Be sure the oxygen therapy, IV infusions, and thermal environment are not interrupted.

The heartbeat should be monitored throughout the procedure with an electronic cardiac monitor and oxygenation monitored with a pulse oximeter.

Increase the inspired oxygen concentration and provide additional supportive care if the baby's condition deteriorates.

Actions	Remarks

Preparing the Baby (continued)

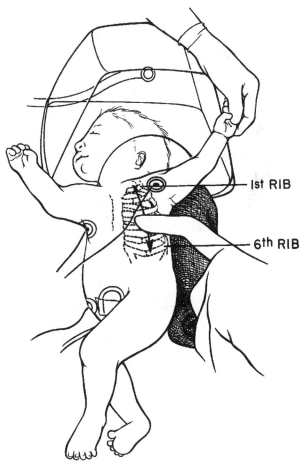

1st RIB

6th RIB

9. Locate the baby's fourth intercostal space and sixth rib at the mid-axillary area.

   This should be well away from the nipple area. Inappropriate placement of chest tubes has been known to interfere with later breast development.

   Note: For illustration purposes, the ribs have been drawn larger than is anatomically correct.

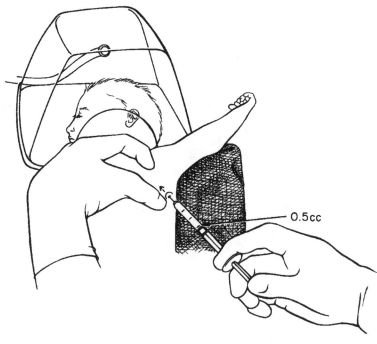

0.5cc

10. Draw up 1% xylocaine into a syringe. Clean the skin with alcohol and then inject the xylocaine to raise a small intradermal "button" over the sixth rib at the mid-axillary point. Infiltrate the xylocaine into the subcutaneous tissue in a track up to the fourth intercostal space.

    To avoid overdose, do not use more than 0.5 mL of 1% xylocaine.

Actions	Remarks

Preparing the Baby (continued)

11. Put on the sterile gloves and mask.

12. Scrub a generous area of skin from below the sixth rib to above the fourth intercostal space with antiseptic solution.

   Allow the povidone-iodine or chlorhexidine to dry, then remove it *completely* from the baby's skin by wiping with alcohol or sterile water swabs. If left in place, either of these antiseptics can cause marked skin irritation.

13. Cover the area around the prepped skin with sterile drapes.

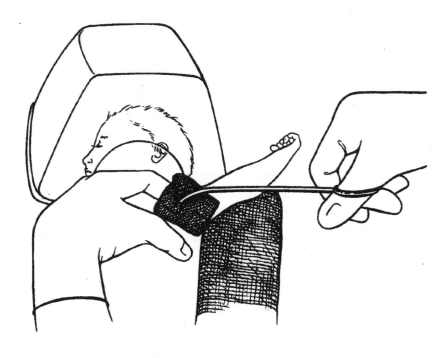

Inserting the Chest Tube

14. Attach the knife blade to the knife handle and make a 3- to 4-mm (1/4 inch) full-thickness skin incision over the xylocaine "button" at the sixth rib.

   The incision in the skin should go completely through the skin but should be no longer than 3 to 4 mm (1/4 inch).

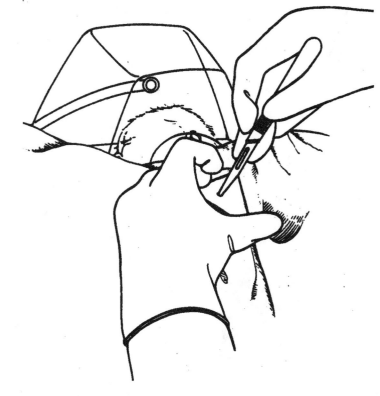

Actions	**Remarks**

Inserting the Chest Tube (continued)

15. Take the chest tube and slide the trocar up and down inside it to be sure it moves freely.

    If the trocar does not slide easily within the chest tube, "rinse" the chest tube with sterile saline.

16. Look at the baby's chest to estimate the length of chest tube to insert. The correct length is from the sixth rib to the fourth intercostal space and then across to the sternum. Note where this length falls in comparison with the black marks on the chest tube.

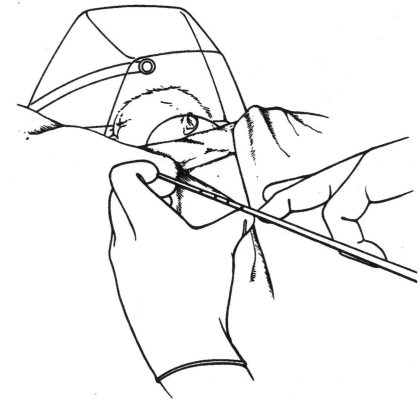

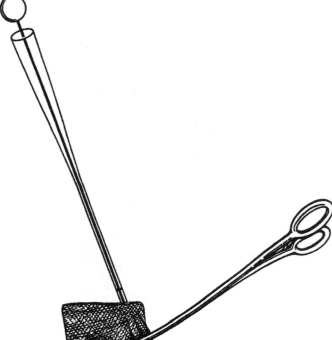

17. Take the chest tube and trocar and measure 2 cm (3/4 inch) (or shorter distance for tiny babies) from the tip of the chest tube.

18. Take a small piece of sterile gauze and wrap it once around the chest tube at this point.

19. Take the Kelly clamp and apply it firmly across the chest tube over the gauze 2 cm (or shorter distance for tiny babies) from the tip of the tube.

Note: After preparing the chest tube in this manner, set it aside (with clamp applied) until you create the skin tunnel (steps 20–24).

Actions   **Remarks**

Inserting the Chest Tube (continued)

20. Take the small curved hemostat and insert the closed tip into the skin incision.

21. By repeatedly spreading and closing the hemostat, create a tunnel from the sixth rib to the fourth intercostal space.

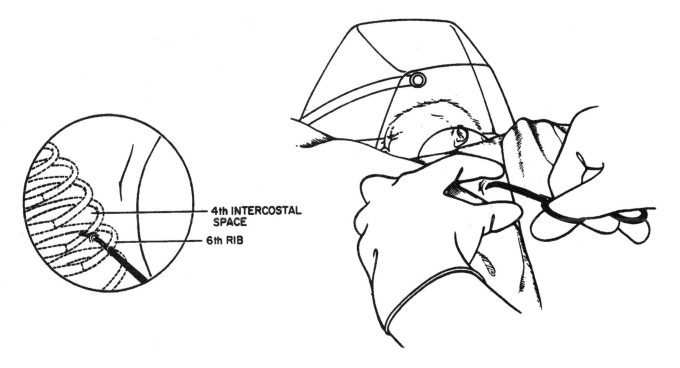

4th INTERCOSTAL SPACE

6th RIB

22. Slide the tip of the hemostat over the top of the fifth rib and into the fourth intercostal space.

Slide the hemostat just over the top of the rib to avoid hitting the intercostal artery that runs along the lower edge of each rib.

23. Now "punch" through the parietal pleura.

    Do not insert the tip of the hemostat any deeper than necessary or you may damage the lung tissue.

The air collection of the pneumothorax provides a small space between the lung tissue and the parietal pleura. This allows you to puncture the parietal pleura without touching the lung, unless you insert the hemostat too far. A rush of air may be heard as you enter the pneumothorax.

24. Remove the hemostat by again repeatedly spreading and closing the tips as you withdraw the hemostat through the tunnel.

Actions   **Remarks**

Inserting the Chest Tube (continued)

25. Place one hand on the baby's chest to steady it. Take the chest tube, with Kelly clamp still applied, in the other hand and hold it firmly, as you would a pencil.

26. Place the tip of trocar and chest tube through the skin incision.

27. "Walk" the tip through the tunnel you previously made with the small hemostat.

    Continue to hold the chest tube perpendicular to the baby's chest. This will cause the skin to "wrinkle" above the chest tube as you walk it through the tunnel.

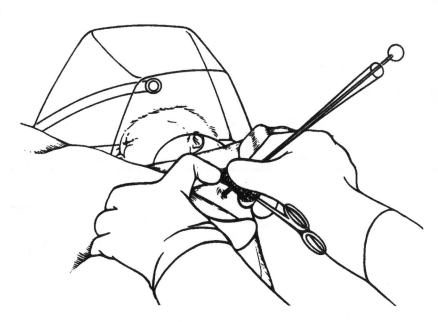

28. When you reach the fourth intercostal space, insert the chest tube until the baby's skin touches the Kelly clamp. You may feel the chest tube "pop" the parietal pleura. The Kelly clamp on the chest tube will prevent the tube and trocar from entering the chest too far.

    You will need to press firmly with the tube to insert it, but never apply insertion pressure higher up on the tube or on the knob of the trocar.

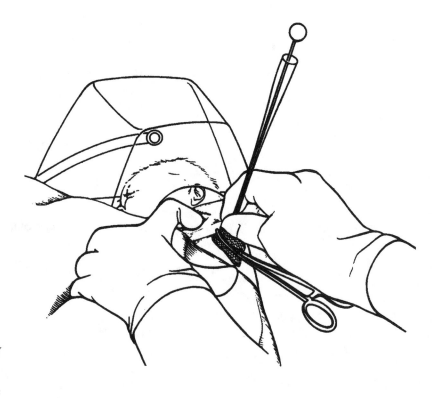

Actions	Remarks

Inserting the Chest Tube (continued)

29. Hold the chest tube in this position as you remove the hemostat and gauze.

30. Hold the tube tip at that level as you swing the tube and trocar downward to an angle that is nearly parallel to the baby's body and pointed toward the baby's opposite shoulder.

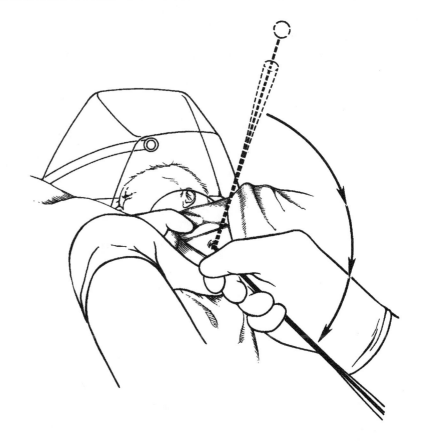

When the tube is in the right position you should feel the tip press firmly against the underside of the fourth rib.

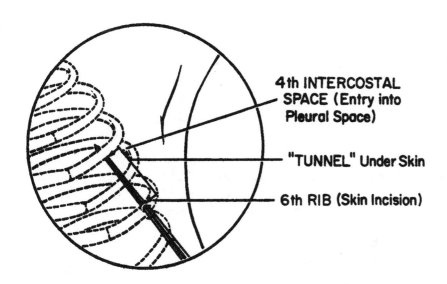

4th INTERCOSTAL SPACE (Entry into Pleural Space)

"TUNNEL" Under Skin

6th RIB (Skin Incision)

Actions   **Remarks**

Inserting the Chest Tube (continued)

31. Hold on to the knob of the trocar and begin to advance the tube as it slips off the trocar.

    Be careful not to advance the trocar.

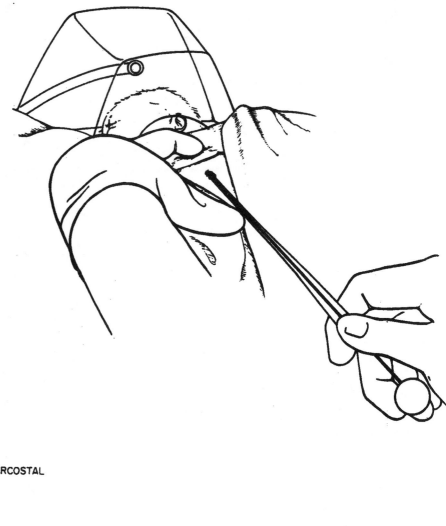

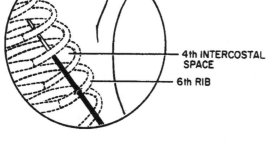

4th INTERCOSTAL SPACE

6th RIB

32. As the tube continues to slip off the trocar, remove the trocar completely.

33. You should see condensation develop within the lumen of the tube and may hear a rush of air.

    You may also see a small amount of straw-colored or blood-tinged fluid in the tube. This is not uncommon in sick babies. More than a small amount of gross blood, however, is abnormal.

34. Advance the tube anteriorly toward the baby's opposite shoulder until you have inserted it the desired length determined earlier. Measure this according to the black marks on the tube.

Actions   **Remarks**

Inserting the Chest Tube (continued)

35. When the tube is inserted the desired distance, have someone promptly connect it to the universal adapter on the patient drainage tubing.

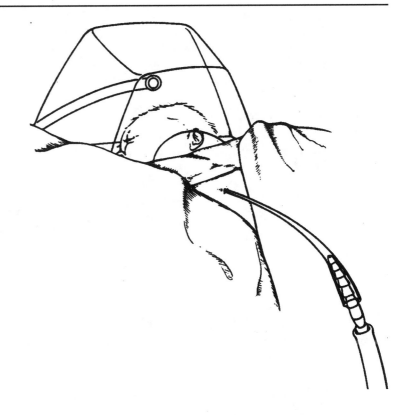

Securing the Chest Tube

36. Be sure there is no tension on the tube while you suture and tape it in place.

Check the location of the black marks frequently to be sure that the tube has not slipped.

37. Place a full-thickness skin suture next to the skin incision. Then take several tight wraps around the tube. Avoid excessive suturing because it doesn't make the tube any more secure and may cause a constriction in the lumen of the tube if the sutures are too tight.

You may use the same suturing technique that is described in securing umbilical catheters (Book II: Neonatal Care, Umbilical Catheters, skill), except that you would delete the purse-string step.

38. Take two 4-inch pieces of 1/2-inch adhesive tape.

39. Split each piece half the length of the tape.

Actions   **Remarks**

Securing the Chest Tube (continued)

40. Take one piece of tape and apply the base and half of the split section to the baby's skin. Wrap the other half of the split section in a spiral around the chest tube.

    Some people prefer to put clear adhesive dressing on the baby's skin, and stick the adhesive tape to that rather than directly to the baby's skin.

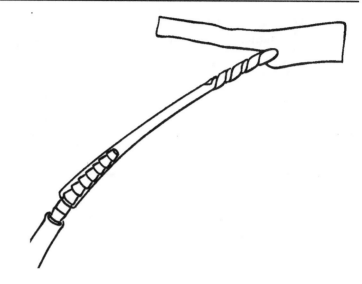

41. Take the other piece of tape and apply it in a similar manner to the chest tube but from a different angle.

    Because the chest tube has been tunneled under the baby's skin, an occlusive dressing is not needed. The skin will close tightly over the chest tube and prevent any air entering the chest cavity from the outside.

    A transparent film adhesive dressing may be placed over the tube and entry site. Large occlusive dressings should be avoided because they can delay recognition of a slipped chest tube.

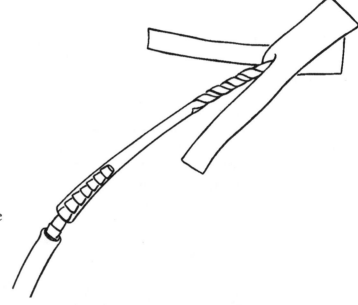

42. As soon as possible, return the baby to a supine position.

    This is to avoid compromise of the baby's "good" lung, which is the one the baby has been lying on during the procedure.

Actions	Remarks

Maintaining Chest Tube Suction

43. Turn on the suction until minimal to moderate bubbling is seen in the suction control chamber.

Rapid, vigorous bubbling should be avoided.

44. Be sure that all connections in the tubing are secure. Tape each connection with a *single* piece of tape wrapped in a spiral fashion (see illustration).

Do *not* over-tape the connections. An unreliable connection will be covered up but not secured by excessive tape.

Some people prefer, therefore, not to tape the connections at all, with the thought that if they come loose, tape may mask the leak.

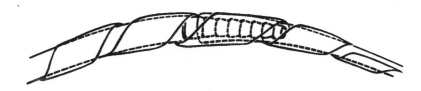

45. Bubbling in the water seal chamber indicates air is being evacuated from the baby's chest or there is a leak in the system.

Check for leaks in the system.

- Disconnect the suction tubing from the suction source.

- Observe the water seal chamber for fluctuations that occur with the baby's respiration.

- If fluctuations occur with respirations, then there are no leaks in the system. Bubbling in the water seal chamber indicates air is being evacuated from the baby's chest.

- If fluctuations do not occur with respiration, there is a leak in the system (check all connections) or the chest tube is blocked.

Actions   **Remarks**

Checking Chest Tube Placement

46. Obtain a chest x-ray anterior-posterior view. Reposition the tube as indicated.

Note: A chest x-ray should include the periphery of the lungs. The illustration may be misleading because the beam is shown as a circle, but really forms a rectangular pattern, and should be wider than shown to include both sides of the chest.

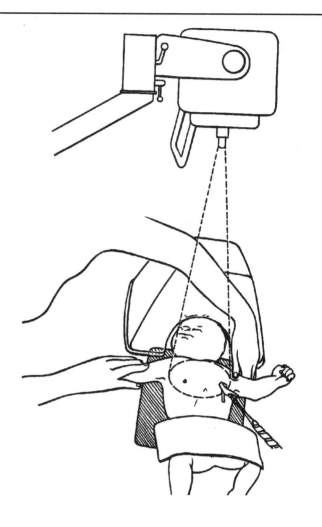

Removing the Chest Tube

47. Periodically change the baby's position to facilitate relocation of any air that might be trapped. This then allows evacuation by the chest tube.

48. A baby with a pneumothorax generally requires a chest tube for several days. During this time make frequent, regular observations of the baby and chest tube system.

Actions	Remarks

Removing the Chest Tube (continued)

49. When bubbling is no longer seen in the water seal chamber, turn the suction off but keep the 3-bottle system intact.

Discontinuing the suction simply converts the system to a 3-bottle water seal system. This allows passive evacuation of air from the chest, rather than active evacuation that occurs when suction is used.

Do *not* clamp the chest tube until it is ready for removal.

If you have been mistaken and the baby still has an active pneumothorax, clamping the chest tube will cause reaccumulation of the pneumothorax and collapse of the lung again. This danger is avoided when the chest tube is kept open to the water seal system for passive evacuation of air.

50. Observe the baby for several hours. Obtain chest x-ray(s), arterial blood gases, and other laboratory tests and procedures as indicated by the baby's condition.

51. If the baby's condition remains stable, obtain another chest x-ray several hours after the suction has been discontinued.

During this time the baby must be watched closely for reaccumulation of the pneumothorax.

52. If there is no evidence of a pneumothorax, clamp the chest tube and get another x-ray 1 to 2 hours later.

53. If there is still no evidence of a pneumothorax, remove the tape, cut the sutures, and slip the chest tube out.

Occasionally, removal of the tube will cause another pneumothorax to appear. Be prepared to transilluminate and perhaps to insert another tube.

54. Dress the wound with a small dressing, if necessary.

If the tube has been in for longer than 24 to 48 hours, a track may have formed. If so, a small Vaseline occlusive dressing may be required to prevent air from entering the chest through the incision.

55. Continue to observe the baby carefully and be alert for the possibility of the development of another pneumothorax.

Unit 4   Umbilical Catheters

Objectives

In this unit you will learn

A. The definition of an umbilical catheter

B. The difference between venous and arterial catheters

C. When and how to use an umbilical *venous* catheter

D. When and how to use an umbilical *arterial* catheter

E. Where to position the tip of either a venous or an arterial umbilical catheter

F. How to maintain umbilical catheters

G. Complications associated with umbilical catheters

Unit 4 Pretest

Before reading the unit, please answer the following questions. Select the **one best** answer to each question (unless otherwise instructed). Record your answers on the answer sheet that is the last page in this book **and** on the test.

1. Below is an illustration of an umbilical cord. What is the structure labeled X?

   A. Umbilical artery
   B. Umbilical vein

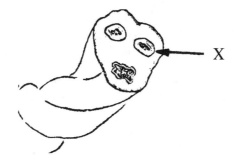

2. If a baby needed emergency medication in the delivery room, you would give the medication through an

   A. Umbilical venous catheter
   B. Umbilical arterial catheter

3. If a baby needed monitoring of blood oxygen, carbon dioxide, and pH, you would obtain blood samples from an

   A. Umbilical venous catheter
   B. Umbilical arterial catheter

4. Which of these dangers are possible with an umbilical venous catheter?

Yes	No	
___	___	Thrombosis
___	___	Blood infection
___	___	Brain damage
___	___	Kidney damage
___	___	Loss of toe from embolus

5. **True   False**   An umbilical *venous* catheter should be left in place until a baby is well.

6. **True   False**   If a constant infusion is to be given through an umbilical *arterial* catheter, an infusion pump must be used.

7. Umbilical *venous* catheters are *most* appropriately used for

   A. Administration of emergency medications
   B. Routine intravenous fluid therapy
   C. Obtaining blood samples for blood gas analyses
   D. Measuring central blood pressure

8. You are inserting an umbilical *arterial* catheter in a baby. The baby's toes on his right foot suddenly turn white. What should be done?

   A. Apply warm compress to the right foot.
   B. Increase the amount of oxygen the baby is receiving.
   C. Remove the catheter.
   D. Observe the baby to see how long the toes stay white.

For each question, please make sure you have marked your answer on the test and on the answer sheet (last page in book). The test is for you; the answer sheet will need to be turned in for continuing education credit.

1. What Is an Umbilical Catheter?

Immediately after birth, or within the next few days, a slender catheter may be inserted into an umbilical artery or the umbilical vein of a newborn. Typically there are 2 umbilical arteries and 1 vein.

An umbilical catheter should have a rounded tip with a single hole in the center. This is to avoid formation of tiny clots that are associated with catheters that have multiple side holes.

A catheter should also be radiopaque (visible on x-ray). This is needed to determine the exact position of the catheter after it has been inserted.

A baby's umbilical cord looks like this.

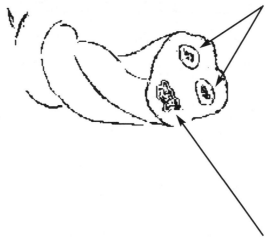

Umbilical arteries have relatively thick, muscular walls with pinpoint-sized lumens. In an umbilical cord cut close to the stump, they can generally be found toward the baby's feet. The presence of only one artery is uncommon. A single artery is sometimes (not always) associated with certain anomalies, particularly renal malformations.

Umbilical vein is a relatively thin-walled vessel, larger than an artery, and usually located toward the baby's head.

2. Where Should the Tip of an Umbilical Catheter Be Positioned?

Umbilical venous catheter (UVC) is inserted into the umbilical vein and then advanced into the inferior vena cava. We recommend that the catheter tip be located at or just above the level of the diaphragm.

Umbilical arterial catheter (UAC) is inserted into either 1 of the 2 umbilical arteries and then advanced into the abdominal aorta. We recommend that the catheter tip be located at a level between the third and fourth lumbar vertebrae. This location can be expected to be below the point where the renal arteries branch from the aorta.

Note: Some experts prefer to locate the tip of a UAC at a level between the sixth and ninth thoracic vertebrae (T6-9), rather than between the third and fourth lumbar vertebrae (L3-4). Locating the tip in the region between these 2 levels (L3-4 and T6-9) should be avoided because this would place the tip at the level of the main arteries feeding vital abdominal organs.

3. When Is an Umbilical Catheter Used?

A. Umbilical Venous Catheter

- Emergency administration of medication
- Exchange transfusions
- Emergency estimation of PCO_2 and pH (not PO_2)
- Fluid administration during the first few days in extremely preterm babies

Venous catheters are generally not used for routine fluids, unless another intravenous (IV) route is not available. If a peripheral IV (PIV) is not available, however, many experts feel it is preferable to give fluids and medications through a UVC positioned above the liver (tip located at or just above the level of the diaphragm), rather than through a UAC.

B. Umbilical Arterial Catheter
- Drawing blood for blood gas analyses (the most common use for UAC)
- Obtaining central arterial blood pressure measurements

Infusion of blood, medications, or maintenance fluid solutions through an arterial catheter is controversial. Insertion of an arterial catheter *solely* for infusion of routine IV fluids is not recommended. However, if a UAC is in place for the purpose of arterial blood sampling and/or central blood pressure monitoring, and another IV route is not available, routine IV fluids may be administered through a UAC.

Table 4.1. Uses for Umbilical Catheters

Catheter Location		
Use	Venous (UVC)	Arterial (UAC)
1. Emergency medications or blood	Yes, especially soon after birth	Not recommended
2. Exchange transfusions	Yes	Not recommended **Note:** UAC may be used to *withdraw* blood with continuous technique, when a UVC or PIV is used to infuse blood.
3. Central blood pressure measurements	Not applicable	Yes
4. Blood gas sampling • Emergency pH and PCO_2 estimation	Yes, especially soon after delivery	Not practical
• Routine PaO_2, $PaCO_2$, pH	Not applicable	Yes, especially if supplemental oxygen is needed for a prolonged period
5. Routine fluids • Extremely preterm babies	Yes, especially during first few days after birth	Not recommended, unless UAC needed for arterial blood gases and/or central blood pressure, and a PIV is not available
• Other babies	Not recommended, unless a PIV is not available	

Note: See Book II: Neonatal Care, Intravenous Therapy.

Now answer these questions to test yourself on the information in the last section.

A1. Label the 3 blood vessels in the diagram below.

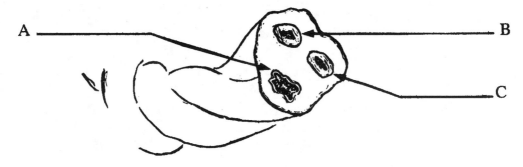

A2. Which of these features should an umbilical catheter have?

Yes	No	
___	___	Radiopaque
___	___	Beveled tip
___	___	Rounded tip
___	___	Single hole in tip center
___	___	Multiple tiny side holes near catheter tip

A3. Name at least 2 uses of umbilical *venous* catheters.

_____

_____

A4. What are 2 uses that are *not* recommended for umbilical arterial catheters?

_____

_____

A5. What is the most common use of an umbilical *arterial* catheter?

_____

A6. What is the recommended location for the tip of an umbilical

Arterial catheter: _____

Venous catheter: _____

Check your answers with the list that follows the Recommended Routines. Correct any incorrect answers and review the appropriate section in the unit.

4. How Should Umbilical Catheters Be Maintained?

A. Umbilical Venous Catheter

A UVC may be required for medication administration during a delivery room resuscitation or for an exchange transfusion. Occasionally, a UVC may be placed for a longer period of use, such as when another exchange transfusion is anticipated within a few hours or another route for administration of fluids is impractical. In such cases, one of the following procedures should be used to ensure that the catheter does not become clotted.

1. Heparin Lock

   - **Heparin concentration:** Large doses of heparin or an excessive number of flushes can result in systemic blood clotting problems in newborns, particularly very small babies. The dosage of heparin that is hazardous is not well defined, but 1 to 2 units of heparin per milliliter of fluid is considered safe, if amounts and frequency of flushes are kept to a minimum.

   - **Flush volume:** Depending on catheter size, 0.5 to 1.0 mL of 1 to 2 U/mL heparin solution is flushed through the UVC and the stopcock is turned off to the catheter. After a blood sample is drawn or any other solution is given through the catheter, the catheter should be flushed again with the heparin-containing solution.

   - **Record fluid given:** Care must be taken to avoid using more flush solution than necessary or the baby may receive too much heparin or too much IV fluid. Each time the catheter is flushed, record the amount of flush solution used on the baby's "intake" record.

2. Continuous Infusion

   - **Infusion *not* containing heparin:** Intravenous fluid (see Book II: Neonatal Care, Intravenous Therapy) without heparin may be infused through a UVC. An infusion pump is used to ensure a constant, correct volume infused and to prevent back up of blood into the catheter.

     After any blood sample is withdrawn, the catheter is flushed with 0.5 to 1.0 mL of either the IV fluid or the 1 to 2 U/mL heparin solution, and then reconnected to the constant infusion. Be sure to record the amount of flush solution used.

   - **Infusion containing heparin:** Heparin may also be added to a continuous infusion solution, but in a concentration lower than that used for a heparin lock. For a continuous infusion, a heparin concentration of 0.5 to 1.0 U/mL of solution is used.

B. Umbilical Arterial Catheter

If a UAC is to be left in place to obtain frequent arterial blood samples for blood gas analyses, either one of the techniques described previously for UVCs may be used to keep a UAC open.

Note: Some experts believe only a continuous infusion, *not* a heparin lock, should be used with a UAC.

If the continuous infusion method is used for a UAC, because of the higher arterial pressure, an infusion pump must be used or blood will back up into the catheter.

C. Either Type of Catheter (UVC or UAC)

- *Air Bubbles*

    Care must be taken to remove all air bubbles from infusion tubing and/or umbilical catheter. If present in an IV line or catheter, air bubbles will enter the bloodstream and can cause severe tissue damage. This can be a particularly severe complication of a UAC.

- *Clotted Catheter*

    You should always be able to get an *instantaneous* blood return from a UAC or UVC. If blood does not return easily, do not push fluid into the catheter. There may be a clot in the catheter, or the catheter tip may be wedged against the side of the vessel.

    After the sterile field used during catheter insertion has been removed, do not advance the catheter farther because that would be putting an unsterile section of the catheter into the umbilical cord. You may withdraw the catheter about 1 cm and try again. If blood still does not return, remove or replace the catheter.

- *Disconnected Catheter*

    If either type of catheter becomes disconnected or gets pulled out, massive blood loss can occur within a few seconds (particularly true of UAC). Catheter connections must be secure. Use Luer-lok connectors, or another system for locking stopcock, tubing, and catheter connections.

    If blood loss occurs, immediately take the baby's blood pressure. If necessary, give an appropriate volume of normal saline, until compatible blood can be obtained (Book II: Neonatal Care, Blood Pressure).

- *Excess Fluid*

    The volume and type of all constant infusion and flush solutions should be recorded so that the amount of fluid a baby receives will be known. The following volumes of flush solution are all that is needed to flush catheters of different sizes completely:

Catheter Size	Flush Volume
3 1/2F	0.4 mL
5F	0.6 mL
8F	1.0 mL

- *Rapid Fluid Infusion*

    Relatively large amounts of fluid can be infused quickly through a UVC or UAC. This should be avoided. Rapid infusions of fluid can cause sudden, dangerous shifts in blood pressure and temporarily alter normal blood flow. All infusions and flush solutions through umbilical catheters should be given slowly and steadily, generally at a rate no faster than 1 to 2 mL/kg/minute.

In summary

- *Remove all air bubbles from infusion tubing and umbilical catheter.*
- *Never push fluid into a catheter that does not have an immediate blood return.*
- *Never advance a catheter when it is no longer sterile.*
- *Use Luer-lok or other system of locking connectors.*
- *Record the volume of all flush solutions given.*
- *Give infusions and flush solutions through a UVC or UAC slowly and steadily. A rate no faster than 1 to 2 mL/kg/minute is recommended.*

5. What Complications Are Associated With Umbilical Catheters?

Umbilical arterial and venous catheters are extremely valuable tools, often required for the care of sick babies. As with any medical treatment, complications are possible. With care, these complications can almost always be avoided.

A. Flow Pathways Determine Many Possible Complications

1. *Umbilical Venous Catheter:* Solutions infused through catheters placed at or just above the level of the diaphragm flow into the inferior vena cava. Solutions infused through a UVC placed below the level of the diaphragm flow through the venous circulation of the liver. Alternatively, when a UVC tip is too high above the level of the diaphragm, infusions flow directly into the heart or into veins that enter the heart.

2. *Umbilical Arterial Catheter:* Solutions infused through catheters placed at a level between the third and fourth lumbar vertebrae flow to the legs. Solutions infused through a UAC placed above the third lumbar vertebra may flow to the liver, spleen, pancreas, kidneys, intestines, spinal cord, and legs.

B. Possible Complications

1. *Umbilical Venous Catheter*

   - **Blood loss** from loose connections between the catheter and stopcock, etc.
   - **Liver damage** from infusion of hypertonic solution into the venous circulation of the liver.
   - **Perforation of the vein** if a catheter is inserted too vigorously.
   - **Thromboses (clots)** may occur when blood backs up into the catheter. The clot that forms may then extend beyond the tip and into the vessel. Thromboses are more likely to occur when catheters with side holes, instead of a single hole in the center of a rounded tip, are used.
   - **Sepsis** (blood infection).
   - **Air embolus** can occur with accidental infusion of air bubbles with fluid or medication. Air embolus also may be formed by air drawn into the circulatory system, if a baby inhales when a UVC is accidentally opened to the atmosphere.

191

2. *Umbilical Arterial Catheter*
- *Massive* **blood loss** from a loose connection between catheter and stopcock.
- **Blocked blood flow** during or following catheter insertion, as shown by blanching of a leg (turning white). The catheter must be immediately withdrawn to prevent permanent damage.
- **Thrombi or emboli,** which may form from small blood clots on the catheter tip that may break off to embolize to one of the legs or vital organs located downstream from the catheter tip. Air bubbles pushed through the catheter will also form emboli.

  An embolus to a leg will cause one or more toes or the foot on the affected side to become cyanotic or blanched (white). Permanent damage may occur. Emboli to one of the abdominal organs will not cause visible changes but can cause permanent damage, often to the kidneys or intestines. Great care must therefore be taken with all infusions through a UAC.
- **Sepsis**
- **Hypoglycemia** can occur with catheters located above the third lumbar vertebra, near the tenth thoracic vertebra, and used for continuous infusion. The pancreas may respond to the glucose concentration in an IV fluid, rather than the baby's true blood glucose, and produce additional amounts of insulin. This increased insulin results in hypoglycemia.

6. How Long Can Umbilical Catheters Be Left in Place?

While extremely valuable, UVCs and UACs are associated with possible complications and, therefore, should be removed as soon as possible.

A. Umbilical Venous Catheter

UVC should be removed as soon as the emergency is over, exchange transfusion is completed, or another route of IV therapy is established.

B. Umbilical Arterial Catheter

UAC should be removed as soon as frequent sampling of arterial blood gases or central arterial blood pressure monitoring is no longer required.

Because the risks associated with umbilical catheters are greater than those associated with PIVs, umbilical catheters should not be used as merely convenient routes for long-term fluid administration. Whenever possible, routine fluids should be infused through PIVs or, in babies requiring long-term venous access, through central venous catheters. These catheters are placed percutaneously or surgically, and are not discussed here.

Now answer these questions to test yourself on the information in the last section.

B1. Identify the following complications as being associated with an umbilical venous catheter (UVC) or an umbilical arterial catheter (UAC), or both.

UVC UAC

___	___	Blood loss from loose connections
___	___	Liver damage from infusion of hypertonic solutions
___	___	Sepsis
___	___	Blanching of a leg
___	___	Thrombosis

B2. **True False**   It is generally recommended to leave an umbilical catheter in place once it has been inserted, because it may be needed for long-term fluid therapy.

B3. What are 2 methods for maintaining an umbilical catheter?

_____

_____

B4. What equipment is required for continuous infusion through an umbilical *arterial* catheter?

_____

B5. Medications, flush solutions, and all infusions through an umbilical venous or arterial catheter should be given

A. As quickly as possible

B. Slowly and steadily

B6. A 1,600-g preterm baby will require intravenous fluids for several days. What is the best route to use for this baby?

_____

Check your answers with the list that follows the Recommended Routines. Correct any incorrect answers and review the appropriate section in the unit.

Recommended Routines

All of the routines listed below are based on the principles of perinatal care presented in the unit you have just finished. They are recommended as part of routine perinatal care.

Read each routine carefully and decide whether it is standard operating procedure in your hospital. Check the appropriate blank next to each routine.

Procedure Standard in My Hospital	Needs Discussion by Our Staff	
_____	_____	1. Establish a policy to ensure the presence of a sterile umbilical catheter tray in each delivery room and in the nursery at all times.
_____	_____	2. Establish a policy of inserting an umbilical venous catheter during delivery room resuscitation when emergency medications are required.
_____	_____	3. Establish a routine to consider insertion of an umbilical arterial catheter in any newborn anticipated to require significant amounts of supplemental oxygen for longer than a short period.

These are the answers to the self-test questions. Please check them with the answers you gave and review the information in the unit wherever necessary.

A1. A. Umbilical vein
     B. Umbilical artery
     C. Umbilical artery

A2. Yes No
     _x_ ___ Radiopaque
     ___ _x_ Beveled tip
     _x_ ___ Rounded tip
     _x_ ___ Single hole in tip center
     ___ _x_ Multiple tiny side holes near catheter tip

A3. Any 2 of the following:
     • Administration of emergency medications, especially in the delivery room
     • Exchange transfusions
     • Emergency estimation of PCO_2 and pH (not PO_2)
     • Fluid administration during the first few days in extremely preterm babies

A4. 1. Not used for exchange transfusions (unless an umbilical arterial catheter used for withdrawal of blood with an umbilical venous catheter, or peripheral intravenous line used for infusion)
     2. Not used for medications or fluids, unless an umbilical arterial catheter is already in place (for blood gas sampling and/or central blood pressure monitoring) and another intravenous route is not available.

A5. Drawing blood for arterial blood gas tests

A6. Umbilical *arterial* catheters: at a level between the third and fourth lumbar vertebrae (some experts prefer T6-9)
     Umbilical *venous* catheters: at or just above the level of the diaphragm

B1. UVC UAC
     _x_ _x_ Blood loss from loose connections
     _x_ ___ Liver damage from infusion of hypertonic solutions
     _x_ _x_ Sepsis
     ___ _x_ Blanching of a leg
     _x_ _x_ Thrombosis

B3. False Except in special circumstances, routine fluid administration through either an umbilical arterial catheter or umbilical venous catheter should be avoided.

B3. 1. Heparin lock
     2. Continuous infusion

B4. An infusion pump

B5. B. Slowly and steadily

B6. Peripheral intravenous line

Unit 4 Posttest

Without referring back to the information in the unit, please answer the following questions. Select the **one best** answer to each question (unless otherwise instructed). Record your answers on the answer sheet that is the last page in this book *and* on the test.

1. Below is an illustration of an umbilical cord. What is the structure labeled "X"?
    A. Umbilical artery
    B. Umbilical vein

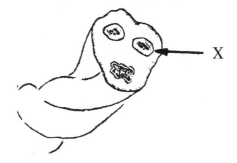

2. A baby needs emergency medications at delivery. You would give the medications through an
    A. Umbilical venous catheter
    B. Umbilical arterial catheter

3. The main purpose of an umbilical *arterial* catheter is for
    A. Exchange transfusions
    B. Arterial blood gases
    C. Giving medications
    D. Administering fluids

4. You are inserting an umbilical arterial catheter. The baby's leg turns white. What should you do?
    A. Apply steady pressure to the catheter for 30 seconds.
    B. Infuse fluid slowly until leg color improves.
    C. Give additional oxygen.
    D. Remove the catheter.

5. **True   False**   If blood cannot be withdrawn from an umbilical arterial catheter, the catheter should be advanced slightly and intravenous fluid gently pushed through the catheter.

6. **True   False**   If fluid is not being infused through an umbilical catheter, the catheter may be filled with a heparinized solution and turned off.

7. **True   False**   The main danger of a disconnected umbilical catheter is that infection may be introduced.

8. Which of these dangers are possible with an umbilical *arterial* catheter?

    Yes   No
    ___ ___   Thrombosis
    ___ ___   Sepsis
    ___ ___   Brain damage
    ___ ___   Kidney damage
    ___ ___   Loss of toe from embolus

For each question, please make sure you have marked your answer on the test and on the answer sheet (last page in book). The test is for you; the answer sheet will need to be turned in for continuing education credit.

Inserting and Managing Umbilical Catheters

This skill unit will teach you how to insert umbilical arterial and venous catheters. Not everyone will actually be required to learn and practice umbilical catheterization. However, everyone should read this unit and attend a skill session to learn the equipment and sequence of steps to assist effectively with umbilical catheterization.

The staff members who will be asked to master all aspects of this skill will need to demonstrate correctly each of the following steps:

1. Restrain and measure "baby" for catheter insertion.

2. Collect the equipment and prepare the "sterile" tray.

3. Prepare catheter, stopcock, and heparin solution.

4. Cleanse the umbilical cord and surrounding skin, loosely tie umbilical tape around stump.

5. Cut cord to appropriate length.

6. Identify umbilical vessels.

7. Dilate umbilical artery and insert catheter (you may also be asked to demonstrate venous catheterization).

8. Check blood return and flush catheter with heparinized solution, turn stopcock off to the catheter.

9. Suture catheter in place (or temporarily tape in place until location is confirmed by x-ray).

10. Tape catheter in place after x-ray taken, catheter location confirmed, and catheter sutured in place.

11. Begin infusion or maintain catheter with heparin lock.

12. Use sterile technique and standard precautions throughout the procedure.

13. Illustrate the techniques to stop bleeding from an umbilical artery and from the umbilical vein.

The staff members who will be asked to master the assistant components of this skill will need to demonstrate correctly each of the following steps:

1. Restrain "baby" for catheter insertion.

2. Collect the equipment and prepare the "sterile" tray.

3. Hold the distal section of cord in an elevated position until it is cut off.

4. Hold instruments to stabilize the umbilical cord and/or expose the artery or vein for catheterization, as needed by the person inserting the catheter.

5. Tape catheter temporarily until placement is confirmed by x-ray (unless catheter was initially sutured in place).

6. Tape catheter in place after x-ray taken, catheter location confirmed, and catheter sutured in place.

7. Begin infusion or maintain catheter with heparin lock.

8. Use sterile technique and standard precautions.

9. Illustrate the techniques to stop bleeding from an umbilical artery and from the umbilical vein.

In addition to the practice session(s) scheduled by your coordinators, a special joint physician-nurse practice session may be arranged for nurses and perinatal care physicians in your hospital.

Note: The graphs that accompany Steps 9 and 27 in this skill unit are adapted with permission from Klaus MH, Fanaroff AA. *Care of the High-Risk Neonate*. Philadelphia, PA: WB Saunders Co.; 2001.

Inserting and Managing Umbilical Catheter

Note: The information presented in this skill unit pertains to the insertion of umbilical arterial catheters (UACs), as well as to umbilical venous catheters (UVCs) to be used for exchange transfusions.

Umbilical venous catheters, needed in the delivery room for administration of emergency medications, may be inserted with minimal preparation by one member of the resuscitation team.

Actions	Remarks

Preparing the Equipment and Baby

1. With patience and careful preparation, the insertion of an umbilical catheter can be accomplished quite easily. Failure occurs most often when there is inadequate preparation or the operators are trying to rush.

   Two people, working together, make the job of inserting an umbilical catheter much easier, particularly an arterial catheter. The procedure will generally take about 30 minutes.

2. During insertion of an umbilical catheter, a baby must be maintained in a properly heated, oxygenated environment. The baby should also be attached to a cardiac monitor.

   Temperature control can best be maintained during catheterization if the baby is under a radiant warmer.

3. Restrain the baby gently but firmly. Restraint is necessary because any movement by a baby will interfere with the procedure, and lengthen the time needed to accomplish catheterization.

   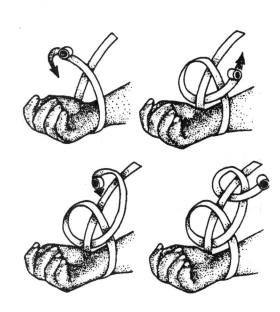

   Double half-hitch knots (shown right), tied with gauze bandage around the baby's arms and legs and taped to the edges of the bed, work well. This knot will secure a baby's hand or foot but will not tighten further or constrict blood supply to the extremity.

   Prefabricated restraints, typically with Velcro closure, may also be used.

   After the procedure, and an x-ray taken to confirm location of the catheter tip, return the baby to a more comfortable position.

Actions   **Remarks**

Preparing the Equipment and Baby (continued)

4. When the restraints have been tied and taped in place, the baby should be in a "spread eagle" position.

   Even the tiniest babies generally need some form of restraint.

   To accomplish umbilical catheterization quickly and easily there must be

   • Excellent view of and access to the umbilicus

   • Good lighting

   • No risk of interference by movement of the baby during isolation of an umbilical vessel and delicate insertion of a catheter

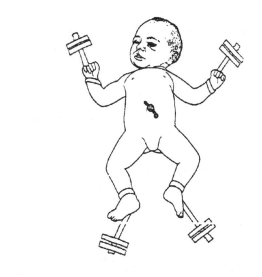

5. Certain instruments are especially helpful for umbilical catheterization. These are

   • One or 2 pairs of curved iris forceps

   • A pair of straight iris forceps

Note: Forceps used should have smooth or serrated tips to grip the vessel firmly, but *not* toothed tips. Toothed tips will shred the edges of a vessel.

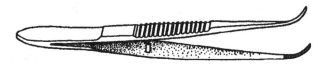

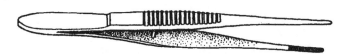

Curved and Straight Iris Forceps
(shown actual size)

6. Other instruments for umbilical catheterization include

   • 1 pair iris scissors
   • 1 pair surgical scissors
   • 1 needle holder
   • 2 curved mosquito clamps
   • 2 straight mosquito clamps
   • 1 knife handle and blade
   • 2-0 silk suture
   • Umbilical tape
   • 3-way Luer-lok (or similar) stopcock

7. The catheter should be sterile and radiopaque.

   Size of the catheter used depends on the size of the baby and the purpose of the catheter.

Actions   **Remarks**

Preparing the Equipment and Baby (continued)

Catheter Size for UAC

- 3 1/2F for tiny babies (<1,000 g)
- 5F for all other babies

Catheter Size for UVC

- 5F for all size babies when UVC used **for** emergency medications
- 5F for exchange transfusion for small babies
- 8F for exchange transfusions for large babies

Determining Catheter Insertion Distance

8. Using a tape measure marked in centimeters, measure from the shoulder to a point equal to the level of the umbilicus (shown by dashed line).

   Do *not* measure from the shoulder on a diagonal to the umbilicus (not shown, but a common mistake).

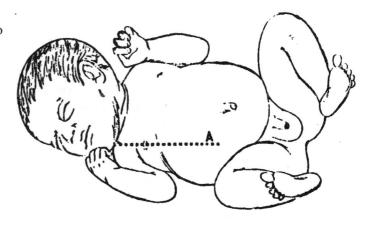

To determine shoulder-umbilicus length, measure along line A.

9. This measurement, when plotted on the graph opposite, will indicate the proper distance to insert a catheter.

   - **Dashed** line is for **venous** catheters.
   - **Solid** line is for **arterial** catheters.

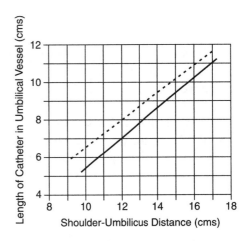

- - - - - - umbilical vein to junction of inferior vena cava and right atrium

———— umbilical artery to bifurcation of aorta

Actions	Remarks

Determining Catheter Insertion Distance (continued)

Example: A baby's shoulder-umbilicus distance is 13 cm.

Step 1. Find this shoulder-umbilicus distance on the horizontal scale (marked with vertical arrow).

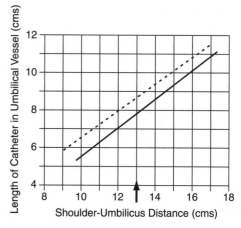

- - - - - - umbilical vein to junction of inferior vena cava and right atrium

———— umbilical artery to bifurcation of aorta

Step 2. Find where this distance intersects each of the black lines on the graph.

Step 3. Read where this point falls on the chart's vertical scale.

For the sample baby, this point is at 8 cm for an arterial catheter.

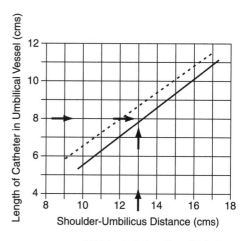

- - - - - - umbilical vein to junction of inferior vena cava and right atrium

———— umbilical artery to bifurcation of aorta

10. It generally is recommended to insert a catheter approximately 2 cm farther than is indicated by the vertical scale.

For the sample baby, with a shoulder-umbilicus distance of 13 cm, the arterial catheter should be inserted 10 cm (8 cm from the chart, plus 2 cm).

An x-ray should be obtained to confirm catheter position. The extra 2 cm will allow the catheter to be *withdrawn* slightly, if repositioning is needed.

A catheter should *never* be inserted farther after sterile drapes have been removed or the exposed part of the catheter has been contaminated. If a catheter was not inserted a sufficient length, and drapes have been removed or the catheter contaminated, the catheter should be removed and a new catheter inserted under sterile conditions.

If a catheter must be repositioned, a repeat x-ray should be obtained to confirm correct position of the catheter.

Actions	**Remarks**

Preparing a Catheter

11. The first operator should put on a cap and mask, scrub, and put on sterile gown and gloves.

12. Check the heparin solution.

A solution of 1 to 2 units heparin per 1 mL of fluid is an appropriate concentration during catheter insertion, or if the catheter is maintained as a heparin lock.

A lower concentration of heparin (0.5–1.0 U/mL) is recommended if a slow continuous infusion will be given through the catheter, such as when it is used for central blood pressure monitoring.

13. Prepare the catheter, using sterile technique.

    • Connect the catheter to a 3-way stopcock, which has been connected to a syringe containing heparinized solution.

    • Fill the catheter, and the stopcock, with the heparinized solution.

    • Turn the stopcock *off* to the catheter.

Different stopcocks indicate the "off" direction in different ways.

You must be thoroughly familiar with the type of stopcock used in your hospital.

To avoid possible confusion, it is recommended that only one type of stopcock be used in all newborn care areas in your hospital.

14. Umbilical catheters are marked in various ways, depending on the manufacturer.

    Be sure to note the number and spacing of marks before inserting a catheter. Use these marks to help determine when the catheter has been inserted the appropriate distance.

    For the sample baby, the catheter should be inserted approximately 10 cm.

Actions	**Remarks**

Preparing the Umbilical Cord

15. Clean the baby's umbilical cord, stump, and surrounding skin using a surgical prep solution, such as povidone-iodine or chlorhexidine.

    The second operator should hold up the umbilical cord by the cord clamp.

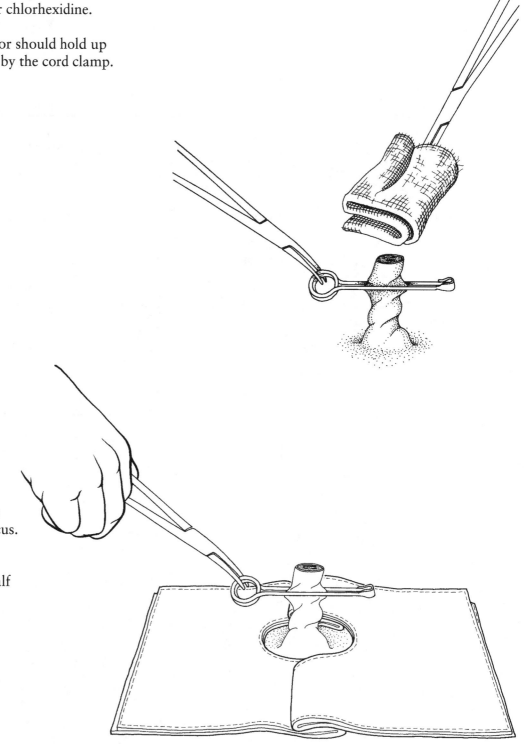

16. Place sterile drapes around the umbilicus.

    Two circumcision drapes folded in half work well for this.

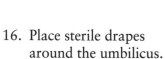

Actions   **Remarks**

Preparing an Umbilical Cord (continued)

17. Loosely tie umbilical tape around the base
of the umbilicus. The umbilical tape should
not be knotted. Rather, it should be wrapped
just once on itself (see illustration).

   This is done so the umbilical tape can be pulled
tight very quickly, in the event that one of the
vessels bleeds when the cord is cut below the
umbilical clamp.

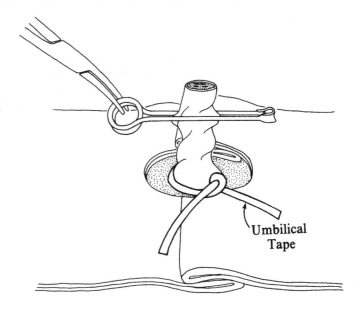

18. While the second operator continues to hold up
the baby's umbilical cord, cut the cord as evenly
as possible with a knife blade. To do this, press
the knife blade firmly against the side of the
cord and use just 1 or 2 passes of the knife
blade to cut cleanly across the cord. A stump of
approximately 1.5 cm should be left.

   To avoid contamination of the sterile
instruments and drapes, discard the cord
remnant and clamp clear of the sterile field.

Avoid multiple back-and-forth sawing motions with
the knife blade because these will lead to a ragged
cord stump. If the stump is ragged, it will be more
difficult to identify the vessels.

Cutting across the cord with scissors is also not
recommended because doing so can crush the
vessels.

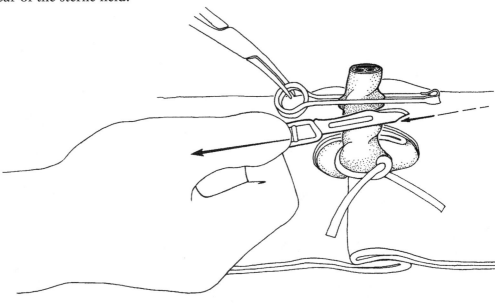

Actions	**Remarks**

Preparing an Umbilical Cord (continued)

19. Now identify the umbilical vessels.

    There should be one vein, usually located toward the baby's head, and 2 arteries, usually located toward the baby's feet.

The vein is thin-walled and larger than the arteries. The arteries are thick-walled and the lumen is pin size.

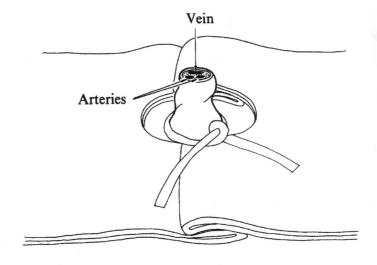

20. If you cannot determine the vessels by visual inspection, rub the flat side of an instrument gently across the top of the cord stump.

The resistance offered by the muscular tips of the arteries can be felt. The vein cannot be felt in this manner.

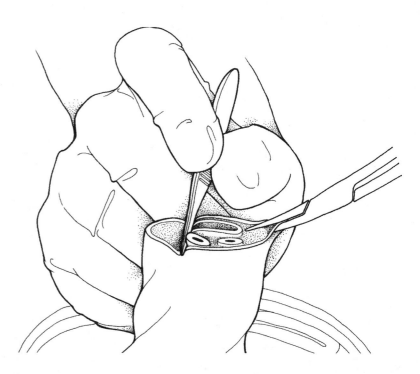

Actions	Remarks

Inserting an Umbilical Catheter

21. The second operator now puts on a cap and mask, scrubs, and puts on a sterile gown and gloves.

    The second operator then holds the edges of the cord stump with the mosquito clamps.

    Note: **Information about umbilical *venous* catheterization is given on the last few pages of this skill unit.**

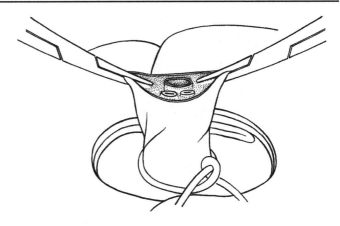

22. Select one artery for catheterization. The first operator should pick up the edge of the selected artery with the straight iris forceps.

    Note: Illustration shows one forceps tip inside the artery and the other on the outside of the umbilical cord. This is recommended for UVC placement (see description later in this skill unit), but is seldom used with UAC placement. Typically, only the artery is grasped with forceps for UAC insertion.

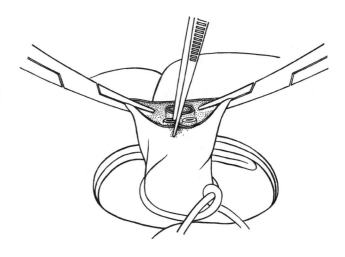

23. The first operator then inserts one tip of the curved iris forceps into the lumen of the artery.

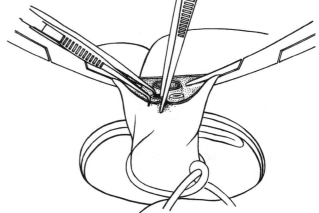

Actions	**Remarks**

Inserting an Arterial Catheter

24. Repeat step 23 several times. When the vessel has begun to dilate, insert both tips of the curved iris forceps.

    Insert only the tips of the forceps. Do *not* attempt to probe deeply into the artery.

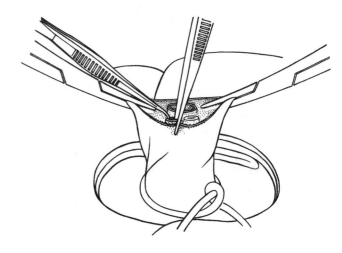

25. Repeat step 24 several times, *slowly and patiently*, to dilate the entrance to the artery. Each time spread the forceps a bit wider inside the artery, and hold the forceps open while sliding them out of the artery.

    Use the instruments firmly but gently. *Never tug on the vessels*, but once you have the proper grip on an artery, hold it tightly.

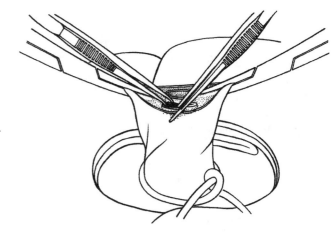

26. Now, with one iris forceps holding one edge of the artery and the curved iris forceps dilating the inside of the artery, the second operator should lay down one of the mosquito clamps holding the edge of the cord and use that hand to insert the catheter (using either your gloved fingers as shown, or with a pair of forceps).

    Grip the catheter near the tip. If held too far from the tip, the catheter will buckle and not enter the artery easily.

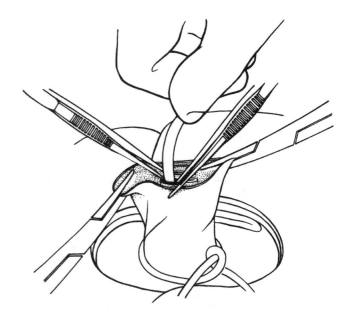

Actions	Remarks

Inserting an Arterial Catheter (continued)

27. The umbilical arteries curve toward the feet before curving upward toward the head. Therefore, it may be helpful to aim the tip slightly toward the baby's feet when first inserting a catheter.

28. After 2 or 3 cm of the catheter have passed into the vessel, the curved iris forceps may be removed from the opening of the artery. Continue to grip the edge of the artery with the other iris forceps and the edge of the cord with the mosquito clamps.

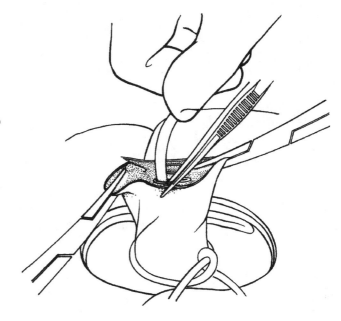

29. Keep a *constant grip* on the catheter (with an instrument or your fingers) and continue to insert the catheter.

   Be sure the cord stump is not pulled toward either the left or right side of the baby because that may make it more difficult to insert the catheter.

   • *UVC insertion,* however, is sometimes helped by pulling the cord stump slightly toward the baby's feet.

   • *UAC insertion* is sometimes aided by pulling the stump slightly toward the baby's head.

30. As you insert the catheter, resistance may be met at 2 points.

   • At the level of the abdominal wall, after the catheter has been inserted approximately 2 cm

   • At the level of the bladder after the catheter has been inserted approximately 5 to 7 cm

Never let go of the catheter until you have inserted it as far as you want to.

Once the catheter has been inserted the desired distance, it will stay there while it is being sutured and taped in place. However, if you let go of it after it has been inserted only a few centimeters, the pressure of the muscular artery may push the catheter out, forcing you to locate the artery once more, dilate it, and reinsert the catheter.

Actions	Remarks

Inserting an Arterial Catheter (continued)

31. If resistance does occur, apply only gentle, steady pressure to the catheter. With gentle, steady pressure, the artery will often relax enough to allow passage of the catheter.

    Do not probe, pry, or repeatedly or forcefully push with the catheter.

If gentle, steady pressure on the catheter does not work, you may do 2 things.

- Remove the catheter and try a smaller size (3.5F is the smallest size).

- Attempt catheterization of the other artery.

Avoid repeated unsuccessful attempts at catheterization. Seek another skilled person to insert the catheter, or plan to use a peripheral arterial puncture to determine blood gases.

32. Insert the catheter the predetermined distance.

Use the marks on the catheter to estimate the proper distance.

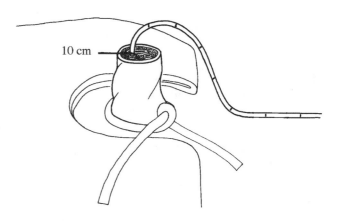

For the sample baby, it was determined that the catheter should be inserted 10 cm. The type of catheter illustrated has black marks spaced every centimeter from the tip.

33. Turn the stopcock so that it is open between the catheter and the syringe containing the heparinized flush solution.

34. Pull back on the syringe. You should obtain an *immediate* blood return in the catheter.

If you do not obtain an immediate blood return, the catheter is placed incorrectly.

Never, at any time, push fluid into a catheter that does not have an instantaneous blood return.

Actions	Remarks

Inserting an Arterial Catheter (continued)

35. After obtaining blood return in the catheter, pull any air bubbles into the syringe. Pull back only enough for air bubbles to enter the syringe. Generally this can be done with little or no blood getting into the syringe.

    Be careful not to infuse any air bubbles. Keep the syringe upright so air bubbles will not enter the catheter.

36. Refill the catheter with the heparinized flush solution. Turn the stopcock off to the catheter.

Note: If a significant amount of blood entered the syringe, hold it upright so the blood will stay near the stopcock and can be given back to the baby without also infusing the full amount of flush solution.

37. One operator and the instrument tray should remain sterile.

    The second operator removes the sterile drapes and tapes the catheter in place.

- OR -

    The catheter is sutured in place (see Step 44) and a sterile drape is placed over the sterile field and catheter while an x-ray is taken.

    If the catheter is taped, this is not the final taping. This temporary taping is done so the catheter will not become dislodged while catheter placement is checked by x-ray.

    A small rectangle of clear adhesive film may be used to protect the baby's skin (shown with dotted lines) before taping with adhesive tape, particularly if the baby is extremely preterm.

    Whether tape or suture is used, the catheter must be firmly secured in place before the x-ray is taken.

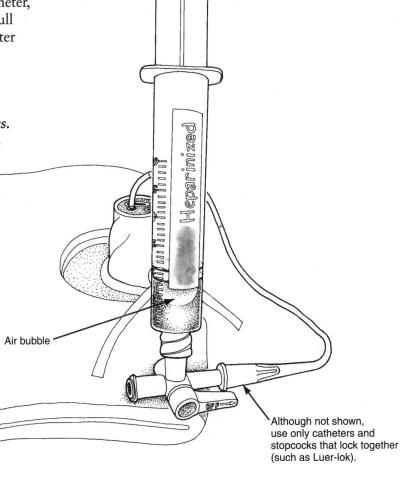

Air bubble

Although not shown, use only catheters and stopcocks that lock together (such as Luer-lok).

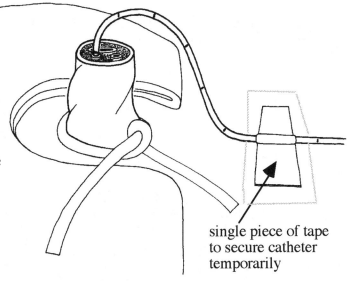

single piece of tape to secure catheter temporarily

Actions	**Remarks**

Checking Catheter Placement

38. Obtain a portable x-ray that includes the baby's abdomen and chest.

The baby should be kept in the same heated and oxygenated environment throughout the entire x-ray procedure.

39. The x-ray may be either an anterior-posterior view or a lateral view.

An anterior-posterior view (shown) will indicate reliably the placement of a catheter. In a sick baby, it is more easily obtained than a lateral view.

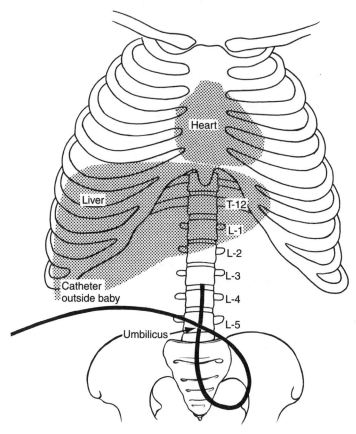

40. Umbilical *arterial* catheters

When a catheter has been inserted the measured distance, the tip of the catheter should be at the level of the aortic bifurcation, below all the major aortic vessels.

This location is preferred for 2 reasons.

- Hypertonic solutions infused through the catheter will not enter the major aortic vessels directly.

- Clots or air bubbles accidentally infused through a catheter probably will not go directly into the major aortic vessels, and therefore will not go directly to the abdominal organs.

On x-ray, the catheter tip of a UAC should be between the level of the third and fourth lumbar vertebrae (L3-4).

Note: Some experts prefer the catheter tip to be between the 6th and 9th thoracic vertebrae (not shown).

Hypertonic solutions can irritate the lining of the blood vessels. Administration of such solutions through a UAC is controversial. Some experts advise it is best *not* to administer hypertonic fluids through a UAC, regardless of tip location.

Clots or air bubbles infused through a catheter may lodge in a blood vessel and occlude the blood supply to the tissues nourished by that vessel. This can cause severe tissue damage.

Actions	Remarks

Checking Catheter Placement (continued)

41. Umbilical *venous* catheters

    When the catheter has been inserted the proper distance, the tip of the catheter should be at the junction of the inferior vena cava and the right atrium.

    This location is used because infusions of hypertonic solutions through a catheter in a lower position may go into the circulation of the liver and cause liver damage.

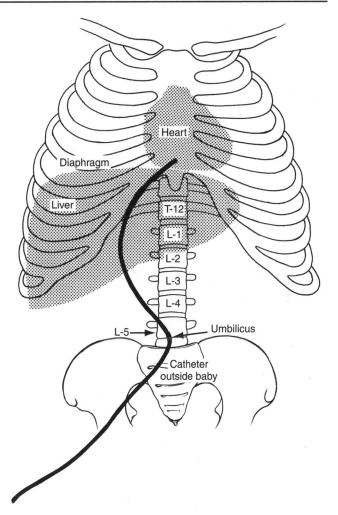

On x-ray, the catheter tip of a UVC should be at or just above the level of the diaphragm.

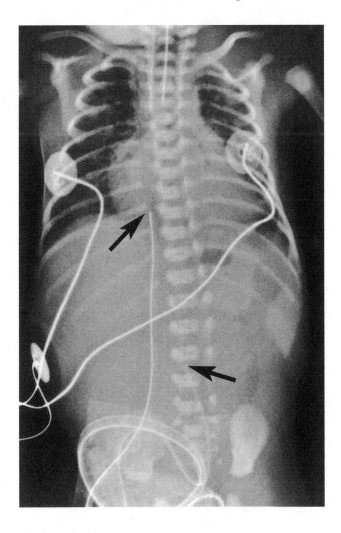

Correct Placement of Umbilical Catheters
Tip of UAC is at the level of L3-4 interspace.
Tip of UVC is just above the level of the diaphragm.

Actions	Remarks

Checking Catheter Placement (continued)

42. When the results of the x-ray are known, reposition the catheter (if necessary).

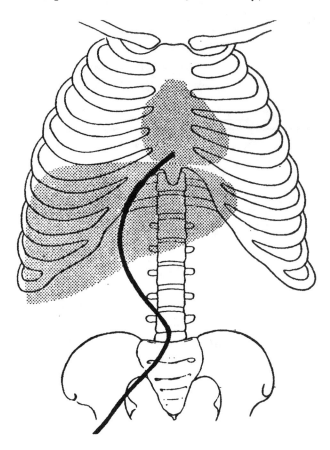

Correct Location: UVC

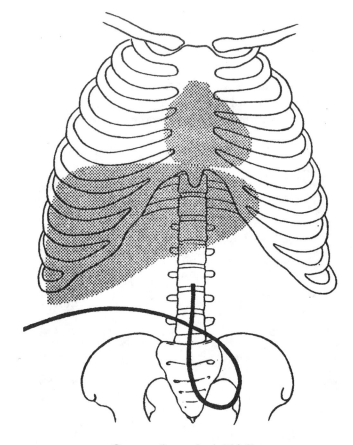

Correct Location: UAC

43. To determine how far to withdraw or insert a catheter that needs to be repositioned, measure on the x-ray

    UVC: from the catheter tip to the diaphragm

    UAC: from the catheter tip to the third or fourth lumbar vertebra

    Using the marks on the catheter as a guide, reposition the catheter the distance you determine from the x-ray.

    If the catheter is repositioned, obtain another x-ray to check the location of the catheter tip.

*If you **removed the sterile drapes** and temporarily taped the catheter in place (see Step 37), you may **only withdraw** a catheter to reposition it. If it needs to be inserted farther, the catheter in place should be removed and a new catheter inserted, using the same procedure and sterile technique used with the first catheter.*

*If you **kept the sterile field intact**, sutured the catheter to secure it while the x-ray was taken (see Steps 37 and 44), you may cut the suture and **either withdraw or insert** the catheter farther to reposition it, then secure the catheter with a new suture. When you cut the first suture, take great care not to nick the catheter.*

Actions   **Remarks**

Securing a Catheter

44. Now suture and tape the catheter in place.

   A. ***Tie a purse-string suture around the wall of the vessel.***

      This is done so there can be no oozing of blood around the catheter (common with a UVC, much less common with a UAC).

      A.1. Take a stitch through the umbilical cord stump and tie this in place.

      Be sure not to sew through any of the vessels.

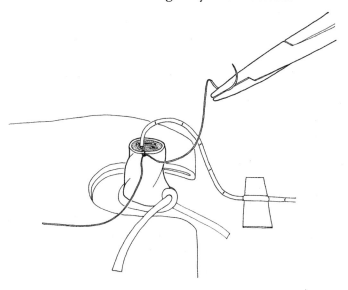

      A.2. Take several stitches around the vessel.

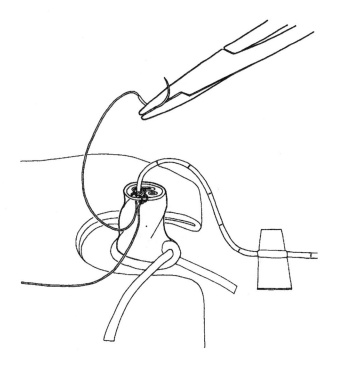

Actions	Remarks

Securing a Catheter (continued)

A.3. Cut off the needle and tie the suture to the original knot, pulling the suture tight around the vessel and catheter as you do so.

A.4. Tie a knot to keep the purse-string tight.

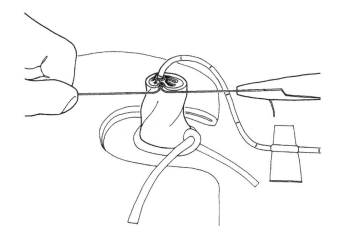

B. Tie the suture to the catheter.

B.1. Wrap one end of the suture around the needle holder.

B.2. Put the needle holder on one side of the catheter and the end of this *same* piece of suture around the other side of the catheter.

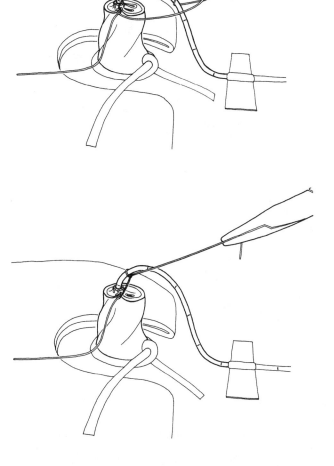

B.3. Pick up the free end of this suture with the needle holder and draw the suture down tight on the catheter.

Actions **Remarks**

Securing a Catheter (continued)

B.4. Repeat this with the other end
of the suture from the purse-
string knot.

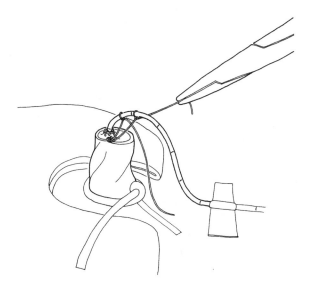

B.5. Finally, tie together both ends of
the suture that have been knotted
around the catheter.

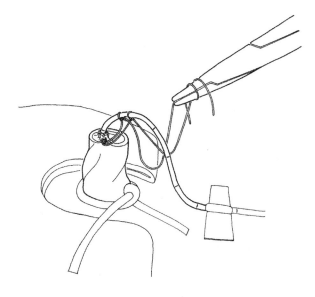

B.6. Cut off the loose ends of the
suture, just beyond the knot.

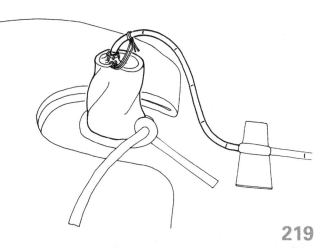

Actions	Remarks

Securing a Catheter (continued)

C. *Remove the povidone-iodine or chlorhexidine, used to prep the umbilical area, completely from the baby's skin by wiping with alcohol or sterile water swabs.*

If left in place, either of these antiseptics can cause marked skin irritation.

D. *After the catheter is sutured and the surgical prep antiseptic removed from the baby's skin, tape the catheter in place with a "tape bridge."*

Clear adhesive dressing can be used to protect the skin, especially if a baby is extremely preterm.

Commercial devices are available to replace tape bridges. Follow the manufacturer's application instructions.

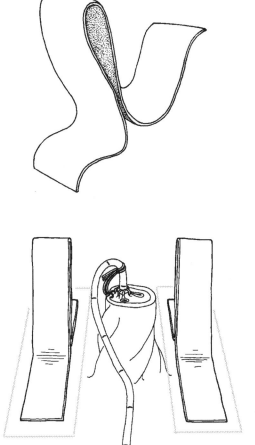

D1. Cut 2 strips of clear adhesive dressing, 2 to 3 inches long by 3/4 of an inch wide.

D2. Place these on either side of the umbilicus (shown by the dotted lines in the illustration).

D3. Take a 4-inch strip of 1/2-inch adhesive tape and fold the center section on itself.

D4. Tape this to one of the clear adhesive strips.

D5. Repeat this with another piece of 1/2-inch adhesive tape and the other clear adhesive strip.

Actions   **Remarks**

Securing a Catheter (continued)

D6. Next, wrap another piece of 1/2-inch adhesive tape from one side of the bridge to the other side, catching the catheter in the center.

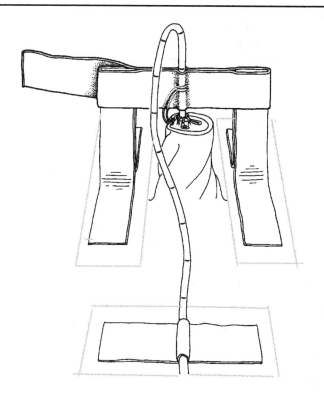

D7. Then loop the catheter over and catch a second section of the catheter with the adhesive tape.

With the catheter secured in this manner, any traction exerted on the catheter will not pull directly on the suture.

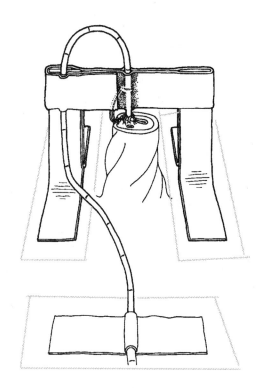

Actions	Remarks

Securing a Catheter (continued)

E. *Gauze dressings are not required and may, in fact, delay recognition of bleeding, catheter displacement, or infection around the umbilicus.*

In almost all cases, the loop of umbilical tape can be removed after the catheter is taped in place. This is desirable because umbilical tape left around the cord for a prolonged period can become an area for bacterial growth.

Only in rare situations will one of the umbilical vessels continue to ooze blood and require umbilical tape to be kept tightly pulled around the cord stump. In such cases, be sure the circulation to the skin at the base of the stump is not compromised.

F. *Use Luer-lok or other system of locking connections between the tubing, stopcock, and catheter.*

This is done to minimize the risk of disconnection, which could result in massive loss of blood from the baby.

G. *Attach only locking syringes to the stopcock. These are syringes that twist into place and provide a more secure connection than syringes that fasten by simply being inserted into a stopcock.*

Take this extra precaution because a loose connection may result in the baby losing a large amount of blood very quickly.

Adapting the Procedure for Umbilical Venous Catheterization

When an umbilical venous catheter is inserted in an emergency for the administration of medications, it may be done with minimal preparation. In such situations there is generally only enough time to put on a pair of sterile gloves, insert the catheter 2 to 3 cm, check for blood return, and then begin administration of emergency drugs.

When the insertion of a UVC is not for emergency purposes, a procedure similar to the one outlined for UAC should be followed. In fact, steps 1 through 21 and 33 through 44 are the same. The differences occur in steps 22 through 32 of the arterial catheterization skill. The corresponding steps for venous catheterization follow.

Actions	Remarks

Inserting an Umbilical Venous Catheter

22. The first operator should pick up the edge of the vein and the side of the umbilical cord with straight iris forceps.

    The vein is thin-walled and easily torn. To avoid this, pinch the side of the vein *and* the side of the umbilical cord together in the forceps.

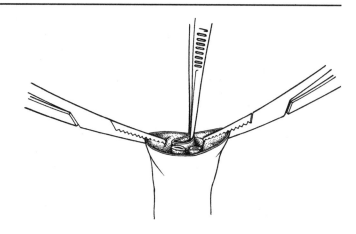

23. The first operator now gently grasps the opposite side of the vein with another pair of iris forceps.

    Because the vein is not a muscular vessel, it is not necessary to dilate it. Simply hold it open with the iris forceps.

    The vein may bleed when first opened. If this happens, apply firm pressure on the baby's abdomen, just above the umbilicus.

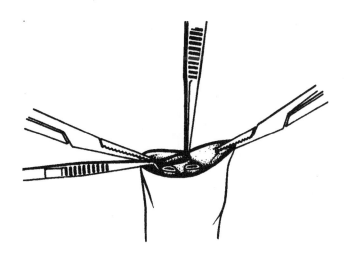

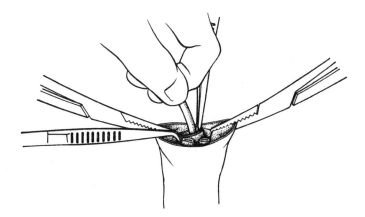

24. The second operator should now lay down one of the mosquito clamps holding the edge of the cord and use that hand to insert the catheter.

Actions   **Remarks**

Inserting an Umbilical Venous Catheter (continued)

25. The umbilical vein curves toward the baby's head and runs superficially under the skin several centimeters before curving downward toward the baby's spine. Therefore, it will be helpful to aim the tip of the catheter toward the baby's head.

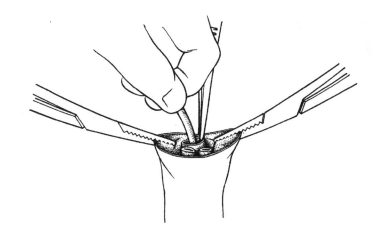

26. Continue to insert the catheter while always keeping a grip on it with forceps or with your fingers.

27. Insert the catheter the desired distance, as measured on the graph (see steps 9–10 earlier in this skill), but use the **dashed** line to determine the distance for a **venous** catheter.

    Example: If the shoulder-umbilicus length for a specific baby is 15 cm, you would insert the catheter 12 cm (10 cm from the chart, plus 2 cm in case catheter withdrawal for repositioning is needed).

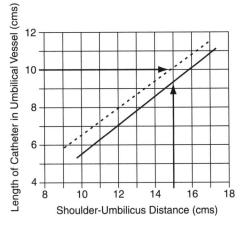

- - - - - - umbilical vein to junction of inferior vena cava and right atrium

———— umbilical artery to bifurcation of aorta

Actions	Remarks

Inserting an Umbilical Venous Catheter (continued)

28. If resistance is met, do *not* try to insert the catheter farther.

Resistance indicates that the tip of the catheter has entered one of the small veins in the circulation of the liver.

29. Withdraw the catheter 1 or 2 cm and twist it slightly in an attempt to aim the tip in a different direction. Gently attempt to insert the catheter the desired distance.

Sometimes it is necessary to undertake this maneuver several times before the catheter will pass through the ductus venosus so that the tip can be placed above the diaphragm.

30. *If repeated attempts to insert the catheter fail, seek another skilled person to attempt the procedure.*

In some cases, trying a different size catheter may be helpful.

31. If the catheter still cannot be inserted so that the tip is above the level of the diaphragm, either remove the catheter or withdraw it until 2 to 3 cm remain within the umbilical vein.

Check to be sure that an instantaneous blood return can be obtained with the catheter tip in this location.

32. Leave the catheter in this position but be aware that hypertonic solutions infused through the catheter will enter the circulation of the liver and may cause irritation.

If possible, location of the catheter tip below the level of the diaphragm should be avoided.

The exception to this is an emergency situation, when there is insufficient time to obtain an x-ray. In an emergency, insert a UVC just far enough to obtain a blood return (2–3 cm), before infusing medication or fluid.

Note: Now return to the basic skill and follow steps 33 through 44 to complete the procedure for UVC. Information about UVCs is also included in the "What Can Go Wrong?" and "Removing an Umbilical Catheter" sections that follow.

Actions	Remarks

What Can Go Wrong?

1. During attempted UAC insertion, you mistakenly insert the catheter into the vein instead of into the artery.

   This will be apparent on x-ray. Also, because arterial pressure is much greater than venous pressure, if the catheter is in an artery and is opened to a column of intravenous (IV) solution, the arterial pressure will cause the blood to back up into the catheter and to pulsate.

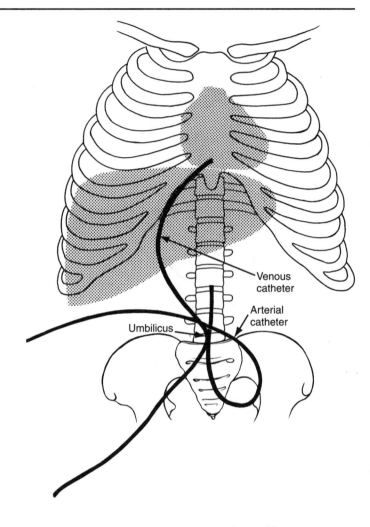

Venous catheter

Arterial catheter

Umbilicus

2. You measure incorrectly.

   The catheter may not be inserted a sufficient distance. If the sterile field has been broken, a new catheter will need to be inserted.

3. When inserting a *venous* catheter you meet resistance but continue to try to insert the catheter.

   The catheter should be withdrawn 1 to 2 cm when resistance is met, twisted slightly, and reinsertion attempted. (See steps 28–31 of the previous venous catheterization section.)

4. When inserting an *arterial* catheter you probe instead of using gentle, steady pressure to overcome resistance.

   Forceful probing may perforate the side of the vessel and cause internal bleeding and/or a failed catheterization.

   For both venous and arterial catheters, you should never probe forcefully if you feel resistance.

   If the catheter is not in a vessel, you will not get a blood return when the stopcock is opened between the catheter and syringe containing flush solution. When you aspirate (pull back) on the flush syringe, you should always get an *immediate* blood return.

Actions	Remarks

What Can Go Wrong? (continued)

5. You do not insert the catheter into the artery but rather create a false lumen or false tunnel through which you may be able to insert a catheter several centimeters.	You will not get a blood return if the catheter is in a false lumen. *Never infuse fluids through a catheter that does not have an instantaneous blood return.*
6. The baby loses blood if one of the vessels in the cord bleeds when you cut the cord in preparation for inserting the catheter.	Remember to always make a loose tie of umbilical tape around the base of the umbilicus before cutting the cord. After the catheter is inserted, a purse-string suture will almost always prevent any oozing of blood from around the vessel.

If the cord bleeds despite these measures, you should know how to stop the bleeding quickly.

Umbilical Artery

If an umbilical artery bleeds, the arterial pressure will cause the blood to spurt out very rapidly, perhaps as high as several feet into the air.

Because the arteries curve toward a baby's feet and then posteriorly toward the spine, pressing downward on the umbilicus will not exert enough pressure on the artery to stop the bleeding.

To stop an umbilical artery from bleeding, quickly grasp the baby's umbilicus and surrounding skin and pinch it tightly. Continue to pinch this handful of the baby's skin for at least 5 minutes.

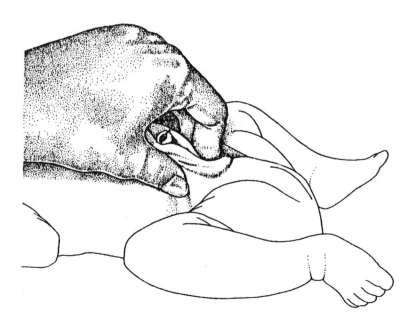

Umbilical Vein

If the vein bleeds, the baby also may lose a large amount of blood fairly quickly. Venous blood will flow steadily, but without spurting or pulsating.

The umbilical vein travels toward a baby's head, directly underneath the abdominal skin. Bleeding from the vein can be stopped by simply pressing downward on a baby's abdomen, just above the umbilicus.

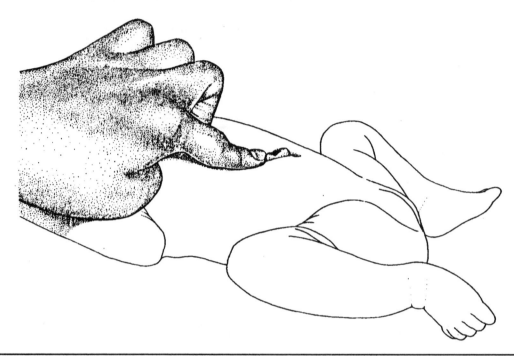

What Can Go Wrong? (continued)

7.	You use the instruments roughly and tear the edge of the umbilical cord or the edge of a vessel.	Do not use toothed forceps and do not tug on the artery, vein, or cord. Do not pick repeatedly at a vessel; rather, grasp the cord and vessel firmly but gently.
8.	A baby may lose blood quickly if there is a loose connection between the catheter, the stopcock, the IV, or the syringe.	Make sure all connections are tight. Use only Luer-lok, or other system of locking connections, and syringes that twist and lock into place.
9.	You infuse an air bubble or blood clot through the catheter.	Always be sure that the IV line is free of air bubbles. When blood samples are withdrawn, be certain no air is injected when the catheter is flushed with the flush solution.
10.	The catheter becomes clotted.	If a *heparin lock* is used, be sure to flush the heparin solution (1–2 units/mL) entirely through the catheter after each blood sample is withdrawn. If a *constant infusion* is used, an infusion pump is needed to ensure a consistent infusion rate and prevent clot formation in the catheter. When a slow infusion is used, heparin is generally added at a concentration of 0.5 to 1.0 units/mL.

Actions	Remarks

Deciding When to Remove a Catheter

1. An arterial catheter should be removed immediately if a baby's foot or leg blanches white while the catheter is being inserted.

   Remark: This means that the artery has gone into spasm, and the white areas are not receiving any blood supply.

2. An arterial catheter should be removed if the baby's toe, foot, or leg turns bluish or white after the catheter has been inserted.

   Remark: This generally means that an air bubble or a clot from the catheter has passed to one of the vessels in the leg, occluding the blood supply to the leg.

3. An *arterial* catheter should be removed as soon as a baby no longer requires a significant amount of supplemental oxygen or central arterial pressure monitoring.

4. A *venous* catheter should be removed as soon as a baby has been resuscitated and stabilized, and emergency medications are no longer needed; an exchange transfusion has been completed; or another IV line has been established.

Removing an Umbilical Catheter

Removal of a Venous Catheter

- Cut the suture that holds the catheter.

- Gradually withdraw the catheter 1 to 2 cm at a time over a period of few minutes.

- After withdrawing the catheter, prevent any bleeding from the vein by placing gentle pressure on the baby's abdomen just above the umbilicus for several minutes.

Removal of an Arterial Catheter

- Cut the suture that holds the catheter.
- Open the stopcock to the catheter.

  Remark: Do not leave the baby's bedside during this time as the unsutured catheter may slip out and result in significant blood loss.

- Draw just enough blood into the catheter to see the blood pulsate within the catheter.
- Close the stopcock to the catheter again.
- Gradually withdraw the catheter until only 2 to 3 cm of the catheter are left in the artery.

  Remark: This step may take 5 to 10 minutes. You need to allow time for the artery, beyond the catheter tip, to constrict. Do not wait so long, however, that blood clots in the catheter.

- When the blood no longer pulsates within the catheter, remove the catheter completely.

Unit 5   Low Blood Pressure

Objectives

In this unit you will learn to

A. Identify infants at risk for low blood pressure, including which babies are at risk for blood loss.

B. Recognize the complications of hypotension.

C. Identify normal and abnormal blood pressure measurements for babies of different birth weight and age categories.

D. Recognize and treat a newborn in shock.

E. Take accurate blood pressure measurements.

Note: Blood pressure graphs in this unit were created from data published in Zubrow AB, Hulman S, Kushner H, and Falkner B. Determinants of blood pressure in infants admitted to neonatal intensive care units: a prospective multicenter study. *J Perinatol.* 1995;15:470.

Before reading the unit, please answer the following questions. Select the *one best* answer to each question (unless otherwise instructed). Record your answers on the answer sheet that is the last page in this book *and* on the test.

1. Blood pressure is a result of

    A. Pumping action of the heart
    B. Volume of blood
    C. Tone of the blood vessels
    D. All of the above

2. A palpation blood pressure most closely approximates the

    A. Mean blood pressure
    B. Diastolic blood pressure
    C. Systolic blood pressure
    D. Pulse blood pressure

3. What is the recommended initial dosage of fluids to increase the blood volume of a 2,000-g (4 lb, 6 1/2 oz) baby who is in shock?

    A. 10 mL
    B. 20 mL
    C. 50 mL
    D. 100 mL

4. Which of the following amounts is the *best* estimate of the total blood volume of a 2,000-g (4 lb, 6 1/2 oz) infant?

    A. 180 mL (6 oz)
    B. 250 mL (8 1/3 oz)
    C. 300 mL (10 oz)
    D. 420 mL (14 oz)

5. What minimum amount of blood loss would put a 2,000-g (4 lb, 6 1/2 oz) baby into shock?

    A. 15 mL (1/2 oz)
    B. 25 mL (5/6 oz)
    C. 45 mL (1 1/2 oz)
    D. 75 mL (2 1/2 oz)

6. Which of the following is the *best* fluid to use to restore a baby's blood volume?

    A. 5% dextrose in water
    B. Sodium bicarbonate
    C. 10% dextrose in water
    D. Normal saline

7. What can happen to babies with low blood pressure?

    A. Acidosis can develop.
    B. Vital organs can be damaged.
    C. Rapid respirations can develop.
    D. B and C.
    E. A, B, and C.

8. **True   False**   If a term baby is born with a blood pressure of 26 mm Hg by palpation, the first action should be to crossmatch the baby's blood and give compatible blood.

9. Low blood pressure in newborns is associated with all of the following, *except*

    A. Poor oxygenation
    B. Polycythemia
    C. Sepsis
    D. Central nervous system insult

10. An infant weighing 1,800 g (4 lb) has a blood pressure of 32/12 mm Hg at 30 minutes of age. How would this infant's blood pressure be described?

   A. Hypertension

   B. Normal

   C. Hypotension

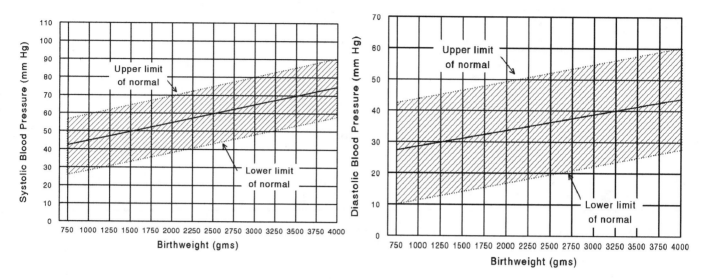

For each question, please make sure you have marked your answer on the test and on the answer sheet (last page in book). The test is for you; the answer sheet will need to be turned in for continuing education credit.

1. What Is Blood Pressure?

Blood pressure is the amount of force pushing blood through the circulatory system. This force is determined by 3 factors: the pumping action of the heart, the tone of the blood vessels, and the amount of blood or blood volume.

- The *systolic* pressure occurs at the end of each heart contraction. It is the higher number in a blood pressure measurement.

- The *diastolic* pressure occurs immediately before each contraction (resting period). It is the lower number in a blood pressure measurement.

- The *mean* pressure is about half way between the systolic and diastolic pressure.

Hypotension means low blood pressure. *Hypovolemia* means low blood volume, which is one cause of hypotension.

2. How Do You Check an Infant's Blood Pressure?

The auscultation (listening with a stethoscope) method used for adults is not appropriate for babies. Palpation or oscillometry methods may be used for babies. Other methods for measuring infant blood pressure are also available (eg, Doppler and central arterial) but require more specialized equipment and are not discussed in this unit.

Palpation measurement gives a single value that is slightly lower than the systolic pressure. Measurement is obtained using a blood pressure cuff, manometer, and the care provider's index finger. The palpation method gives reliable readings if the pressure is greater than 20 mm Hg.

Oscillometric measurement is obtained by detection of oscillations in the arterial wall caused by pressure changes within the artery and gives accurate readings even if the blood pressure is below 20 mm Hg. Separate machines may be used, or some cardiac monitors have a blood pressure channel and cable that connects between the blood pressure cuff and the monitor. In either case, oscillometric measurements are displayed as systolic, diastolic, and mean blood pressure values.

3. Which Babies Should Have Their Blood Pressure Taken?

All babies can have their blood pressure checked as a routine vital sign. Some babies will require more frequent blood pressure readings because they are at risk for low blood pressure.

A. Babies With Signs of Low Blood Pressure (hypotension)

- Rapid respirations

- Paleness and/or mottled coloring of skin

- Weak pulses and rapid heart rate

- Slow capillary refill time

Note: To test *capillary refill time,* press firmly for several seconds over one of the long bones in a baby's arm or leg. After the pressure is released, the blanched fingerprint area should disappear in 1 to 2 seconds as the skin capillaries refill with blood. If the fingerprint remains longer than 1 or 2 seconds, the baby has slow capillary refill time.

B. Babies With Suspected Blood Loss (hypovolemia)

- Tear in an umbilical vessel (inspect cord closely because a tear may not be obvious)

- Cord clamped incompletely

- Accidental cutting of the placenta during cesarean delivery

- Placenta previa or abruptio placentae (risk of fetal blood loss is significantly higher with placenta previa than with abruptio placentae, but can occur with either condition)

- Internal bleeding caused by trauma (difficult delivery)

C. Babies Suspected of Having Congenital Heart Disease

For these babies, blood pressures should be taken in all 4 extremities. Differences in pressures among the extremities may suggest specific cardiac defects. The interpretation of these is not discussed in this program.

D. Babies Born From a Multifetal Pregnancy

In pregnancies with more than one fetus, there is sometimes an abnormal connection between the placental circulation of one fetus and the placental circulation of another fetus, if placentas become fused together. This happens when a blood vessel from the placental circulation of one fetus and a blood vessel from the placental circulation of another fetus grow together. Fetal-fetal transfusion may result, with one fetus becoming the "blood donor" to the other "recipient" fetus.

Usually this is a chronic process that allows the donor fetus to compensate for loss in blood volume, but not for loss of red blood cells. Therefore, a donor fetus is usually not hypovolemic, but is often anemic. If the abnormal connection is long-standing the donor fetus may become severely anemic, which may lead to the development of hydrops (generalized fetal edema that occurs as a result of extreme, chronic anemia). A recipient fetus is typically a ruddy red color from polycythemia.

Blood pressure and hematocrit should be checked in twins and triplets, etc. (See Book III, Review: Is the Baby Sick? for information about hematocrit values.)

E. Babies Born Following Fetal-Maternal Transfusion

Sometimes an abnormal connection occurs between the fetal and the maternal circulation in the placenta, which results in fetal-maternal transfusion. The reverse direction of maternal-fetal transfusion apparently does not occur, probably because the pressure gradient in the intervillous space in the placenta favors a flow direction from the fetus to the woman.

When fetal-maternal hemorrhage occurs, the newborn may present with findings similar to the "donor" fetus described previously in fetal-fetal transfusion.

If fetal-maternal transfusion is suspected, the mother's blood can be tested for the presence of fetal cells with the Kleihauer-Betke test.

F. All At-Risk and Sick Babies

Now answer these questions to test yourself on the information in the last section.

A1. **True** **False** Blood pressure depends entirely on how hard the heart pumps blood through the circulatory system.

A2. **True** **False** A transfusion from the fetus to the mother can occur in utero.

A3. Which of the following methods is/are being recommended in this unit for taking infant blood pressures?
   A. Oscillometric
   B. Palpation
   C. Auscultation
   D. Doppler

A4. Which babies should have their blood pressures checked?

_____

_____

_____

_____

_____

A5. Hypotension means low blood _____, while hypovolemia means low blood

_____.

A6. If a fetus-to-fetus transfusion develops in utero, it can cause _____

in the donor fetus and _____ in the recipient fetus.

Check your answers with the list that follows the Recommended Routines. Correct any incorrect answers and review the appropriate section in the unit.

4. What Is a Normal Infant Blood Pressure?

The blood pressure range for newborn babies is much lower than the blood pressure ranges for older children or adults. In addition, neonatal blood pressure varies, according to a baby's birth weight and age. Blood pressure rises with increasing birth weight, advancing gestational age, and days and weeks since birth.

At birth, blood pressure is closely related to birth weight and gestational age. The graphs below show the normal range of systolic and diastolic pressures for babies of different birth weights during the first day after birth.

Figure 5.1. Blood Pressure During First Day After Birth

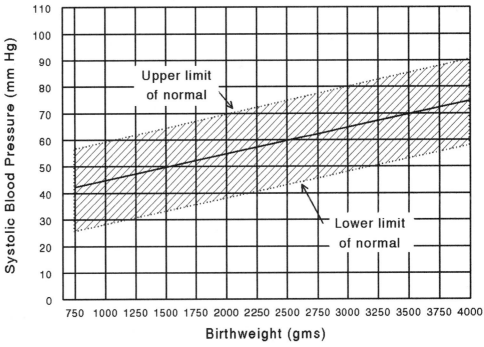

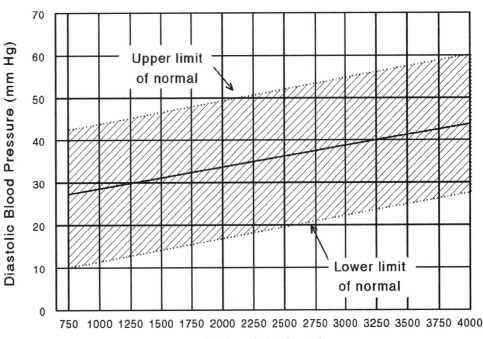

During the first 5 days after birth there is a predictable rise in blood pressure for babies of all birth weights and gestational ages. The graphs below show the rise in systolic and diastolic blood pressure during that time, for babies of 4 different gestational age groups (≤28 weeks, 29 to 32 weeks, 33 to 36 weeks, and ≥37 weeks).

After 5 postnatal days there is a much slower, but also predictable, rise in blood pressure for all babies.

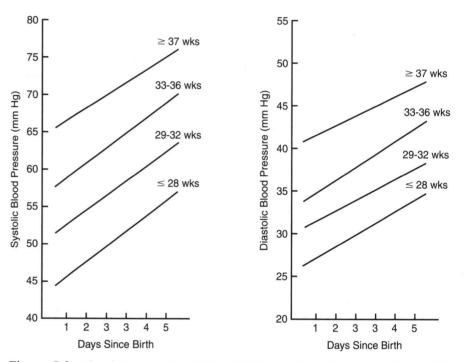

Figure 5.2. Blood Pressure for Babies of Different Gestational Ages During First 5 Days After Birth

Blood pressure for babies older than 5 days is closely related to postmenstrual age. Postmenstrual age is a baby's gestational age at birth, plus the number of weeks since birth. For example, a 2-week-old baby born at 32 weeks' gestation has a postmenstrual age of 34 weeks. The graphs on the next page show the normal range of systolic and diastolic pressures for babies of different postmenstrual ages.

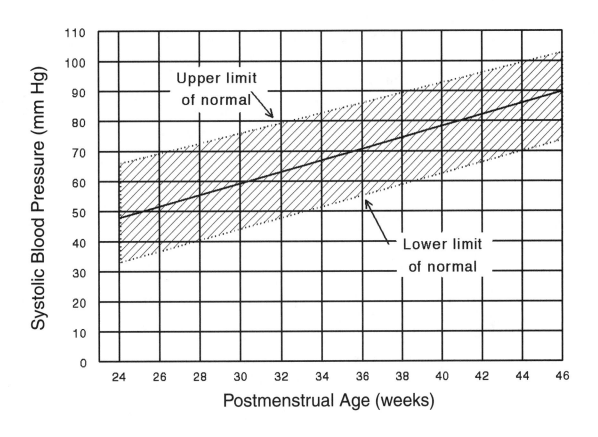

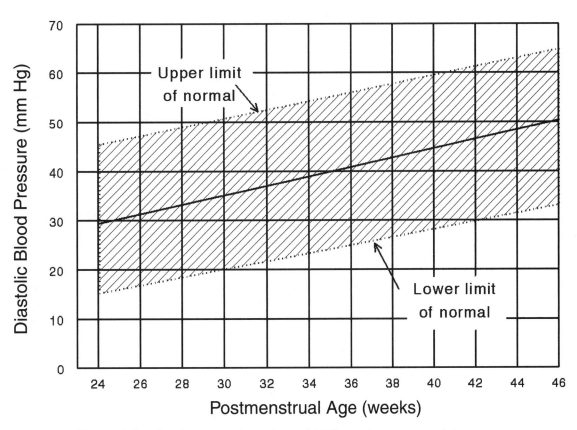

Figure 5.3. Blood Pressure for Babies of Different Postmenstrual Ages

5. What Is Normal Infant Blood Volume?

Babies have only about 90 mL of blood per kilogram of weight (about 40 mL/lb).

Example: A 1,500-g (3 lb, 5 oz) baby has only about 135 mL of blood.

90 mL × 1.5 kg = 135 mL (4.5 oz)

Example: A 7 lb (3,170 g) baby has only about 280 mL of blood.

40 mL × 7 lb = 280 mL (9.33 oz)

6. How Much Blood Loss Will Cause Shock?

 Babies in shock require immediate treatment.

If babies lose 25% or more of their blood volume, they probably will go into shock.

Example: A baby is born weighing 2,000 g (4 lb, 6 1/2 oz)

- What is the baby's normal blood volume?

2 kg × 90 mL/kg = 180 mL

- How much blood would this baby need to lose to go into shock?

180 mL × 25% = 45 mL (about 3 tablespoons)

If this same baby were born to a woman with placenta previa or abruptio placentae, the woman may easily lose 1,000 mL of blood during delivery. If only 5% (50 mL) of this blood is the infant's, the infant will go into shock.

Note: Babies also lose blood when it is taken for laboratory tests. It is recommended to

- Take the minimum amount of blood required for the test(s).

- Keep a record of the amount withdrawn for each test and a tally of the total amount of blood withdrawn.

Critically ill babies usually need periodic blood replacement for the volume withdrawn for laboratory tests. Many clinicians recommend replacing with transfused blood whenever the cumulative total of blood withdrawn for tests reaches 10% of a baby's blood volume.

Now answer these questions to test yourself on the information in the last section. Refer to the graphs or charts in the unit, as necessary, to answer these questions.

B1. Of the following, which value(s) is/are within normal limits for *systolic* blood pressure for a newborn with a birth weight of 6 lb, 10 oz (3,000 g)?

    A. 36 mm Hg

    B. 42 mm Hg

    C. 56 mm Hg

    D. 72 mm Hg

B2. A 2,100-g (4 lb, 10 oz) baby is born at your hospital. His initial blood pressure is 60 mm Hg by palpation. How would his blood pressure be described?

    A. Normal

    B. Hypertensive

    C. Hypotensive

B3. What is the normal blood volume of a newborn infant?

    _____ mL/kg or _____ mL/lb.

B4. What minimum blood loss would put a normal 2,400 g (5 lb, 4 1/2 oz) infant into shock?

    A. 14 mL

    B. 54 mL

    C. 108 mL

    D. 216 mL

B5. Why is a baby at risk for low blood pressure if the mother loses a large volume of blood during delivery?

    _____

    _____

B6. What is the possible consequence of frequent sampling of blood for laboratory tests in infants?

    _____

B7. The normal diastolic blood pressure range for a 1-day-old, 1,750-g (3 lb, 14 oz) baby is approximately _____

    mm Hg to _____ mm Hg. The normal systolic blood pressure range for the same baby is approximately

    _____ mm Hg to _____ mm Hg.

Check your answers with the list that follows the Recommended Routines. Correct any incorrect answers and review the appropriate section in the unit.

7. What Happens to Babies With Low Blood Pressure?

A baby's body will try to adjust so that vital organs receive adequate blood flow and oxygen from the available blood volume. As a result, the following complications may occur:

A. Inadequate Oxygenation

Loss of blood volume also means a loss of red blood cells. The remaining red blood cells may not be able to carry sufficient oxygen to the brain and other vital organs. A baby may try to compensate for this by breathing fast. Babies may not, however, be able to take in enough oxygen to maintain normal blood oxygen levels.

B. Acidosis (low blood pH)

Low blood pressure will result in the closing off or constriction of the smaller blood vessels to less vital organs (skin, muscles) in an effort to preserve blood flow to more vital organs (brain, heart, lungs). The consequences of this restricted blood flow include

- *Increased production of lactic acid:* Restricted oxygen supply forces a less-efficient, more acid-producing form of metabolism to be used.

- *Reduced removal of lactic acid:* Restricted blood flow limits the amount of metabolic waste products that can be removed.

The lactic acid that accumulates in the tissues may result in lowering the pH of the blood.

 In addition to the clinical appearance of rapid respirations, pale and/or mottled skin color, weak pulses, rapid heart rate, and slow capillary refill time, hypotensive babies are likely to be hypoxic and develop metabolic acidosis.

8. What Are the Causes of Low Blood Pressure in the Newborn?

Hypovolemia is only one of many reasons for low blood pressure. It is important to make every attempt to establish the cause of the hypotension and treat it appropriately. For example, an infant may be hypotensive because of poor oxygenation, which will cause the heart to beat poorly and blood vessels to dilate. The appropriate treatment, therefore, would be to give oxygen and/or assist the baby's ventilation. The following causes of hypotension should be considered:

- Blood loss (hypovolemia)

- Poor oxygenation

- Severe acidosis

- Sepsis (blood infection)

- Poor cardiac output

- Severe central nervous system insult

Sick babies may be hypotensive due to a combination of 2 or more factors. If not corrected, these factors may lead to a worsening cycle of acidosis and hypoxia.

9. What Do You Do for Babies With Low Blood Volume?

As mentioned earlier, infants may have low blood pressure from blood loss. The general treatment for hypovolemia is to give a blood volume expander to increase the baby's blood volume.

Theoretically, crossmatched whole blood is the best blood volume expander. Whole blood, however, is usually not immediately available and carries a higher risk of infection than other volume expanders. **Do *not* wait.**

In the past, 5% albumin or plasma protein fraction were recommended as blood volume expanders. Recent evidence, however, indicates that normal saline is equally effective in restoring blood volume, and costs significantly less than plasma-based products. Ringer's lactate IV solution may also be used for emergency blood volume expansion. Packed red blood cells may be administered later, if indicated.

A. Take Baby's Blood Pressure to Confirm It Is Low

If blood pressure is low, leave the deflated blood pressure cuff in place.

B. Choose Appropriate Blood Volume Expander

Normal saline (0.9% sodium chloride concentration) is recommended for immediate treatment. If large volumes are required, or if the baby is subsequently found to be anemic, packed, washed red blood cells may be given

C. Give 10mL/kg (4mL/lb) Intravenously

Although it is important to begin infusion of a blood volume expander immediately, the fluid should be given *slowly and steadily*. Sudden shifts in blood volume place a baby at risk for an intraventricular hemorrhage (bleeding in the brain), particularly if the baby is significantly preterm.

If blood is given for any other reason to a baby with normal blood pressure, the rate of administration should be slower than the rate used for emergency blood volume expansion.

 If volume expansion is needed, treatment should start immediately. A volume expander, however, should be given slowly and steadily, over 5 to 10 minutes.

Fluids given for any reason other than volume expansion should be given more slowly, especially in preterm infants.

D. Check Baby's Blood Pressure

- *If Normal:* Continue taking the baby's blood pressure (every 10 minutes for a while and then at longer intervals) to ensure that the blood pressure has stabilized.

- *If Still Low:* Administer another dose of volume expander and recheck baby's blood pressure frequently.

E. Investigate Other Possible Causes of Hypotension

10. What Do You Do for Hypotensive Babies if You Do *Not* Suspect Blood Loss?

Always look for the cause of low blood pressure. (See section 8.) Frequently, in infants who have had significant perinatal compromise, the initial blood pressure reading may be low as a result of severe hypoxia and acidosis. The most important treatment for these infants is to perform rapid and efficient resuscitative measures. These measures alone will usually restore an infant's blood pressure to the normal range. If they do not, special drugs, such as dopamine or dobutamine, may be required to increase cardiac output.

Septic infants may also be hypotensive. If sepsis is suspected as the cause of the low blood pressure, the baby's blood should be cultured and the baby started promptly on antibiotics.

Self-Test

Now answer these questions to test yourself on the information in the last section.

C1. List the fluid(s) recommended as an emergency blood volume expander.

_____

C2. What is the recommended starting amount of volume expanders?

_____ mL/kg (_____ mL/lb)

C3. What is the recommended rate of administration of volume expanders?

_____

C4. How is low blood volume treated?

    A. Administer blood volume expander to increase blood volume.

    B. Administer caffeine to improve cardiac output.

    C. Administer epinephrine to increase the tone of the blood vessels.

C5. Physical examination and blood pressure measurement show a baby is in shock. Blood loss is suspected. What should be done?

    A. Send blood for crossmatching and give blood as soon as it is available.

    B. Give normal saline immediately.

C6. List 3 of the possible causes of hypotension in a baby.

_____

_____

_____

Check your answers with the list that follows the Recommended Routines. Correct any incorrect answers and review the appropriate section in the unit.

Recommended Routines

All of the routines listed below are based on the principles of perinatal care presented in the unit you have just finished. They are recommended as part of routine perinatal care.

Read each routine carefully and decide whether it is standard operating procedure in your hospital. Check the appropriate blank next to each routine.

Procedure Standard in My Hospital	Needs Discussion by Our Staff	
_____	_____	1. Consider including blood pressure as a part of the initial assessment for all newborns.
_____	_____	2. Require repeated blood pressure measurements for babies at risk for hypotension.
_____	_____	3. Be sure sterile normal saline (0.9% NaCl) for intravenous use is always immediately available in each delivery room and each nursery.
_____	_____	4. Check all blood pressure cuffs to ensure availability of appropriate-sized cuffs for newborns of all sizes.

These are the answers to the self-test questions. Please check them with the answers you gave and review the information in the unit wherever necessary.

A1. False In addition to the pumping action of the heart, blood pressure also depends on the tone of the blood vessels and the volume of blood.

A2. True

A3. A. Oscillometric
    B. Palpation

A4. All of the following babies:
- Babies with suspected blood loss
- Babies with signs of low blood pressure
- Babies suspected of having heart disease
- Babies born from multifetal pregnancies
- All at-risk and sick babies

Note: A baby with fetal-maternal transfusion would fall into the "at-risk and sick" group of babies above because such babies are likely to have signs similar to a "donor" fetus in fetal-fetal transfusion. After immediate treatment and stabilization of the baby, a Kleihauer-Betke test of the mother's blood might then be done to document or rule out fetal-maternal transfusion.

A5. Hypotension means low blood *pressure*, while hypovolemia means low blood *volume*.

A6. *Anemia* in the donor fetus and *polycythemia* in the recipient fetus

B1. C and D

B2. A. Normal

B3. 90 mL/kg or 40 mL/lb

B4. B. 54 mL (2.4 kg × 90 mL/kg = 216 mL; 216 mL × 0.25 = 54 mL)

B5. If only a small fraction of the blood lost is the baby's blood, the baby can go into shock.

B6. Low blood volume and low blood pressure. A running total of the amount of blood withdrawn should be kept and the baby transfused with replacement volume before symptoms develop.

B7. Normal diastolic range is approximately 16 to 48 mm Hg; normal systolic range is approximately 36 to 68 mm Hg for a 1-day-old baby with a birth weight of 1,750 g.

C1. Normal saline; Ringer's lactate may also be used.

C2. 10 mL/kg 4 mL/lb

C3. Over 5 to 10 minutes (volume expansion begun immediately but fluid given slowly and steadily)

C4. A. Administer blood volume expander to increase blood volume.

C5. B. Give normal saline immediately. The baby should not be left in shock while waiting for blood to be crossmatched.

C6. Any 3 of the following:
- Low blood volume or blood loss
- Poor oxygenation
- Severe acidosis
- Severe central nervous system insult
- Poor cardiac output
- Sepsis

Unit 5 Posttest

Without referring back to the information in the unit, please answer the following questions. Select the **one best** answer to each question (unless otherwise instructed). Record your answers on the answer sheet that is the last page in this book *and* on the test.

1. What problems can result from low blood pressure in infants?
   - **A.** Acidosis can develop.
   - **B.** Vital organs can be damaged.
   - **C.** Sepsis can develop.
   - **D.** A and B.
   - **E.** A, B, and C.

2. Which of the following is the *best* fluid to use in an emergency to increase a baby's blood volume?
   - **A.** 5% dextrose in water
   - **B.** Normal saline
   - **C.** Quarter-normal saline
   - **D.** 25% albumin

3. A 2,000-g (4 lb, 6 1/2 oz) infant is born in your hospital following emergency cesarean delivery for placenta previa. The baby's blood pressure is taken and reads 24 mm Hg by palpation. Which action should be taken *first*?
   - **A.** Give oxygen and recheck blood pressure in 30 minutes.
   - **B.** Administer 45 mg of caffeine citrate.
   - **C.** Send blood for crossmatch.
   - **D.** Begin infusion of 20 mL of normal saline.

4. A 4,200-g (9 lb, 4 oz) infant is born in your hospital, with Apgar scores of 5 and 7 at 1 and 5 minutes respectively. She is mottled and pale with rapid respirations and a blood pressure of 42/22 mm Hg. Which of the following actions is *best* for this infant?
   - **A.** Recheck blood pressure in 30 minutes.
   - **B.** Administer caffeine sodium benzoate to increase heart rate.
   - **C.** Start administering 40 mL of volume expander intravenously. Recheck blood pressure every 15 minutes.
   - **D.** Obtain blood sample for type and crossmatch. Transfuse baby as soon as compatible blood is available.

5. Which of the following amounts is the *best* estimate of the total amount of blood a 3,000-g (6 lb, 10 oz) infant has?
   - **A.** 325 mL
   - **B.** 270 mL
   - **C.** 200 mL
   - **D.** 75 mL

6. **True   False**   Measuring blood pressure in a newborn infant can be done only with special electronic equipment.

7. What minimum amount of blood loss would put a preterm 1,300-g (2 lb, 14 oz) baby into shock?
   - **A.** 10 mL
   - **B.** 30 mL
   - **C.** 50 mL
   - **D.** 120 mL

8. What is the recommended initial dosage of fluids to treat low blood volume?
   - **A.** 5 mL/kg (2 mL/lb)
   - **B.** 10 mL/kg (4 mL/lb)
   - **C.** 25 mL/kg (10 mL/lb)
   - **D.** 50 mL/kg (20 mL/lb)

9. Low blood pressure in newborns is associated with all of the following, *except*

   A. Antenatal steroids
   B. Severe acidosis
   C. Poor cardiac output
   D. Sepsis

10. An infant is born weighing 1,500 g (3 lb, 5 oz). Her systolic blood pressure is 30 mm Hg. How would this infant's pressure be described?

   A. Hypertensive
   B. Normal
   C. Hypotensive

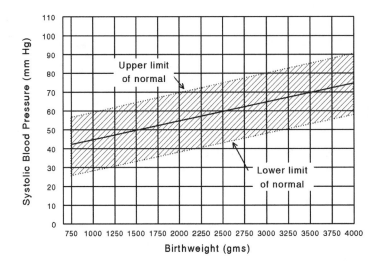

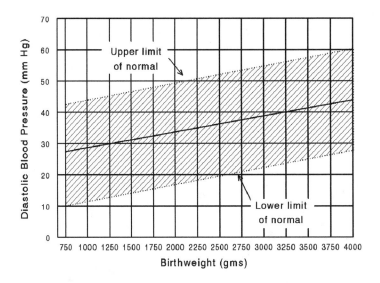

For each question, please make sure you have marked your answer on the test and on the answer sheet (last page in book). The test is for you; the answer sheet will need to be turned in for continuing education credit.

Skill Unit   Measuring Blood Pressure

This skill unit will teach you how to take oscillometric and palpation blood pressure measurements on a baby.

Study this skill unit, then attend a skill practice and demonstration session.

To master the skill, you will need to demonstrate correctly each of the steps listed below. At least one of the blood pressure measurement techniques needs to be demonstrated on 3 different babies.

Oscillometric Blood Pressure Measurement

1. Select cuff.
2. Set monitor to manual mode; set monitor for automatic mode and determine cycle time*.
3. Position cuff around baby's arm or leg.
4. Activate operation of the machine or oscillometric blood pressure mode on the cardiac monitor.
5. Record baby's systolic, diastolic, and mean blood pressure.
6. Set alarm limits for a specific baby (when automatic mode used)*, as appropriate.

Palpation Blood Pressure Measurement

1. Select cuff.
2. Wrap cuff around the baby's arm or leg.
3. Connect gauge to cuff; check to see that the gauge reads zero.
4. Palpate artery, inflate cuff.
5. Release cuff pressure at an appropriate rate.
6. Determine when arterial pulsation first occurs, deflate cuff.
7. Record palpation blood pressure.

---

*Automatic mode will not be used for all babies. It is most useful for babies who require frequent blood pressure measurements. You will need to know how to obtain oscillometric measurements in manual and automatic mode.

Actions	Remarks

Deciding to Take a Baby's Blood Pressure

1. Ask yourself, "Is there a reason why this baby's blood pressure might be low?"

   • Is/was there a cause for blood loss? ⟶ Neonatal blood loss can occur with
   • Umbilical cord tear
   • Incomplete clamping of umbilical cord
   • Placenta previa or abruptio placentae
   • Accidental cutting of the placenta during cesarean delivery
   • Trauma to the infant with internal bleeding

   • Was the baby born from a high-risk pregnancy?

   • Is the baby sick for any reason, such as perinatal compromise, acidosis, suspected sepsis, or other illness?

   • Does the baby have signs of shock? ⟶ Babies who are hypotensive (in shock) typically have
   • Rapid respirations
   • Rapid heart rate
   • Weak pulses
   • Pale or mottled appearance
   • Slow capillary refill time

   • Is a cardiac abnormality suspected?

   • Was the baby born from a multifetal pregnancy (twin, triplet, etc)?

   Yes: Take the blood pressure as soon as possible. (This may be done in the delivery room.)

   No: Blood pressure measurement may be taken as a part of routine vital signs

Preparing to Obtain an Oscillometric Blood Pressure

2. Collect the appropriate equipment
   • Oscillometric blood pressure machine or appropriate cable for the cardiac monitor

   Proper operation of an oscillometric device or of the peripheral blood pressure mode on a cardiac monitor is specific to each brand of equipment. Detailed knowledge of equipment used in your hospital is essential.

   • Appropriate-sized blood pressure cuff

   Cuffs are usually disposable and should be either used once and then discarded, or kept at the baby's bedside and used only for that baby.

   Cuffs may be sized according to the baby's weight; follow manufacturer's guidelines for selecting size.

   Size of the cuff is important. A cuff that is either too large or too small will give inaccurate readings.

3. If using a separate machine, plug the monitor into a grounded outlet and turn on the power.

Actions	Remarks

Deciding Which Mode of Operation to Use

4. Ask yourself
   - Is the baby's condition unstable, requiring frequent blood pressure measurements?

If frequent measurements are needed, select the automatic mode. This means that the monitor will automatically reinflate the blood pressure cuff and obtain a new measurement once every cycle period. Some monitors have preset cycle periods; for other monitors, you program the specific cycle time you want.

   - Is the baby's blood pressure being taken as a part of routine vital signs?

If blood pressure measurements are needed infrequently, select the manual mode. This means that the monitor will measure the baby's blood pressure only when you activate it.

5. If the automatic mode is selected, determine the cycle period to be used.

   Rotate cuff location.

   When an arm or leg repeatedly receives, over an extended period, the inflation pressures needed to obtain blood pressure readings, the baby's extremity can be bruised, especially if the baby is significantly preterm.

Generally, an automatic cycle time of 3 minutes or less does not provide sufficient deflation time to allow adequate circulation to the extremity between cuff inflations.

Cycle periods of 5 to 10 minutes are usually appropriate for unstable babies. However, be sure to change cuff location periodically.

Obtaining an Oscillometric Blood Pressure Measurement

6. Wrap the cuff around the baby's extremity so that it fits snugly, but does not constrict blood flow.

The baby's upper or lower arm, thigh, or calf may be used.

   Some cuffs are designed to be positioned in a particular way.

For example, an arrow may indicate the point that should be positioned over the artery.

7. Connect the blood pressure cuff to the machine or cardiac monitor channel and begin operation.

8. Read the blood pressure values off the monitor. Systolic, diastolic, and mean arterial values are measured.

For example, if a baby's blood pressure is registered as 64 systolic, 40 diastolic with a mean arterial pressure (MAP) of 52, record this as

   64/40 mm Hg, MAP 52 mm Hg

9. Set the upper and lower alarm limits 10 mm Hg higher and 10 mm Hg lower than the baby's initial systolic blood pressure reading. If a baby is hypotensive, readjust the alarm limits as the blood pressure is corrected.

Actions	Remarks

What Can Go Wrong?

Actions	Remarks
1. The monitor is out of calibration and does not give accurate values.	Follow manufacturer's recommendations regarding calibration and maintenance. Any time you are in doubt about the values given by the monitor, double-check your findings with another monitor or with a palpation blood pressure measurement. Remember, palpation gives a single value that is slightly lower than the baby's systolic pressure.
2. The baby wiggles while you are taking the blood pressure. The values given are inaccurate or the machine does not register any blood pressure.	The baby needs to be quiet while the cuff is inflated and the measurements are taken or the extremity needs to be held still during this time.
3. The circulation in the baby's extremity is compromised and/or the skin is bruised.	Be sure that the time between automatic cycles is 5 minutes or longer. Observe the baby's extremity for signs of circulatory compromise. Rotate location of cuff placement.
4. The monitor gives a blood pressure reading but the simultaneous heart rate it records is significantly different than the baby's heart rate.	This is almost surely *not* an accurate blood pressure measurement. Take the blood pressure again. If the baby is crying, calm the baby before rechecking the measurement.

Actions	**Remarks**

Preparing to Take an Infant's Blood Pressure by Palpation

1. Does the baby need a blood pressure measurement?

    See the beginning of the oscillometric section.

2. Collect the proper equipment.

    Blood pressure gauge, inflator, and cuff are the only items needed.

    - A standard mercury or aneroid manometer (blood pressure gauge) with bulb inflator

    - Appropriate-sized blood pressure cuff

    The inflatable part of the cuff, called the bladder, should be long enough to wrap entirely around the baby's arm or leg. This means the ends of the bladder must meet or overlap.

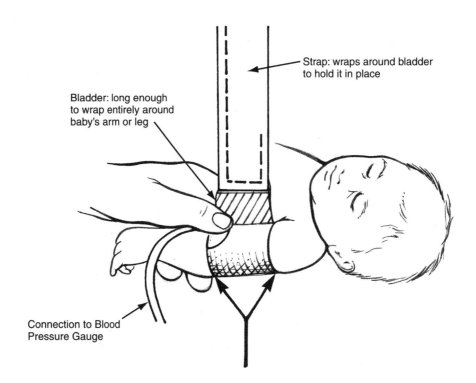

Strap: wraps around bladder to hold it in place

Bladder: long enough to wrap entirely around baby's arm or leg

Connection to Blood Pressure Gauge

3. Do you have the correct-sized cuff?

    Yes: Go ahead with taking the blood pressure.

    No: Get the correct-sized cuff.

    Cuffs with bladders too small (especially if it does not fully encircle baby's arm or leg) may give extremely inaccurate readings, which are usually much higher than the true blood pressure. Cuffs with bladders that are too large will often give inaccurate low readings.

Actions	Remarks

Preparing to Take an Infant's Blood Pressure by Palpation (continued)

4.	Wrap the blood pressure cuff around the baby's upper arm or thigh.	The cuff should be neither loose nor tight. A cuff too tight will give a falsely low blood pressure reading because it will restrict the blood flow.
5.	Connect the cuff to the blood pressure gauge.	
6.	Check to see that the gauge reads zero.	If the gauge does not read zero, adjust it or get a different gauge.

Obtaining a Palpation Blood Pressure Measurement

7.	Hold the baby's arm straight, with the palm and inner part of the arm facing you.	
8.	Using your index finger of this same hand, feel for the pulse in the baby's brachial artery.	You can usually palpate the artery (feel the pulse) just above the crease of the elbow and slightly toward the inside of the arm.

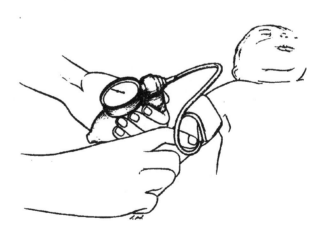

9.	When you feel the pulse well, keep your index finger lightly pressed over this spot.	
10.	Using your other hand, pump up the cuff until the mercury or needle reads approximately 100 mm Hg.	
11.	Release the screw clamp and let the mercury or needle fall fairly quickly until it reaches about 80 mm Hg, then *slow* the rate of fall to approximately 2 mm Hg per second.	*It is important that the mercury or needle falls <u>slowly</u>. If allowed to fall too quickly, the blood pressure reading will be falsely low.*

Actions	Remarks

Obtaining a Palpation Blood Pressure Measurement (continued)

12. Watch the top of the mercury column or needle as it drops. Note the reading on the blood pressure gauge when you first begin to feel the artery pulsate beneath your index finger.

   The blood pressure reading when you first feel the baby's pulse is slightly less than the systolic blood pressure.

13. After the arterial pulsation has been felt, the cuff may be rapidly deflated.

14. Record the blood pressure reading and the method used.

   For example, if the arterial pulsation was first felt at 48 mm Hg, the blood pressure reading may be abbreviated and recorded as

   48 mm Hg/palpation (or 48 mm Hg/P)

What Can Go Wrong?

1. You press your index finger too firmly over the brachial artery.

   You will restrict the blood flow through the artery and get a falsely low blood pressure reading.

2. You are not certain when you first feel the pulse.

   A very sick baby may have weak pulses, making it difficult to obtain an accurate palpation blood pressure reading.

3. You may perform the blood pressure measurement correctly, but not take the blood pressure often enough.

   A sick and unstable infant needs frequent blood pressure determinations. One normal reading does not mean the baby's blood pressure will stay within the normal range.

4. The strap may be wrapped too tightly or the cuff may be left inflated.

   This may restrict the blood flow to the baby's limb for a long time and cause tissue damage.

5. The bladder of the cuff is too small.

   Readings will be falsely high.

6. The bladder of the cuff is too large.

   Readings will be falsely low.

7. You may release the pressure in the cuff too fast.

   Readings will be falsely low.

Unit 6

Hypoglycemia

Objectives

In this unit you will learn to

A. Understand the hazards of hypoglycemia.

B. Identify infants at risk for hypoglycemia.

C. Institute monitoring and preventive measures for infants at risk for hypoglycemia.

D. Recognize the signs of hypoglycemia.

E. Obtain accurate blood glucose screening test results.

F. Treat hypoglycemia and monitor babies receiving treatment.

Unit 6 Pretest

Before reading the unit, please answer the following questions. Select the *one best* answer to each question (unless otherwise instructed). Record your answers on the answer sheet that is the last page in this book *and* on the test.

1. **True** **False** Untreated hypoglycemia in a newborn can cause mental retardation.

2. **True** **False** Intravenous therapy for hypoglycemia should be stopped as soon as the blood glucose screening test results become normal.

3. **True** **False** A baby who is hypoglycemic may have a seizure.

4. **True** **False** Large for gestational age infants are at risk for the development of hypoglycemia.

5. **True** **False** Infants of diabetic women also have diabetes mellitus and, therefore, are at risk for hypoglycemia.

6. **True** **False** A newborn's blood glucose screening test result of 32 mg/dL requires evaluation and treatment.

7. Which of the following term babies is at *highest* risk for hypoglycemia?
    A. Infant whose mother last ate 14 hours prior to delivery
    B. Infant with intrauterine growth restriction
    C. Breastfed infant
    D. Infant who was delivered by planned cesarean section

8. The legs of a term, appropriate for gestational age baby shake uncontrollably for a minute or two. What should you do?
    A. Begin intravenous therapy with 25% glucose.
    B. Wrap the baby in an extra blanket.
    C. Obtain a blood glucose screening test.
    D. Watch the baby to see if the shaking happens again.

9. A baby weighing 3,780 g (8 lb, 5 oz) is born at 38 weeks' gestation to a woman with diabetes mellitus. What is the most appropriate time for this baby's *first* feeding?
    A. 1 to 2 hours of age
    B. 4 to 6 hours of age
    C. 8 to 10 hours of age
    D. On demand

10. A baby is being treated for hypoglycemia. The baby's intravenous (IV) infiltrates at 3:00 am. What should you do?
    A. Pull out the IV and have a new one started immediately.
    B. Leave the IV in and slow the rate.
    C. Pull out the IV and have a new one started when rounds are made at 8:00 am.
    D. Pull out the IV and feed the baby 15% glucose by mouth.

11. A baby has a blood glucose screening test result of 10 mg/dL. What should you do next?
    A. Start feedings of formula or breast milk immediately.
    B. Give 2 mL/kg of 25% glucose intravenously, then run a 10% glucose infusion at 5 mL/kg per hour.
    C. Draw a blood sample for laboratory analysis of blood glucose. Start treatment, if the test confirms low blood glucose, as soon as the test result is known.
    D. Give 2 mL/kg of 10% glucose intravenously, then run a 10% glucose infusion at 5 mL/kg per hour.

For each question, please make sure you have marked your answer on the test and on the answer sheet (last page in book). The test is for you; the answer sheet will need to be turned in for continuing education credit.

1. What Is Hypoglycemia?

Hypoglycemia means low blood sugar (glucose). The blood glucose level is maintained by the body converting glycogen stores to glucose. When glycogen reserves are used up, the blood glucose level drops.

 Untreated hypoglycemia in babies can result in death or permanent neurological damage, including mental retardation.

2. Which Babies Are Likely to Develop Hypoglycemia?

A. Infants of Diabetic Mothers (IDM)

Women with diabetes mellitus often have elevated blood glucose levels. This high blood glucose is passed to the fetus through the placenta.

The fetus is not diabetic and, therefore, increases insulin production to counteract the high blood glucose levels. At delivery, the baby is suddenly separated from the woman's glucose supply. The baby still has very high insulin levels. This causes hypoglycemia to develop in the baby.

Very tight control of maternal diabetes throughout pregnancy may minimize, or eliminate, these effects on the fetus and newborn.

B. Large for Gestational Age (LGA) Babies

Some women develop gestational diabetes mellitus (GDM), a condition unique to pregnancy. This may not be detected. Babies born to women with abnormal glucose tolerance, whether they have diabetes mellitus or GDM, are often LGA. Therefore, all LGA babies should be considered at risk for developing hypoglycemia.

C. Small for Gestational Age (SGA) Babies

These babies have been malnourished in utero and, therefore, have not built up glycogen stores. Their meager glycogen stores are quickly used up after birth. SGA babies also have a relatively greater metabolic rate and, therefore, use more glucose than appropriate for gestational age babies of the same size.

D. Preterm Babies

These babies have not had time to build up glycogen stores. They are also likely to be more stressed at birth than term infants. Their small glycogen reserves may be quickly exhausted after birth.

E. Post-term Babies

Placental function may begin to deteriorate in post-term gestation. This limits the supply of nutrients from the pregnant woman to the fetus. The fetus may then begin to use fetal glycogen stores to meet metabolic demands. Therefore, when the baby is born there is a reduced glycogen reserve, which may be used up quickly.

F. Sick or Stressed Babies

Babies may be stressed because the woman has problems during pregnancy (eg, pregnancy-specific hypertension). Babies may also be stressed if problems develop during labor and/or delivery (eg, abruptio placentae). Babies are stressed after birth if they are sick or have been chilled.

Sick or stressed babies have a higher metabolic rate and need extra energy to keep their body functions as close to normal as possible. Babies use glucose and glycogen stores to produce this extra energy. This may deplete the glycogen stores more quickly than normal and hypoglycemia may develop.

G. Fasted Babies

Babies who must be kept NPO or who cannot take adequate amounts orally may become hypoglycemic as their glycogen stores are depleted. Supplementation with glucose-containing intravenous (IV) fluids is essential for all sick babies and for many at-risk babies.

H. Babies With Polycythemia

Babies whose hematocrit exceeds 65% to 70% are at risk for hypoglycemia, although the mechanism is unclear.

Self-Test

Now answer these questions to test yourself on the information in the last section.

A1. **True False** Babies with hypoglycemia often have low glycogen reserves.

A2. What can happen to a baby who develops hypoglycemia and is not treated properly?

_____

A3. Name 8 categories of babies who are at risk for hypoglycemia

A. _____

B. _____

C. _____

D. _____

E. _____

F. _____

G. _____

H. _____

A4. Infants of diabetic women often have adequate glycogen stores but are at risk for hypoglycemia because

of the high _____ levels they develop in response to their mothers' high blood glucose levels.

Check your answers with the list that follows the Recommended Routines. Correct any incorrect answers and review the appropriate section in the unit.

3. How Is Hypoglycemia Detected?

A. Babies With Signs of Hypoglycemia

The most common signs of hypoglycemia include the following, either individually or in combination:

- *Jitteriness:* The baby is hyperreactive to sudden stimuli.
- *Tremors:* An arm or leg shakes uncontrollably.
- *Seizures:* A part of the body shakes rhythmically or becomes rigid.
- *Lethargy:* The baby responds sluggishly or not at all to normal stimuli.
- *Apnea:* Breathing stops suddenly; the baby may turn blue.
- *No signs:* Blood glucose can be very low without giving any clinical indication.

 Some babies with hypoglycemia will not show any signs.

If a baby displays any signs of hypoglycemia, a blood glucose screening test should be obtained *immediately.* A variety of small, handheld blood glucose screening instruments are available for this purpose.

B. Babies With Risk Factors for Hypoglycemia

Newborns at risk for hypoglycemia should have a blood glucose screening test obtained within 1 hour after birth. Even if the first test result is normal, these at-risk babies should have tests repeated until there is adequate glucose intake (feedings and/or IV fluids) and at least 3 hourly test results have been 45 mg/dL or higher.

4. How Is Hypoglycemia Treated in Babies?

There is some controversy about the specific blood glucose value that should be used to define hypoglycemia. Most experts agree, however, that blood glucose in newborns should be maintained above 40 mg/dL and that a screening test value below 45 mg/dL requires evaluation and some form of treatment.

A low screening test result should be confirmed with an actual blood glucose level.

 However, <u>do not wait</u> for the blood glucose result before starting therapy. All low blood glucose screening test results should be treated promptly.

Appropriate treatment depends on the degree of hypoglycemia. Early, frequent feedings are used to prevent hypoglycemia in at-risk babies. Early, frequent feedings are also used to treat slightly low blood glucose in any baby. If blood glucose falls, or if a baby develops signs of hypoglycemia, IV infusion of glucose is required.

267

A. Prevention of Hypoglycemia for At-Risk Babies

Treatment for at-risk babies is aimed at *prevention* of hypoglycemia. In some cases, hypoglycemia will still develop. It is, therefore, important to *continue to monitor blood glucose screening tests.*

- Start early, frequent feedings. Give the first feeding *within* 4 hours after birth. For some babies, it may be appropriate to start feedings less than 1 hour after birth.

- Use formula (not glucose water) if a baby is able to tolerate nipple or tube feedings.

- Put breastfed babies to the breast frequently, and follow blood glucose screening tests closely.

- Continue to check blood glucose screening tests for at-risk babies until formula or breast milk feedings are well established.

- Give 10% glucose intravenously to babies who are NPO or are unable to tolerate nipple or tube feedings.

B. Treatment for Babies Who Have Developed Hypoglycemia

 Low blood glucose must be brought up quickly. The longer a baby is left with hypoglycemia, the greater the chance of brain damage.

- *Treatment Recommendations* are given in the chart below, according to blood glucose screening test results.

Table 6.1. Treatment Recommendations

Screening Test Results	*Actions*
<20–25 mg/dL	1. Draw blood glucose. 2. Start IV with 10% glucose. Give 2 mL/kg over 5 minutes. 3. Run IV at 5 mL/kg/hour 4. Obtain another screening test or blood glucose level within 15–30 minutes. If test result remains <20–25 mg/dL, 15% glucose may be needed. 5. Keep NPO initially. Begin frequent feedings as soon as blood glucose is normal, baby is stable, and baby is able to feed. 6. Monitor with frequent blood glucose screening tests.

Between 20–45 mg/dL	1. Draw blood glucose.
	2. Begin early, frequent feedings (within 4 hours of birth).
	3. Supplement with 10% glucose intravenously if
	  • Feedings are not tolerated.
	       or
	  • Blood glucose screening test remains 20–45 mg/dL.
	4. Monitor with frequent blood glucose screening tests.

- *Highly Concentrated Glucose:* When bringing blood glucose levels up quickly, **do *not* use highly concentrated glucose** solutions (such as 25% or 50% glucose). Rapid infusions of such concentrated glucose may cause brain damage in small babies.

- *Infusion of Glucose Higher Than 12.5%:* If continuous infusion of glucose in a concentration higher than 12.5% is needed, infusion through a peripheral IV should be avoided. Infiltration of IV fluids containing concentrated glucose can cause severe tissue damage.

  Infusions of concentrated glucose should be through a central line, such as an umbilical venous catheter (UVC). If a UVC is used, the tip should be placed above the diaphragm to avoid infusion of concentrated glucose solutions into the circulation of the liver. (See Umbilical Catheters in this book.) When an umbilical catheter is in place, it is generally recommended that a baby be kept NPO.

  The concentration of glucose can usually be decreased gradually so that a peripheral infusion of glucose can be used, the UVC removed, and then feedings started.

- *Stopping IV Glucose:* As feedings are tolerated, the infusion should be tapered gradually as blood glucose screening tests are checked frequently. The glucose infusion may be required for 24 to 48 hours or longer.

 Low blood glucose must be <u>treated quickly</u>, but IV glucose therapy should be <u>terminated gradually</u>, or hypoglycemia may recur.

5. Do Some Babies Need Additional Blood Glucose Monitoring?

Certain babies may need blood glucose monitoring for several days after birth. Babies treated for hypoglycemia may have an undetected recurrence if monitoring is stopped too soon. At-risk babies with low glucose stores may do well initially but develop late-onset hypoglycemia at several days of age, particularly if a baby becomes sick or stressed or eats poorly.

A. Monitoring Babies At Risk for Hypoglycemia

- Continue to obtain blood glucose screening tests until full feedings are well established. This is especially important for breastfed babies because the actual volume of milk a baby takes is unknown.

- Obtain the blood glucose screening tests before the baby eats because blood glucose is likely to be lowest just prior to a feeding.

- Consider supplemental feedings for at-risk babies who are being breastfed, if they cannot maintain their prefeeding blood glucose in the normal range.

B. Monitoring Babies Treated for Hypoglycemia

- After beginning IV glucose therapy, frequently check the placement and flow of a baby's IV. If the IV becomes infiltrated, another one should be started without delay.

- Even if a baby is receiving treatment for hypoglycemia, screening test values or blood glucose levels must be checked within 15 to 30 minutes of starting therapy and frequently thereafter. This is done to be sure the baby is receiving enough glucose.

- If a baby has a blood glucose (or blood glucose screening test) less than 20 to 25 mg/dL or has signs of hypoglycemia, oral feeding should be delayed until blood glucose has been increased by IV therapy. A hypoglycemic baby may not be able to coordinate swallowing and breathing and therefore may aspirate feedings.

- Obtain blood glucose screening tests frequently while the glucose infusion is being tapered and until full feedings become established.

The flow chart on the next page summarizes the detection, prevention, and treatment of hypoglycemia. Review the chart, then answer the questions on the following page.

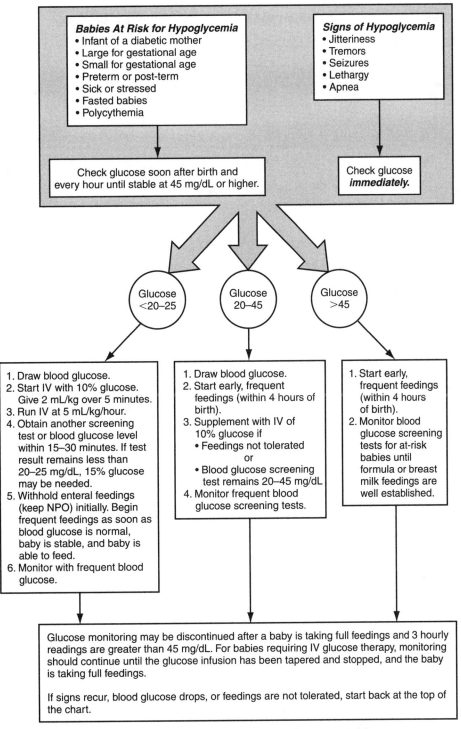

Babies At Risk for Hypoglycemia
- Infant of a diabetic mother
- Large for gestational age
- Small for gestational age
- Preterm or post-term
- Sick or stressed
- Fasted babies
- Polycythemia

Signs of Hypoglycemia
- Jitteriness
- Tremors
- Seizures
- Lethargy
- Apnea

Check glucose soon after birth and every hour until stable at 45 mg/dL or higher.

Check glucose *immediately.*

Glucose <20–25

Glucose 20–45

Glucose >45

1. Draw blood glucose.
2. Start IV with 10% glucose. Give 2 mL/kg over 5 minutes.
3. Run IV at 5 mL/kg/hour.
4. Obtain another screening test or blood glucose level within 15–30 minutes. If test result remains less than 20–25 mg/dL, 15% glucose may be needed.
5. Withhold enteral feedings (keep NPO) initially. Begin frequent feedings as soon as blood glucose is normal, baby is stable, and baby is able to feed.
6. Monitor with frequent blood glucose.

1. Draw blood glucose.
2. Start early, frequent feedings (within 4 hours of birth).
3. Supplement with IV of 10% glucose if
   - Feedings not tolerated
     or
   - Blood glucose screening test remains 20–45 mg/dL
4. Monitor frequent blood glucose screening tests.

1. Start early, frequent feedings (within 4 hours of birth).
2. Monitor blood glucose screening tests for at-risk babies until formula or breast milk feedings are well established.

Glucose monitoring may be discontinued after a baby is taking full feedings and 3 hourly readings are greater than 45 mg/dL. For babies requiring IV glucose therapy, monitoring should continue until the glucose infusion has been tapered and stopped, and the baby is taking full feedings.

If signs recur, blood glucose drops, or feedings are not tolerated, start back at the top of the chart.

Low blood glucose must be *brought up quickly.*
IV glucose infusion should be *tapered gradually.*

Figure 6.1. Prevention, Detection, and Treatment of Neonatal Hypoglycemia

Now answer these questions to test yourself on the information in the last section.

B1. What are 5 of the most common signs of hypoglycemia?

    A. _____

    B. _____

    C. _____

    D. _____

    E. _____

B2. A baby has a blood glucose screening test value of 40 mg/dL. What would you do?

    A. Prepare for a blood glucose determination.

    B. Begin early feedings and repeat the blood glucose screening test in 1 hour.

    C. No action indicated.

B3. A baby with hypoglycemia should have the low blood glucose level brought up

    A. Quickly

    B. Slowly

B4. A baby has a blood glucose of 10 mg/dL. What is the *first* thing that should be done to treat the hypoglycemia?

    A. Intravenous therapy with normal saline

    B. Early feedings

    C. Intravenous therapy with 10% glucose

B5. **True   False**   A blood glucose screening test result of 0 to 25 mg/dL should be confirmed with a blood glucose level.

B6. Which of the following solutions is correct to use for treatment of hypoglycemia?

    A. 10% glucose

    B. 25% glucose

    C. 50% glucose

B7. **True   False**   It is important to obtain blood glucose screening tests even while a baby is receiving intravenous glucose in the treatment of hypoglycemia.

B8. **True   False**   A baby with low blood glucose will always have at least one sign of hypoglycemia.

B9. A 4,000-g (8 lb, 13 oz) baby has a blood glucose screening test result of 20 mg/dL. You draw a blood glucose level, then immediately begin treatment with an intravenous infusion of 10% dextrose.

How much would you give initially? _____

What rate would you set for the infusion? _____

Check your answers with the list that follows the Recommended Routines. Correct any incorrect answers and review the appropriate section in the unit.

Recommended Routines

All of the routines listed below are based on the principles of perinatal care presented in the unit you have just finished. They are recommended as part of routine perinatal care.

Read each routine carefully and decide whether it is standard operating procedure in your hospital. Check the appropriate blank next to each routine.

Procedure Standard in My Hospital	Needs Discussion by Our Staff	
_____	_____	1. Establish standing orders that will ensure blood glucose screening for all babies at risk for hypoglycemia.
_____	_____	2. Establish a policy of starting feedings at • No more than 4 to 6 hours of age for well babies • Less than 4 hours of age for babies at risk for hypoglycemia
_____	_____	3. Establish a policy of regular calibration and quality control measures for the bedside glucose screening instrument(s) used in your hospital. This procedure should follow manufacturer's instructions and be in accordance with your hospital's policy regarding point-of-care tests.

These are the answers to the self-test questions. Please check them with the answers you gave and review the information in the unit wherever necessary.

A1.   True

A2.   Death or permanent neurological damage, including mental retardation.

A3.   A.   Infants of diabetic mothers
      B.   Large for gestational age babies
      C.   Small for gestational age babies
      D.   Preterm babies
      E.   Post-term babies
      F.   Sick or stressed babies
      G.   Fasted babies
      H.   Babies with polycythemia

A4.   Insulin

B1.   A.   Jitteriness
      B.   Tremors
      C.   Seizures
      D.   Lethargy
      E.   Apnea
      - OR -
      F.   No signs

B2.   A and B

B3.   A.   Quickly.

B4.   C.   Intravenous therapy with 10% glucose

B5.   True   However, treatment for the hypoglycemia should begin immediately, before the result of the blood glucose level is known.

B6.   A.   10% glucose

B7.   True

B8.   False   Some babies with hypoglycemia may not have any signs. Lack of signs does not mean the baby's hypoglycemia is less significant.

B9.   *Initial dose* is 2 mL/kg given slowly: 2 mL × 4.0 kg = 8 mL.
      Continuous infusion is 5 mL/kg/hr: 5 mL × 4.0 kg = 20 mL/hr
      You would give 8 mL of 10% glucose intravenously over 5 to 10 minutes. This should be followed by a continuous infusion of 10% glucose at a rate of 20 mL per hour.

Unit 6 Posttest

Without referring back to the information in the unit, please answer the following questions. Select the **one best** answer to each question (unless otherwise instructed). Record your answers on the answer sheet that is the last page in this book **and** on the test.

1. **True** **False** All babies with hypoglycemia severe enough to require treatment will show one or more of the clinical signs of hypoglycemia.

2. **True** **False** Intravenous glucose therapy for a baby with proven hypoglycemia should be stopped as soon as the baby's blood glucose level reaches 45 mg/dL.

3. **True** **False** It is rarely necessary to continue blood glucose screening tests after an intravenous infusion of glucose has been started on a baby.

4. **True** **False** Infants of diabetic women are at risk for hypoglycemia after birth.

5. **True** **False** Preterm and post-term infants are at risk for hypoglycemia.

6. **True** **False** It is generally agreed that a newborn's blood glucose should be kept above 40 mg/dL.

7. Which of the following actions may help to prevent hypoglycemia?
   - **A.** Bathe the baby as soon as possible.
   - **B.** Delay feeding for 12 hours.
   - **C.** Lower the baby's inspired oxygen concentration.
   - **D.** Keep the baby at normal body temperature.

8. A vigorous 4-hour-old baby has a blood glucose screening test result of 20 to 40 mg/dL. After drawing blood for glucose determination, what else should you do?
   - **A.** Watch the baby and repeat the test in 1 hour.
   - **B.** No action is indicated.
   - **C.** Feed the baby and repeat the test in 1 hour.
   - **D.** Administer 4 mL of 50% glucose intravenously immediately.

9. A baby weighing 2,400 g (5 lb, 5 oz) is born with an estimated gestational age of 39 weeks. The baby is small for gestational age but is not sick. What would you plan to do for this baby?
   - **A.** Start feedings within 4 hours after birth.
   - **B.** Start feedings between 6 and 8 hours after birth.
   - **C.** Give 6 mL of 25% glucose intravenously.
   - **D.** Begin intravenous therapy with 15% glucose.

10. When hypoglycemia is not treated, which consequence may develop?
    - **A.** Significant weight loss
    - **B.** Brain damage
    - **C.** Partial blindness
    - **D.** Onset of diabetes mellitus

11. A baby born at 43 weeks' gestation has a seizure at 2 hours of age. What should you do *immediately*?
    - **A.** Insert an umbilical venous catheter for medication administration.
    - **B.** Obtain a blood glucose screening test.
    - **C.** Feed the baby.
    - **D.** Draw blood for laboratory determination of blood glucose.

For each question, please make sure you have marked your answer on the test and on the answer sheet (last page in book). The test is for you; the answer sheet will need to be turned in for continuing education credit.

Blood Glucose Screening Tests

This skill unit will teach you how to perform a blood glucose screening test. Several brands of glucose readers are commercially available. If your hospital uses more than one brand of glucometer in the perinatal care areas, you will need to learn how to use each brand.

Study this skill unit, then attend a skill practice and demonstration session.

To master the skill, you will need to demonstrate correctly each of the following steps:

1. Calibrate the electronic reader(s) used in your hospital according to manufacturer's instructions.

2. Milk blood toward baby's heel and/or wrap foot in warm compress (may be optional if using an automated incision device).

3. Prepare heel.

4. Prick heel.

5. Touch drop of blood to reagent strip or microchamber.

6. Record test results.

Perinatal Performance Guide
Blood Glucose Screening Tests

Several different manufacturers produce a variety of electronic instruments designed for bedside screening of blood for blood glucose level. This skill unit will describe the general technique for obtaining a blood sample and delivering it to a glucometer, but details of the procedure are different for different brands of machines. Be sure to follow manufacturer's instructions for the testing materials and device(s) used in your hospital.

Actions	Remarks

Deciding to Use a Blood Glucose Screening Test

1. Ask yourself "Is there any reason to suspect the baby's blood glucose level may be low?"

   - Does the mother have diabetes mellitus?

   - Is the baby small or large for gestational age?

   - Is the baby preterm or post-term?

   - Is the baby sick or been stressed?

   - Does the baby have polycythemia (hematocrit >65%)?

   - Does the baby have any signs of hypoglycemia (lethargic, irritable, tremors, seizures, jittery, unexplained apnea spell)?

   - Is the baby not being fed enterally or not taking adequate feedings?

   Yes: Do a screening test.

   No: There is no indication a blood glucose screening test is needed.

Obtaining a Blood Glucose Screening Test

2. Collect the proper equipment.

   - Reagent test or microchamber strip

   - Alcohol swab

   - Sterile 2 x 2 gauze

   - Adhesive bandage (optional)

   - Heel warmer (optional)

   - Incision device for blood sampling*

   Test strips gradually deteriorate after a container is opened. Always use the original container to store strips, label the bottle with the date first opened, and close the cap tightly immediately after obtaining a strip.

   Select the size that matches the size of the baby.

---

*Tenderfoot, by International Technidyne Corporation (www.itcmed.com), and NeatNick, by Hawaii Medical (www.hawaiimedical.com), are examples.

Actions	**Remarks**

Obtaining a Blood Glucose Screening Test (continued)

3. Prepare the glucose monitor according to the manufacturer's instructions and your hospital's policy regarding tests done at the bedside.

   Electronic readers may require a drop of blood to be absorbed into the microchamber of a disposable test strip. The microchamber is then inserted into the reader, which gives a blood glucose value in a specified number of seconds.

The readers, or glucometers, must be checked against a quality control standard. Usually this check is performed when

- A new bottle of test strips is opened.
- The lid was left off a bottle of test strips.
- The monitor was dropped.
- Test results do not seem to match clinical condition.
- Glucometer batteries were changed.
- A specified period of time (usually 24 hours) has elapsed since the last check was done.

Know the specific quality control procedure for the glucometer you are using.

4. Take the baby's leg in your hand. Gently milk the blood toward the heel, then gently squeeze the foot. Release your squeeze and milk again. Repeat this until the sole of the foot is bright pink.

   Note: This step is generally not needed when an automated incision device is used.

This is to ensure freshly circulated capillary blood in the baby's foot, and that blood will flow readily when the heel is pricked. If time allows, it is preferable to achieve the same effect by wrapping a warm compress or heel warmer around the baby's foot for 5 to 10 minutes.

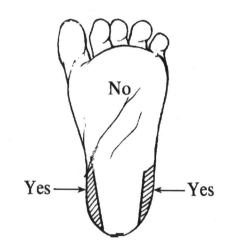

5. Identify the spot to prick to obtain the blood sample.

   Better blood flow is obtained when the inside of the heel is pricked. The outside of the heel may also be used, but do *not* prick the

   - Sole of the foot

   - Center or the back of the heel

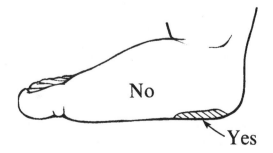

Actions   **Remarks**

Obtaining a Blood Glucose Screening Test (continued)

6. Clean the baby's heel with the alcohol swab.

7. Dry the alcohol with the sterile 2 x 2 gauze.

8. Stick the heel with a quick determined thrust of   If using a microlancet (shown in illustration,
    the microlancet or use an automated incision   below), cautious, tiny jabs may cause trauma to the
    device.   skin but not produce any blood.

    Note: There is evidence that spring-loaded
            automatic microlancets need fewer
            repeat punctures and are associated
            with fewer newborn distress responses
            than manual lancets.

            A manual lancet is illustrated.

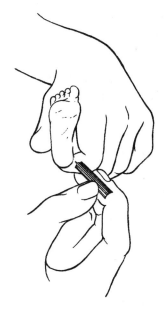

9. Repeatedly milk the baby's leg toward the heel.
    Then gently squeeze the leg and foot until a
    drop of blood appears (shown below, right).

    Note: If using an automated incision device,
            you will generally not need to milk the
            leg because blood usually flows freely.

10. Touch the opening of the microchamber or the
    reagent strip to the drop of blood.

    Capillary action will fill the microchamber with
    blood. Be sure the chamber is completely filled.

    For some strips, additional blood may be
    applied for up to 15 seconds to fill the chamber.
    Be certain you know how the testing materials
    and glucometer(s) used in your hospital work.

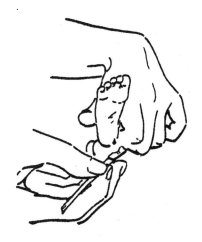

Actions	Remarks

Obtaining a Blood Glucose Screening Test (continued)

11. Put the reagent strip or microchamber into the glucose reader.

The machine will take a specified time (usually a precise number of seconds) to register a reading.

12. Record the glucose screening test result and time in the baby's chart.

If you get a low blood glucose screening test result, you should confirm this by sending a blood sample to the laboratory for chemical analysis of blood glucose. However, do not wait for the laboratory result before starting therapy.

13. Soothe the baby. A variety of comfort measures can be used alone or in combination to manage heelstick pain. These include

Reducing pain and helping a baby to self-regulate following a painful procedure can reduce short-term physiologic and biochemical stress responses.

- Facilitated tucking (extremities flexed and held close to infant's trunk)

- Positioning and nesting

- Gentle, rhythmic stroking, patting, or rocking

- Swaddling

- Pacifier use for nonnutritive sucking

- Pacifier with 24% sucrose solution

What Can Go Wrong?

1. The baby's heel is not dry, thus resulting in diluted blood.

Reading will be low.

2. The test strip has deteriorated.

Reading will be false. Be sure to put the lid tightly on the bottle after obtaining a strip. Label the bottle with the date it is first opened. Discard containers according to manufacturer's recommendations and/or expiration date on the container, whichever comes sooner.

3. You prick the center or back of the baby's heel.

This may have serious, long-term consequences. Repeated pricks over the weight-bearing center of the heel can cause scar tissue formation and result in delayed walking and/or abnormal gait. Pricks over the back of the heel can damage the Achilles tendon.

Numerous repeated blood samples may be safely obtained, however, when the heel is pricked within the shaded areas shown in the illustrations that accompany step 5 of the previous section.

Actions	Remarks

What Can Go Wrong? (continued)

Actions	Remarks
4. The baby's foot or leg is bruised after the procedure.	Excessive squeezing was used to obtain the drop of blood. Bruising should *not* occur. Good blood flow can be obtained by warming the baby's foot and/or by milking the blood in the leg toward the heel, or by correctly using an automated incision device.
5. Quality control checks are not performed regularly.	Be sure to follow the manufacturer's directions for the quality control procedure and recommended frequency of checks for the specific glucose reader used in your hospital. You should also know your hospital's policy regarding point-of-care laboratory tests.
6. You use a manual lancet or an incorrect size of automatic incision device and go too far into the baby's flesh.	The depth of penetration of a manual lancet is variable. Automatic devices enter the skin a controlled, standard depth, but must be the correct device for the size of the baby in your care. Devices for term babies enter the skin farther than devices designed for smaller babies. Devices are generally available in term and preterm neonatal sizes, and sometimes in a third size for extremely preterm babies.

Intravenous Therapy

Objectives

In this unit you will learn

A. The purpose of intravenous therapy

B. Routes and types of fluid therapy

C. What normal and abnormal fluid losses may occur in a baby

D. How to tell if a baby is getting too much or too little fluid

E. When to stop an intravenous infusion

Note: In this unit you will *not* learn the fluid management for complex situations (eg, severely compromised infant, extremely preterm infant, and/or infant requiring parenteral nutrition).

   In any situation in which fluid management seems to be a problem, further consultation should be obtained.

Unit 7 Pretest

Before reading the unit, please answer the following questions. Select the *one best* answer to each question (unless otherwise instructed). Record your answers on the answer sheet that is the last page in this book *and* on the test.

1. Which of the following babies should receive intravenous therapy?

Yes	No	
___	___	A 1,590-g (3 lb, 8 oz) vigorous baby on the first day after birth
___	___	A 3,175-g (7 lb) baby with Apgar scores of 6 at 1 minute and 9 at 5 minutes
___	___	A 3,620-g (8 lb) baby with suspected sepsis who has taken 120 mL (4 oz) of formula during the past 24 hours
___	___	A 2,720-g (6 lb) vigorous baby whose mother was hospitalized with bacterial pneumonia at 20 weeks' gestation

2. An umbilical venous catheter is appropriately inserted when a baby weighing 1,900 g needs

   A. Frequent blood gas determinations
   B. An exchange transfusion
   C. 10 days of intravenous antibiotics
   D. Intravenous fluids to supplement oral intake

3. Which intravenous fluid should be used during the first 24 hours after birth for a baby with no specific complications?

   A. 10% dextrose in water with 10% sodium bicarbonate added
   B. Lactated Ringer's solution
   C. 10% dextrose in 1/4 normal saline with 20 mEq of KCl added to each 1,000 mL
   D. 10% dextrose in water

4. How much fluid does a term baby need after the first 48 hours of postnatal age?

   A. 80 mL/kg/24 hours
   B. 100 mL/kg/24 hours
   C. 120 mL/kg/24 hours
   D. 180 mL/kg/24 hours

5. **True   False**   The specific gravity of a baby's urine is 1.026. This may indicate the baby is receiving too much fluid.

6. A baby who is NPO has been receiving intravenous therapy for 4 days. Which test(s) should this baby routinely receive?

   A. Blood electrolyte values
   B. Hemoglobin and hematocrit
   C. Complete blood count
   D. Serum bilirubin level

7. A 6-day-old, 2,500g (5 lb, 8 oz) baby is receiving adequate fluid. How much would you expect his daily urine output to be?

   A. 40 mL
   B. 100 mL
   C. 140 mL
   D. 200 mL

8. Approximately how much fluid should a 2,700-g (5 lb, 15 oz) baby receive during the third day after birth?

   A. 225 mL/24 hours
   B. 275 mL/24 hours
   C. 325 mL/24 hours
   D. 375 mL/24 hours

For each question, please make sure you have marked your answer on the test and on the answer sheet (last page in book). The test is for you; the answer sheet will need to be turned in for continuing education credit.

1. What Is Intravenous (IV) Therapy?

Intravenous (IV) therapy means fluid, blood, or medication given through a needle or catheter that has been inserted into a blood vessel.

2. What Is the Purpose of Intravenous Therapy

Intravenous therapy has several purposes. They include to

- Replace or maintain body stores of water and electrolytes

- Replenish blood volume

- Give medication

- Provide calories, in the form of glucose (Calories in the form of protein and fat can also be delivered intravenously, but will not be discussed in this unit.)

3. Which Babies Should Receive IV Fluids?

- All sick babies

- Babies with low blood glucose

- All babies who are NPO or who cannot take an adequate amount of fluid with nipple or tube feedings

- All babies weighing less than 1,800 g (4 lb)

It is generally recommended that IV fluids be started early for babies weighing 1,800 g or less. As nipple or tube feedings become established, IV fluids should be tapered.

4. What Routes Are Used for IVs in Babies?

Different intravascular routes are used for different purposes.

- *Umbilical artery*
  — Used for arterial blood gas sampling and/or direct blood pressure monitoring
  — Not used for blood, medications, or fluids unless another IV route is not available

- *Umbilical vein*
  — Used for exchange transfusion, emergency medications, or fluids during the first few days in extremely preterm babies
  — Not used for routine fluids, unless another IV route is not available

- *Peripheral vein* (hand, foot, or scalp vein)
  — Used for maintenance fluids, medications, and/or blood transfusion

Note: Central venous lines, placed either percutaneously or surgically, are often used when long-term IV therapy is needed for sick or small babies, but are not covered in the Perinatal Continuing Education Program (PCEP) books.

Self-Test

Now answer these questions to test yourself on the information in the last section.

A1. Which of these babies should receive intravenous therapy?

    A. A baby weighing 3,175 g (7 lb) with sepsis and unstable heart rate

    B. A baby weighing 3,670 g (8 lb) taking 30 mL of formula per day

    C. A baby weighing 1,500 g (3 lb, 5 oz) on the first day of postnatal life

A2. Describe the route you would use for these purposes.

    A. Give blood to baby with normal vital signs: _____

    B. Draw blood for blood gas analysis: _____

    C. Administer emergency medications during resuscitation: _____

    D. Administer antibiotics: _____

    E. Carry out an exchange transfusion: _____

A3. Name 4 reasons why you might use intravenous therapy for a baby.

    A. _____

    B. _____

    C. _____

    D. _____

A4. A 2-hour-old baby weighing 1,800 g (4 lb) develops hypoglycemic seizures and is given 15% glucose by umbilical vein. Would you start an intravenous line on this baby?

_____

If so, what kind? _____

Check your answers with the list that follows the Recommended Routines. Correct any incorrect answers and review the appropriate section in the unit.

5. How Does a Baby Lose Fluid?

A. Normal Losses

An infant normally loses fluid from the *skin and respiratory passages*. This is called *insensible water loss*. In term infants, insensible losses usually amount to about 35 to 40 mL/kg per day. Insensible water losses may be higher in preterm infants, especially extremely low birth weight babies.

The remainder of a baby's normal fluid losses are in *feces and urine*.

B. Abnormal Losses

- Vomiting
- Diarrhea
- Bleeding
- Excessive urine output
- Frequent blood sampling
- Increased insensible loss
  - *Phototherapy:* May increase insensible loss by as much as 40%.
  - *Radiant warmer:* May increase insensible loss by as much as 100%.
  - *Extremely preterm babies:* Insensible loss may increase by as much as 100%.

6. Which IV Solutions Are Used for Babies?

For simplicity of computation, electrolyte requirements are presented in this unit in terms of electrolyte *concentration* in the IV fluid (eg, 1/4 normal saline). The recommendations will result in delivery of the appropriate amount of electrolytes to babies with normal kidney and heart function. Babies with impaired kidney and/or cardiac function present complex management problems and require frequent adjustment of their IV electrolyte solutions.

While receiving IV therapy, a baby's blood electrolytes and glucose need to be checked. The composition of IV fluid is readjusted if values are not within normal ranges.

The IV solutions described below are suggestions for short-term maintenance therapy. Individualized therapy is needed for babies requiring long-term or complex management.

A. During the First 24 Hours After Birth

10% dextrose in water ($D_{10}W$) for most babies. Some babies will require concentrations of dextrose higher or lower than 10%.

B. After 24 Hours of Postnatal Life

$D_{10}W$ (or other appropriate concentration of dextrose) in 1/4 normal saline with 20 mEq of potassium (as potassium chloride) per 1,000 mL of fluid

C. Unusual Circumstances

- *Sick babies*—These babies may need other solutions such as blood or fluids with higher or lower electrolyte concentration. Long-term fluid management may become complex.

- *Babies with low blood glucose*—These babies may require more glucose than is supplied in $D_{10}W$. Solutions of $D_{12.5}W$, $D_{15}W$, or even $D_{20}W$ are sometimes needed.

- *Extremely preterm infants*—D_5W should be used initially and later changed to fluids containing more glucose. Fluids containing fat and protein will also be needed but fluid therapy and nutrition for tiny babies are not covered in PCEP.

7. How Much Fluid Does a Baby Need?

A. Preterm, Term, and Post-Term Babies

- *During the first 24 hours after birth:* 80 mL/kg/24 hours
  During the first postnatal day, babies need less fluid than later in life. Over the next 2 days infant fluid requirements gradually increase.

- *During 24 to 48 hours after birth:* 100 mL/kg/24 hours

- *More than 48 hours after birth:* 120 mL/kg/24 hours

Frequently an at-risk baby may be able to take nipple or tube feedings but not in sufficient amount to give the volume of fluid the baby needs for a 24-hour period. The additional fluid the baby requires may be supplied by a peripheral IV.

B. Babies Following Resuscitation

Newborns who had low Apgar scores or required prolonged resuscitation may not have normal kidney or heart function. Fluids may need to be restricted to as little as 35 to 40 mL/kg/day (insensible losses) for term babies, or somewhat higher for preterm babies.

C. Extremely Preterm Babies

- *During the first 24 hours after birth,* extremely preterm babies need more fluid. This is because of their proportionately larger surface area compared to body weight, which results in greater insensible water losses through the skin. These babies should receive 100 mL or more of fluid for each kilogram (2 lb, 3 oz) of body weight during the first 24 hours (100 mL/kg/24 hours).

- *After 24 hours of postnatal life,* the fluid management for extremely preterm babies becomes very complex. Insensible water losses are variable and unpredictable. Complications such as patent ductus arteriosus, intraventricular hemorrhage, hyperglycemia, and electrolyte imbalance become much more likely. These conditions mandate special considerations for fluid management, which are not discussed in this program. Consult your regional perinatal center staff.

Example: You are caring for a 3-day-old 3,100-g (6 lb, 13 1/2 oz) baby born at term and being evaluated for neurologic depression.

1. *How much fluid does the baby need per day?*

    - She needs 120 mL per kilogram of body weight per day.
    - Therefore 120 mL $\times$ 3.1 kg = 372 mL needed per day

2. *You find the baby will take only 30 mL every 3 hours by nipple. How much fluid is she getting by nipple per day?*

    - 24 ÷ 3 = 8 feedings per 24-hour period
    - 8 feedings $\times$ 30 mL = 240 mL per day by nipple

3. *You should give the baby more fluids by IV. How much fluid does she need by IV?*

    - 372 mL needed/day − 240 mL received by feedings = 132 mL needed by IV/day

4. *What rate of flow per hour should you use to give the baby 132 mL in 24 hours?*

    - 132 mL ÷ 24 hours = 5.5 mL per hour

Self-Test

Now answer these questions to test yourself on the information in the last section.

B1. What special action will you probably need to take for babies who are under radiant warmers or phototherapy lights?

_____

B2. When is D_5W or $D_{10}W$ (without saline or potassium chloride) usually used as the intravenous fluid for babies?

_____

B3. A newborn baby weighs 3,000 g (6 lb, 10 oz). How much fluid does the baby need during the first 24 hours after birth?

_____

B4. How much fluid should a 2,500-g (5 lb, 8 oz) baby take in each 24 hours *after* the first 48 hours of postnatal life?

_____

B5. The baby in question B4 takes 150 mL/24 hours by bottle feedings. How much intravenous fluid should the baby get to supplement the liquids received from feedings?

_____

B6. What is insensible water loss?

_____

B7. You are caring for a 3-day-old baby being treated with antibiotics for suspected sepsis. The baby weighs 2,600 g (5 lb, 12 oz). The baby is vigorous but takes only 20 mL of formula every 3 hours. How much fluid should the baby be given intravenously?

_____ mL per day

_____ mL per hour

B8. Most babies who have suffered severe perinatal compromise will require _____ fluids during the first few days after birth.

   A. Increased
   B. Decreased

Check your answers with the list that follows the Recommended Routines. Correct any incorrect answers and review the appropriate section in the unit.

8. How Do You Know a Baby Is Getting Too Much or Too Little?

A. Day-to-Day Changes in Body Weight

- *With the exception of extremely post-term or small for gestational age babies, babies normally lose weight during the first few days after birth.* After that, the normal daily weight gain is approximately 20 to 30 g per day. (See the next unit, Feeding, for details regarding caloric requirements and expected weight gain.)

  Obtaining daily weights is not always practical with sick infants. If it is possible to weigh the baby, the most accurate weights are obtained when an infant is weighed on the same scale at the same time of day, before a feeding. It is also important to note if any equipment is weighed with the baby.

- *Excessive weight gain* may mean an infant is receiving more fluid than necessary, that a baby's kidneys are not putting out urine as well as they should, or that a baby is in congestive heart failure.

- *Excessive weight loss* may be due to an inadequate fluid or calorie intake, the kidneys putting out too much urine, or a baby losing extra fluid by some other route.

B. Volume of Urine Output

- *Normal volume of urine output* in a 24-hour period is approximately 40 mL/kg of body weight (1–2 mL/kg/hour).

  1. *Urine may be collected to measure output.*

     A commercially available plastic bag placed over the baby's genitalia with the edges sealed with adhesive may be used to collect urine. To avoid frequent removal and reapplication of the bag and adhesive, a feeding tube may be inserted into the bag through a tiny slit. The tube is sealed in the insertion slit with plastic tape to prevent leaks around the tube. A syringe is attached to the feeding tube and urine aspirated from the bag for measurement and/or analysis.

  2. *Urine output may be estimated by weight.*

     - The dry weight of a diaper is calculated. (If commercial disposable diapers are used, an average dry weight may be determined, rather than weighing each separate diaper.)

     - After a baby voids, the wet diaper is weighed and the difference between the dry and wet weight in grams is determined. This difference is a close estimate of the number of milliliters of urine voided by the baby.

     - If a baby is under a radiant warmer it is important to weigh diapers frequently because urine on a diaper will evaporate quickly under a radiant warmer.

- *Decrease in urine output* may occur when there is inadequate fluid intake or when the kidneys are damaged and unable to make urine normally, especially following an episode of severe hypoxia. Babies with heart disease may have low urine output and retain fluid, as reflected by excessive weight gain.

- *Increase in urine output* may occur when a baby is getting too much fluid or when the kidneys are damaged and unable to conserve fluid appropriately.

C. Concentration of Urine, Measured as Specific Gravity

- *Normal specific gravity range for babies is 1.008 to 1.012.* Only a few drops of urine are needed to obtain a urine specific gravity reading.

- *Increase in specific gravity* occurs when a baby is getting less fluid and the kidneys are trying to conserve fluid, or when there is sugar in the urine.

- *Decrease in specific gravity* occurs when a baby is receiving more fluid than necessary or is unable to concentrate the urine because of kidney damage or diuretic therapy.

Now answer these questions to test yourself on the information in the last section.

C1. What is the normal expected weight gain per 24 hours of an appropriate size for gestational age baby weighing 3,000 g at 5 days of age?

_____

C2. What is the normal urine output of a baby weighing 2,000 g?

_____ mL/24 hours

_____ mL/hour

C3. A baby is receiving intravenous therapy. What would you do to obtain the baby's daily weight?

Yes   **No**

___   ___   Obtain the baby's weight at the same time each day.

___   ___   Remove all equipment attached to the baby.

___   ___   Use the same scale for every weight.

___   ___   Weigh the baby before a feeding.

___   ___   Weigh the baby immediately after a feeding.

C4. What are 2 methods of measuring urine output?

_____ or _____

C5. A 2,500-g baby's daily urine output is 40 mL.

Is this in the normal range? ___ Yes ___ No

If not, what could have caused this? _____

C6. A 2,000-g (4 lb, 6 1/2 oz), 35 weeks' gestation, appropriate for gestational age baby gains 120 g (4 oz) in

24 hours. Is this the same, larger, or smaller than the expected weight gain? _____

Check your answers with the list that follows the Recommended Routines. Correct any incorrect answers and review the appropriate section in the unit.

9. When Are IV Infusions Stopped and Restarted?

A. Infiltration of IV Fluid Into Subcutaneous Tissues

IV infiltration is detected by

- *Significant increase in the pressure registered by the IV pump*

  Many IV pumps indicate the pressure required to infuse an IV solution. If the pump indicates a specific pressure, it should be recorded whenever a new IV is started, and checked every hour throughout the infusion. Whenever a significant increase in pressure is noted, the IV site should be investigated carefully because an infusion pressure increase is often the first sign of an infiltration.

- *Puffiness around the insertion site*

  When puffiness or swelling is present, untape and pull out the IV needle. Insert another IV in a different site.

- *Fluid not pushed easily through the IV*

  To check this, withdraw a small syringe of IV fluid and gently push it through the IV needle. If this fluid flushes easily, with no sign of swelling, the IV almost surely is not infiltrated.

- *No blood return in the IV needle tubing when it is disconnected from the rest of the IV tubing*

  A brisk, definite blood return is a good indication that the IV has not infiltrated. However, blood return is not an entirely reliable indicator. Occasionally, a non-infiltrated IV will not have a blood return, and sometimes a delayed and/or minimal blood return occurs with an infiltrated IV.

- *Persistent fussiness or irritability of the baby* because the infiltrated skin is painful

B. Thrombophlebitis

Thrombophlebitis is detected by

- *Warmth over the insertion site*

- *Redness along the vein*

- *Tenderness around the insertion site*

The baby may become fussy and irritable or cry when the area near the IV is touched.

Thrombophlebitis is an inflammation of a vein associated with the formation of a clot, or thrombus, within the vein. Thrombophlebitis occurs much less often in babies than it does in adults. This is because peripheral IVs generally infiltrate more easily and more often in babies, before thrombophlebitis has time to develop. Therefore, IV sites are not routinely changed in babies. If thrombophlebitis develops, however, the treatment is to remove the IV and insert it at another site.

 It is important to detect thrombophlebitis or infiltration early and discontinue the IV infusion through that insertion site without delay.

Some medications and IV solutions are extremely irritating and may cause severe tissue damage if an infiltrated IV is not removed immediately.

10. When Are IV Infusions Discontinued?

When a baby meets all of the following requirements, infusion of IV fluid may be stopped:

- There is adequate intake of calories and fluid by nipple or tube feedings.

- Baby has recovered from an illness and is stable.

- IV infusion is no longer needed for glucose or medication administration.

11. What Is an IV Lock?

Occasionally stable babies taking full feedings will continue to require IV medications, most commonly antibiotics. These may be given through an IV lock. An IV lock does not require a continuous infusion of IV fluid. Many clinicians add a dilute solution of heparin to the IV lock, in which case it may be called a "heplock."

An IV lock is a regular IV catheter connected to a self-sealing medication port (T-connector). This is flushed periodically with a dilute solution of heparin (1–2 units/mL) or normal saline to keep it patent. It is generally recommended that a small volume (0.5–1.0 mL) of dilute heparin solution or normal saline be flushed through the IV lock after each medication administration and/or every 4 to 6 hours. Between uses, the IV lock should be clamped off, to prevent blood from backing up into the catheter. Despite these precautions, sometimes a clot will develop in the tip of the catheter.

Before each infusion of medication, check the IV lock for patency and for infiltration into the subcutaneous tissues.
- If there is a clot in the tip, it could be dislodged into the baby's bloodstream if flush solution is forced through an IV lock.
- If the IV has become infiltrated, forcing fluid through an IV lock would only put IV solution and/or medication into the subcutaneous tissues.
If the IV lock cannot be flushed *easily*, do not force fluid through it. Remove it and insert a new one in a different site.

12. What Facts Are Important to Remember?

1. **Use IV fluids for all babies less than 1,800 g (4 lb).**

2. **Obtain consultation** for fluid management of infants with severe perinatal compromise and for extremely preterm infants.

3. **Usual IV solutions** (except for extremely preterm babies)
    - *During first 24 hours:* $D_{10}W$
    - *After first 24 hours:* $D_{10}W$ with 1/4 normal saline and 20 mEq potassium chloride per liter

    Adjust the IV dextrose concentration higher or lower than $D_{10}W$ according to a baby's blood glucose level.

4. **Daily fluid requirements**
    - *During first 24 hours:* 80 mL/kg/24 hours
    - *After first 24 hours:* gradually increase to 120 mL/kg/24 hours by 72 hours
    - *Extremely preterm babies (less than 28 weeks' gestation) during first 24 hours:* 100 mL (or more)/kg/24 hours

5. **Daily normal weight gain** (4–6 days or more after birth): about 20 to 30 g/day

6. **Daily normal urine output:** about 40 mL/kg/24 hours, or 1 to 2 mL/kg/hour

7. **Normal urine specific gravity:** 1.008 to 1.012

8. **Normal insensible water loss:** about 35 to 40 mL/kg/24 hours (increase dramatically when a baby is under phototherapy lights or a radiant warmer, or is extremely preterm)

Now answer these questions to test yourself on the information in the last section.

D1. How can you make sure whether or not an intravenous line is infiltrated?

_____

_____

_____

D2. When does a baby no longer need an intravenous infusion?

    A. _____

    B. _____

    C. _____

D3. A baby receiving intravenous fluids begins to fuss and cry and nothing you do will soothe him. What might be the cause of his crying?

_____

Check your answers with the list that follows the Recommended Routines. Correct any incorrect answers and review the appropriate section in the unit.

Recommended Routines

All of the routines listed below are based on the principles of perinatal care presented in the unit you have just finished. They are recommended as part of routine perinatal care.

Read each routine carefully and decide whether it is standard operating procedure in your hospital. Check the appropriate blank next to each routine.

Procedure Standard in My Hospital	Needs Discussion by Our Staff	
_____	_____	1. Arrange staffing patterns to ensure constant availability of personnel with capability of starting and monitoring a peripheral intravenous line in a baby.
_____	_____	2. Establish a policy of delivering intravenous fluids to all babies • Who are sick • Weighing less than 1,800 g (4 lb) • With inadequate intake from nipple or tube feedings
_____	_____	3. Establish a routine of measuring urine volume and daily weights in all babies receiving intravenous fluids.

These are the answers to the self-test questions. Please check them with the answers you gave and review the information in the unit wherever necessary.

A1. All of the babies listed should receive intravenous therapy.
  A. Sick baby
  B. Inadequate fluid intake
  C. Less than 1,800 g and would not yet be on full feedings
A2. A. Peripheral vein intravenous line
  B. Umbilical arterial catheter, or radial artery sampling
  C. Umbilical venous catheter
  D. Peripheral vein intravenous line
  E. Umbilical venous catheter
A3. A. Replace or maintain body stores of water and electrolytes.
  B. Replenish blood volume.
  C. Give medication.
  D. Provide calories, in the form of glucose.
A4. Yes; peripheral intravenous line

B1. Increase fluid intake to account for increased insensible water losses
B2. During the first 24 hours after birth
B3. 240 mL (80 mL $\times$ 3.0 kg)
B4. 300 mL (120 mL $\times$ 2.5 kg)
B5. 150 mL (300 − 150)
B6. Body fluid lost through the skin and respiratory passages
B7. 152 mL intravenously per day; 6.3 mL per hour
      2.6 $\times$ 120 = 312 mL total fluid required per day
      20 mL $\times$ 8 = 160 mL by nipple
      312 − 160 = 152 mL intravenously
      152 / 24 = 6.3 mL per hour
B8. Decreased

C1. Approximately 20 to 30 g/24 hours
C2. Approximately 80 mL/24 hours; approximately 2 to 4 mL/hour (1–2 mL/kg/hour)
C3. Yes No
  _x_ ___ Obtain the baby's weight at the same time each day.
  ___ _x_ Remove all equipment attached to the baby.
  _x_ ___ Use the same scale for every weight.
  _x_ ___ Weigh the baby before a feeding.
  ___ _x_ Weigh the baby immediately after a feeding.
C4. Collecting the urine in a plastic bag or determining the weight (in grams) of the urine by weighing each wet diaper and subtracting the dry diaper weight
C5. No, the baby is getting too little fluid or the baby's kidneys and/or heart are not functioning properly.
C6. Larger

D1. If an intravenous line flushes *easily* with a syringe or has a brisk, definite blood return it is probably not infiltrated. Difficulty in flushing an intravenous line, a significant increase in infusion pressure, or puffiness at the site are each indications that an intravenous line very likely is infiltrated.
D2. A. Adequate intake of calories and fluid by nipple or tube feedings
  B. Recovered from an illness and is stable
  C. No longer needs intravenous line for glucose or medications
D3. The intravenous line is infiltrated.

Unit 7 Posttest

Without referring back to the information in the unit, please answer the following questions. Select the *one best* answer to each question (unless otherwise instructed). Record your answers on the answer sheet that is the last page in this book *and* on the test.

1. Insensible water loss occurs when fluid is lost from the body through
   - **A.** Diarrhea and vomiting
   - **B.** Frequent blood sampling
   - **C.** Urine and feces
   - **D.** Skin and respiratory passages

2. Which intravenous fluid should be used after the first 24 hours of postnatal life for a baby with no specific complications?
   - **A.** 10% dextrose in 1/2 normal saline with 20 mEq of potassium added to each 1,000 mL of fluid
   - **B.** 10% dextrose in 1/4 normal saline with 20 mEq of potassium added to each 1,000 mL of fluid
   - **C.** 10% dextrose with 20 mEq of potassium added to each 1,000 mL of fluid
   - **D.** 10% dextrose in normal saline

3. How much fluid does a term baby need during the first 24 hours after birth?
   - **A.** 80 mL/kg
   - **B.** 100 mL/kg
   - **C.** 140 mL/kg
   - **D.** 200 mL/kg

4. A baby requires 280 mL of intravenous fluid per day. How much intravenous fluid should she receive every hour?
   - **A.** 6 mL to 7 mL
   - **B.** 8 mL to 9 mL
   - **C.** 11 mL to 12 mL
   - **D.** 14 mL to 15 mL

5. Babies who have experienced severe perinatal compromise are *most* likely to require
   - **A.** Additional calories
   - **B.** Additional intravenous fluid
   - **C.** Restricted calories
   - **D.** Restricted intravenous fluid

6. **True   False**   Phlebitis is not an indication for discontinuing an intravenous line in a baby.

7. Which route is preferred to administer intravenous antibiotics to a baby?
   - **A.** Umbilical venous catheter
   - **B.** Umbilical arterial catheter
   - **C.** Peripheral vein
   - **D.** Venous cut down

8. A baby's urine has a specific gravity of 1.028. This may be caused by the baby
   - **A.** Receiving too little fluid
   - **B.** Having immature kidneys
   - **C.** Receiving too much fluid
   - **D.** Having hypoglycemia

For each question, please make sure you have marked your answer on the test and on the answer sheet (last page in book). The test is for you; the answer sheet will need to be turned in for continuing education credit.

Skill Unit   Peripheral Intravenous Infusions

This skill unit will teach you how to start a peripheral intravenous (PIV) line on a baby. Not everyone will be required to start PIVs. Everyone should read this skill unit, however, to learn the equipment and sequence of steps so they can assist with starting a PIV.

Because it is impossible to practice on babies, you will need to demonstrate mastery of the skill by inserting and stabilizing an IV for a baby in your nursery the next time a baby needs an IV. Preliminary practice may be possible on certain manikins.

To master the skill, you will need to demonstrate correctly each of the following steps:

1. Collect and prepare proper equipment.

2. Demonstrate IV insertion technique.

3. Secure IV catheter.

4. Monitor IV site and fluid intake.

Note: Illustrated in this skill unit are conventional IV equipment and insertion devices. More and more, shielded catheters for PIV insertion and IV tubing with needleless access ports are becoming available to protect the practitioner from exposure to blood and needle sticks. Shielded catheters are ones where the needle can be withdrawn into the insertion hub and locked within a cover, once the catheter has been inserted.

Insertion and taping of these devices is essentially the same as shown in this unit, but each brand of IV insertion device requires its own insertion technique. These techniques are very similar to each other but also slightly, but importantly, different from each other. You will need to become familiar with the specific insertion devices used in your hospital and master the specific technique to insert each device.

Inserting and Managing Peripheral Intravenous Infusions

Note: Although the exact technique of PIV insertion and taping may vary, the principles are always the same. The method described below is just one of several that work well. Only PIV insertion into the hand or foot is discussed. Central, long-line catheter insertion and maintenance is not covered.

Whatever method is used, it is important to *expect to succeed* in starting an IV and, therefore, to *have everything ready*. A good IV can be ruined by delay in proper taping or by clotting of the line due to delay in starting infusion of IV fluid.

Actions	Remarks

Collecting the Equipment for a PIV

Actions	Remarks
1. Gather all of these materials.	It is recommended that an IV solution be changed every 24 hours, regardless of the amount of fluid left in the bottle or bag. This is to minimize the chance of an infection being transferred to the baby through the IV fluid. All of the tubing up to, but not including, the IV catheter should be routinely changed at least every 72 hours. Follow your hospital's guidelines for changing IV fluids and equipment.

• **IV solution—check to ensure it is**
  – Prepared as ordered
  – Labeled with this information
    • Solution
    • Electrolytes or other medications, if any, added to the IV fluid
    • Date and time it was prepared	

• **IV pump**	To provide a consistently accurate IV delivery rate, a pump is essential.

• **IV tubing**
  – Tubing with measuring chamber
  – Special tubing needed for specific IV pump being used
  – Appropriate-sized syringe, if using a syringe pump
	A measuring chamber marked in milliliters allows the exact amount of fluid a baby receives to be calculated every hour. Most pumps have a digital readout of the volume infused. However, pumps sometimes malfunction. The measuring chamber serves as a check on the pump readout. The measuring chamber also permits only a limited amount of fluid (rather than all the fluid in the IV bag or bottle) to infuse at one time if the IV rate is accidentally increased or the pump malfunctions.

• **Micropore bacterial filter** (optional for routine IV therapy)	

• **Tape, pre-cut**
  – 1/2 inch tape cut into one 1-inch strip
  – 1/2 inch tape cut into one 3-inch strip
  – Clear adhesive film dressing cut to fit over insertion site	

• **Cotton ball** (optional)	
• **Small tourniquet**	An elastic band is sometimes used as a tourniquet around an extremity.

Actions	**Remarks**

Collecting the Equipment for a PIV (continued)

- **IV board** (optional, for an arm or leg site)

  An extremity board is sometimes used to restrain the limb of a large, vigorous baby.

- **IV catheters**

  #24 for most babies; #22 for large veins

- **Antimicrobial solution**

  Isopropyl alcohol swabs are commonly used. Either povidone-iodine or chlorhexidine is more effective, as well as less drying to the skin, than isopropyl alcohol. If povidone-iodine or chlorhexidine is used, the solution should be allowed to dry and then must be removed *completely* from the skin by wiping the area with alcohol or sterile water swabs. If left in place, these antiseptics can cause marked skin irritation.

- **Sterile 2 x 2 gauze**

- **T-connector**

  This is a short piece of tubing, with a medication port, that is inserted between the catheter and main IV tubing.

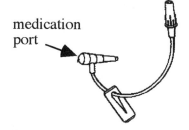

medication port

Preparing the Equipment

2. Run the IV solution through the tubing, taking care to eliminate all air bubbles.

   If using a syringe pump, also draw a specific amount of IV solution into the syringe.

3. Insert the tubing into the pump according to the manufacturer's directions.

4. Set the IV rate but do not start the pump.

5. Draw up a syringe of flush solution.

   Use normal saline, the baby's IV fluid, or a dilute heparin solution (1–2 units/mL).

6. Connect the syringe to the T-connector and fill the connector with the flush solution, leaving 2 to 3 mL of flush solution in the syringe.

   Leave the T-connector and syringe connected.

7. Select an appropriate vein. Choose the largest vein in a convenient, relatively easy place to insert, stabilize, and protect the catheter.

   It is prudent to avoid using a vein in the antecubital space (bend of the elbow). Leave this vein available to obtain blood for laboratory tests, unless no other IV site is available.

Actions	Remarks

Preparing the Equipment (continued)

8. For an ***extremity vein***, consider use of an armboard or legboard to stabilize the extremity.

   Note: *In most situations, an extremity board is not needed. This information is provided in case a board is useful to protect an IV in a large and/or active baby.*

   • Be sure the board is the appropriate length. If the selected vein is in a foot, for example, the board should be short enough not to rub in the popliteal space (bend of the knee), but long enough to stabilize the ankle joint.

   • The extremity may be secured before or after the IV is inserted and taped in place.

   • Check for capillary refill to make sure the tape is not too tight.

9. Restrain the baby.

10. Cleanse the intended insertion site.

11. Wipe alcohol dry with sterile 2 x 2 or wash povidone-iodine or chlorhexidine off with alcohol or sterile water swabs.

Remarks column:

If an extremity board is used, secure the extremity above and below the insertion site. Use Velcro wraps or face a section of adhesive tape with another, shorter piece of tape long enough to go over the top of the extremity, leaving the ends of the longer piece sticky to secure to the underside of the board.

The important thing is to prepare the IV board at this point in the procedure. Actual taping of the arm or leg can be done later, in step 24.

Gently press and release the toes or fingers. Note how quickly the blanched area turns pink again. There should be an almost instantaneous pink flush. If this does not happen, loosen the restraint slightly and check again.

This is always a safe practice, but may not be necessary with very small or sick infants. A mummy wrap, however, is often necessary for large and/or vigorous babies.

See earlier section (step 1, antimicrobial solution) for information about antiseptic agents.

Actions	**Remarks**

Inserting an IV Catheter

12. If starting an arm or leg IV, apply a tourniquet with your fingers (shown in illustration) or with an elastic band.

If using an elastic band, be certain it is removed after the IV is inserted.

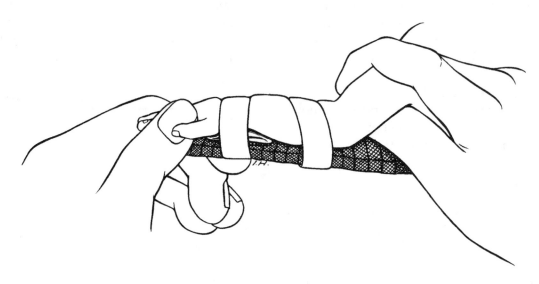

13. Either the person holding the baby or the person inserting the IV may use their fingers to spread the skin over the insertion site to keep it taut.

With the skin taut, the vein will roll less as the catheter and needle are inserted.

14. Take the catheter and hold the hub between your thumb and index finger with the bevel (slanted part) of the needle facing upward.

15. ***Insert the catheter directly into the vein.*** Do not try to thread it through the skin.

Proceed slowly because there is normally a slight delay in the backflow of blood into the catheter hub that indicates the vein has been entered.

16. When backflow of blood is first seen, *stop.*

Care must be taken to avoid puncturing the opposite side of the vein.

backflow of blood

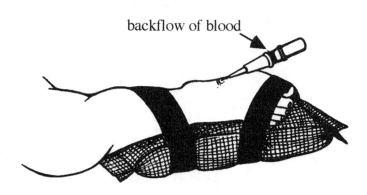

17. Remove the needle from the catheter.

18. Release your squeeze around the baby's arm or leg, or release the elastic band.

Actions	**Remarks**

Inserting an IV Catheter (continued)

19. ***Thread*** the catheter into the vein as far as it will go ***easily***.

20. Stabilize the catheter with a small piece of clear adhesive film dressing over the insertion point.

    Some practitioners cover the insertion point and the catheter hub with the clear adhesive film (not shown).

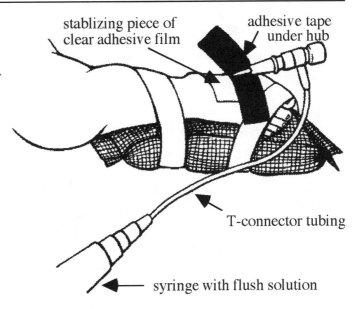

stablizing piece of clear adhesive film

adhesive tape under hub

T-connector tubing

syringe with flush solution

21. Connect the T-connector and syringe with the flush solution to the catheter. Flush a small amount of solution through the catheter.

    If the area in the skin near the tip of the catheter becomes swollen, the catheter is in the subcutaneous tissue and not in the vein. It should be removed immediately.

22. Observe the insertion site and the ease or difficulty of pushing the flush solution.

Securing an IV Catheter

23. When the catheter flushes easily, tape it in that position with the 3-inch piece of adhesive tape.

    - Slide the tape under the catheter hub, with the sticky side facing up.

    - Crisscross the ends over the hub and tape the ends to the clear adhesive dressing that covers the insertion site.

    - A tiny piece of cotton under the hub (not shown) may be useful to protect the baby's skin from the hard hub pressing into it.

      Do not overtape!

    Additional tape will not make the catheter any more secure, but will make early detection of an infiltration more difficult.

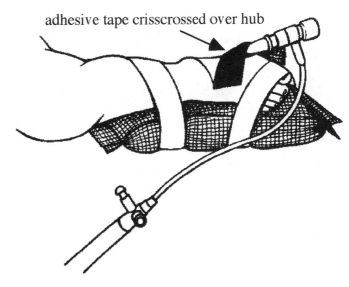

adhesive tape crisscrossed over hub

311

Actions	**Remarks**

Securing an IV Catheter (continued)

24. Recheck the ease with which the catheter can be flushed after it is taped in place. If it continues to flush easily, connect the IV tubing and begin the infusion.	In most cases, an arm or leg restraint is not needed with IV catheters. If one is indicated, and it was not taped in place earlier (step 8), secure the baby's arm or leg to the IV board now, as shown in the previous illustrations.
25. Be sure to include the T-connector tubing under the tape (not shown).	This is extremely important so that any pull on the IV tubing will pull against the tape and not the catheter.

Monitoring an IV Line

26. Record the amount of IV fluid infused during the insertion procedure and the time at which the continuous IV infusion was started.	In addition to IV fluid intake, record the amount of fluid the baby received in • Feedings (if any) • Any other fluid intake (transfusion, etc) Note the baby's output, too, including • Volume of urine output • Blood taken for tests • Any other fluid loss (vomiting, etc)
27. Record the amount of IV fluid infused each hour. Compare this to the ordered amount of IV fluid and the readout on the pump. Adjust the flow rate as necessary. Every 8 hours, total the amount of IV fluid the baby received. Total the baby's IV fluid intake for each 24 hours too.	
28. If the pump you are using measures infusion pressure, record the pressure when the IV is started.	
29. Inspect the insertion site at least every hour for signs of puffiness and increased IV pump infusion pressure.	To minimize possible tissue damage from infiltrated IV fluid, it is important to detect an infiltration as early as possible.

Unit 8   Feeding

Unit 8 Pretest

Before reading the unit, please answer the following questions. Select the *one best* answer to each question (unless otherwise instructed). Record your answers on the answer sheet that is the last page in this book *and* on the test.

1. In which of the following situations is a baby *most* likely to develop feeding problems?

   A. When the baby's mother has ulcers
   B. When there was excess amniotic fluid
   C. When the baby's mother has hypoglycemia
   D. When there was minimal amniotic fluid

2. Which of the following babies is *most* likely to develop feeding problems?

   A. 3-day-old term baby who has not stooled
   B. 3,200-g (7 lb, 1 oz) baby
   C. Baby with a myelomeningocele
   D. Baby with an estimated gestational age of 43 weeks

3. Which of the following characteristics of formula is *most* important for preterm babies?

   A. Low calcium compared to breast milk
   B. Low sodium compared to breast milk
   C. High potassium compared to breast milk
   D. Osmolarity same as breast milk

4. A 2-hour-old, term, appropriate for gestational age baby has rapid, shallow respirations at a rate of 80 breaths/minute. The baby is requiring only 30% oxygen. How would you provide fluids/nutrition for this baby?

   A. Nipple feedings
   B. Nasogastric or orogastric tube feedings
   C. Peripheral intravenous fluids
   D. Delay fluids/feedings until the baby is 24 hours old

5. **True   False**   A 2,000-g (4 lb, 6 1/2 oz) small for gestational age baby will require more calories to grow than a 2,000-g appropriate for gestational baby.

6. **True   False**   Most preterm infants can be expected to lose weight until they are approximately 2 weeks old.

7. **True   False**   Breast milk has sufficient vitamins for a growing preterm infant.

8. Which of the following babies requires tube instead of nipple feedings?

   A. 30-week, appropriate for gestational age baby with a strong suck reflex
   B. 36-week, small for gestational age baby with polycythemia
   C. 40-week baby with hyperbilirubinemia requiring phototherapy
   D. 43-week, small for gestational age baby with a strong suck reflex

9. Which of the following procedures should usually be carried out before each tube feeding?

   A. Aspirate the stomach contents, record the amount, and discard the aspirated fluid.
   B. Aspirate the stomach contents, record the amount, and refeed the fluid to the baby through the tube.

10. **True   False**   Placement of a feeding tube should be checked before every feeding.

11. **True   False**   Term babies who require oxygen may be fed safely by nipple.

12. **True   False**   A combination of nipple and tube feedings may be appropriate for some babies.

13. A baby requires tube feedings of 25 mL of milk every 2 hours. While preparing the baby for the next feeding, you find that the baby has 5 mL of residual milk left in the stomach from the previous feeding. The baby's abdomen is not distended; vital signs, color, and activity are normal. What should you do?

    A. Refeed the residual milk but not give any new milk at this feeding time.
    B. Discard the residual milk and feed the baby 25 mL of new milk.
    C. Refeed the residual milk and feed the baby 20 mL of new milk.
    D. Discard the residual milk and feed the baby 20 mL of new milk.

For each question, please make sure you have marked your answer on the test and on the answer sheet (last page in book). The test is for you; the answer sheet will need to be turned in for continuing education credit.

Feeding Principles

Objectives

In Part 1 of this unit you will learn

A. To recognize the dangers of feedings

B. Which milks are suitable for preterm babies

C. To determine how much and how often a baby should be fed

D. To determine if a baby should be fed by feeding tube or nipple

E. To determine if a preterm baby is gaining weight satisfactorily

Note:
- Throughout this unit, the general term 'milk' is used to indicate either formula or breast milk.
- Kilocalories is often shortened to calories in everyday usage.
- Nutritional management of extremely low birth weight babies (<1,000 g) is not discussed.

1. What Are the Dangers of Feeding?

- Babies may aspirate (inhale) milk into their lungs as they eat.

- Babies may vomit and aspirate the vomitus into their lungs.

- Milk in the lungs can lead to pneumonia.

- Babies with respiratory distress cannot breathe as easily with a full stomach.

- Babies with respiratory distress or other acute illness may not have the energy or coordination to nurse and breathe at the same time.

2. Which Babies Are At Risk for Developing Feeding Problems?

Table 8.1. Feeding Risk Factors and Recommended Responses

Risk Factor	Response
Excessive mucus	• Do *not* feed until a tube is passed into the baby's stomach to rule out tracheoesophageal fistula and esophageal atresia.*
History of maternal hydramnios	• Monitor baby's feeding tolerance carefully. If abdominal distension or vomiting develops, place baby NPO,* insert nasogastric (NG) or orogastric (OG) tube, and obtain abdominal x-ray.
Distended abdomen	• Insert NG or OG tube and withdraw air/fluid to decompress baby's stomach. • Do *not* feed until baby checked for obstruction or ileus.*
Respiratory distress, rapid breathing, or depressed activity	• Do *not* feed by bottle or allow to nurse at breast until respiratory rate is less than approximately 60 breaths per minute and baby can coordinate sucking, swallowing, and breathing.*†
Babies younger than 32–34 weeks' gestation may be able to suck, swallow, and breathe adequately, but *not coordinate* these activities.	• Feed by NG or OG tube or give intravenous fluids until tube feedings can be administered. • Preterm babies also have special nutritional needs.
Vomiting of green material or persistent vomiting or spitting	• Stop feedings.* • Obtain abdominal x-ray to evaluate for possible intestinal obstruction.
No stool by 48 hours of age	• Stop feedings.* • Evaluate for obstruction or ileus.
Prolonged resuscitation (perinatal compromise increases risk for developing an ileus or necrotizing enterocolitis)	• Keep NPO until baby is stable. • Consider keeping NPO for at least 24–48 hours or until bowel sounds are heard.*
Sepsis (increases risk for developing an ileus)	• Keep NPO until baby is stable.*

*Maintain hydration and blood glucose with intravenous fluids.
†Tube feedings may be appropriate for some babies. See Tube Feeding section at the end of this unit.

3. What Type of Milk Should Be Used for Preterm Babies?

Preterm babies have immature gastrointestinal tracts that can easily be injured if given a formula that is too concentrated. The more preterm the baby, the greater the risk of intestinal damage. Therefore, formulas have been developed to have the same osmolarity (particle concentration) as breast milk.

These formulas also have a slightly higher caloric density and more vitamins, minerals, and protein than breast milk. While breast milk and commercial formulas for term infants have a caloric density of 20 kcal/oz, formulas designed for preterm babies contain 24 kcal/oz.

Preterm baby formulas

- Enfamil Premature Formula

- Similac Special Care Formula

The small amount of breast milk* a preterm baby ingests does not contain an adequate amount of vitamins to meet the nutritional requirements of a growing preterm baby. For this reason, additives have been designed to increase the caloric density, mineral, and vitamin content of breast milk without appreciably increasing the osmolarity. These supplements are added to breast milk by different techniques. Follow manufacturer's instructions carefully.

Breast milk supplements

- Enfamil Human Milk Fortifier

- Similac Human Milk Fortifier

The preterm baby formulas and breast milk additives are generally designed to be used for babies born at 34 weeks' gestation or younger. In some cases, they may also be appropriate for preterm babies born between 35 and 37 weeks' gestation, particularly if a baby was sick.

 Preterm babies have immature intestines that are easily damaged. Use only formula designed for preterm babies or breast milk fortified with an appropriate supplement.

4. What Type of Milk Should Babies Who Are Term, Slightly Preterm, or Almost Ready for Discharge Receive?

Breast milk or any one of several standard formulas, all of which have a caloric density of 20 kcal/oz, are appropriate for *babies born at term or near term.* These include

- Breast milk*

- Similac

---

*For information about collection, handling, and storing breast milk, consult the American Dietetic Association, *Guidelines for Preparation of Formula and Breastmilk in Health Care Facilities,* 2003 at www.eatright.org/cps/rde/xchg/ada/hs.xsl/nutrition_5441_ENU_HTML.htm and/or Human Milk Banking Association of North America, *2006 Best Practice for Pumping, Storing and Handling of Mother's Own Milk in Hospital and at Home,* at www.hmbana.org/index.php?mode=pubs.

- Enfamil

- Carnation Good Start

As *babies born significantly preterm approach discharge weight*, they still have unique but changing nutritional requirements.

- *Non-breastfeeding babies* may be switched to a formula intended to meet the special needs of the growing preterm baby after hospital discharge. The commercial formulas Similac NeoSure and Enfamil EnfaCare are designed for this purpose. These formulas contain 22 kcal/oz, plus the mineral, vitamin, and iron concentration of preterm baby formulas. NeoSure and EnfaCare are frequently given to preterm babies until they reach 6 months of age.

- *Breastfeeding babies* receiving unfortified breast milk or nursing at the breast still need additional vitamins and iron (see sections 9 and 10).

5. Are Special Formulas Used for Any Other Babies?

Babies with certain digestive problems may need special formulas that contain only certain sugars or proteins, or contain elemental compounds that can be easily digested. Although the following formulas differ considerably in their composition, all contain 20 kcal/oz:

- Nutramigen

- ProSobee

- Isomil

- Pregestimil

6. How Do You Know How Much Milk an Appropriate for Gestational Age Baby Needs?

A. Determine the Total Daily Volume of Milk Needed

Babies who are appropriate size for their gestational age will generally require a minimum of 120 kcal/kg of body weight to maintain metabolic functions, gain weight, and allow for some losses in the stool. The amount of milk required to achieve this can be calculated by the following formula:

$$30 \times 120 \times \text{baby's weight in kg} \div \text{milk kcal/oz} = \text{mL/day}$$

Example: A baby appropriate for gestational age (AGA) and weighing 1,600 g (1.6 kg) was born at 33 weeks' gestation. His mother decided not to breastfeed, so this baby needs preterm baby formula containing 24 cal/oz. His daily milk requirement is

$$30 \times 120 \times 1.6 \div 24 \text{ cal/oz} = 240 \text{ mL/day}$$

B. Decide on a Feeding Schedule

The Table 8.2 gives *general guidelines* for AGA babies.

Table 8.2. Feeding Guidelines for Appropriate for Gestational Age Babies

Baby's Weight and Estimated Gestational Age (EGA)	Feeding Frequency	Feeding Method
1,000–1,500 g (2 lb, 3 oz–3 lb, 5 oz) EGA below 32–34 weeks	Every 2–3 hours	Nasogastric or orogastric tube
1,500–2,000 g (3 lb, 5 oz–4 lb, 6 1/2 oz) EGA more than 32–34 weeks	Every 3 hours	Bottle or breast (unless contraindicated)
>2,000 g (>4 lb, 6 1/2 oz)	Every 3–4 hours	Bottle or breast (unless contraindicated)
Healthy full term babies	On demand (usually every 3–4 hours)	Bottle
	On demand (usually every 2–3 hours, and at least 8 feedings every 24 hours)	Breast

C. Determine the Target Volume per Feeding

Divide the total daily volume by the number of feedings per day

- every 2 hours = 12 feedings

- every 3 hours = 8 feedings

- every 4 hours = 6 feedings

Example: The 1,600-g baby described earlier would probably be fed every 3 hours, for a total of 8 feedings per day. Therefore, the feeding goal is

240 ÷ 8 = 30 mL per feeding

D. Gradually Increase Feeding Volume to Reach Target Amount

If a baby is preterm or has been sick, work up slowly to the calculated volume of feedings. This may take several days.

 To prevent hypoglycemia and possible brain damage, babies who are not receiving full feedings should receive intravenous fluids until adequate milk intake has been established.

The speed with which full feedings can be achieved depends on the baby's degree of illness and/or prematurity. General guidelines for preterm babies are shown in Table 8.3.

Table 8.3. Guidelines for Increasing Feedings for Preterm Babies

Baby's Weight	Starting Volume	Progression
1,000–1,250 g	2 mL/kg at each feed	1 mL/kg every 12 hours
1,250–1,800 g	2–3 mL/kg at each feed	2–3 mL/kg every 8 hours
>1,800 g	5–10 mL/kg at each feed	5–10 mL/kg every 6–12 hours

Example: The 1,600-g baby described in section C might first be given a feeding of 5 mL. If that is taken well, consider increasing the feeding volume by 5 mL every second or third feeding (every 6 or 9 hours) until the baby is receiving the full, targeted amount of 30 mL every 3 hours.

7. How Do You Know How Much Milk a Small for Gestational Age Baby Needs?

Most babies who are small for gestational age (SGA) need additional kilocalories per kilogram of body weight for achievement of "catch-up" growth. To determine the milk needed, calculate the minimum *expected* weight for the baby's gestational age. To do this, use Figure 8.1 to estimate what the baby's weight would have been if born at the 10th percentile weight for that baby's gestational age.

Example: A 1,700-g (3 lb, 12 oz) baby born at 37 weeks' gestation can be expected to weigh at least (10th percentile) 2,100 g (4 lb, 10 oz). Use this minimum *expected* weight of 2,100 g, rather

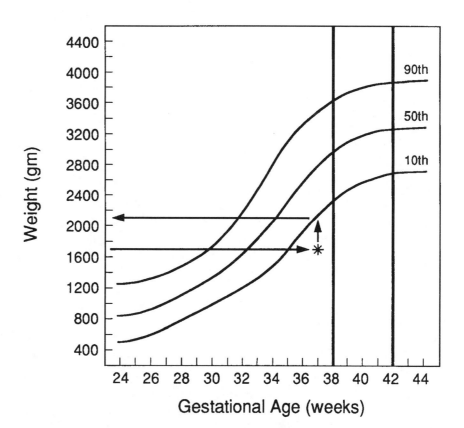

Figure 8.1. Weight by Gestational Age Percentile Curves

than the baby's actual weight of 1,700 g, when calculating the formula needs for this SGA baby.

In general, you should not immediately feed an SGA baby the volume based on the minimum expected weight. Feedings should be increased as tolerated, over several days, until the baby is receiving the appropriate amount for expected weight. If an SGA baby still seems hungry after receiving this calculated amount, more may be given.

Any baby taking enough milk to receive full calories will receive more than enough fluid to meet minimum body fluid requirements (previous unit, IV Therapy).

Self-Test

Now answer these questions to test yourself on the information in the last section. Refer to the graphs or charts in the unit, as necessary, to answer these questions.

A1. What can happen if a baby of 30 weeks' estimated gestational age is fed by nipple?

_____

A2. A woman with hydramnios delivered a full-term, vigorous baby. At 30 minutes of age the baby is noted to have excessive mucus. What would you do before the first feeding?

A. Suction the baby with bulb syringe, then feed.
B. Insert an orogastric or nasogastric tube, and feed the baby with the tube in place.
C. Insert an orogastric or nasogastric tube, and evaluate for obstruction before feeding.

A3. **True   False**   Formulas with high osmolarity are preferred for preterm babies.

A4. A baby weighs 1,800 g (4 lb) and is appropriate size for gestational age. The baby is in no distress. How often would you feed this baby?

_____

A5. A baby weighs 2,300 g (5 lb, 1 oz) at 40 weeks' gestation.

A. How often would you feed this baby?

_____

B. Is this baby small, large, or appropriate weight for gestational age?

_____

C. How much would you eventually give the baby at each feeding?

_____

A6. A 2-day-old baby is requiring 50% oxygen and breathing at a rate of 70 breaths per minute. The baby's estimated gestational age is 36 weeks. This baby should be fed by

A. Intravenous fluids only
B. Nipple feedings while holding the oxygen to the baby's face
C. Nasogastric or orogastric tube feedings

Check your answers with the list that follows the Recommended Routines. Correct any incorrect answers and review the appropriate section in the unit.

8. How Can You Tell if a Baby Is Growing Satisfactorily?

It is normal for AGA babies to lose weight during the first several days after birth. Preterm infants will take longer to regain this weight than will full term babies. Figure 8.2 shows the normal weight gain curves* for preterm and term AGA babies.

Stable SGA babies or post-term babies, however, will frequently start gaining weight immediately after birth. They may continue to gain weight at a faster rate than AGA babies.

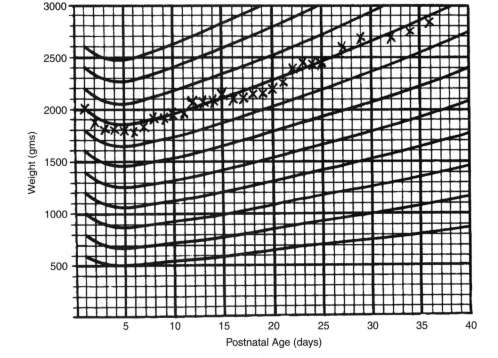

Figure 8.2. Normal Weight Gain Curves for Preterm and Term Appropriate for Gestational Age Babies from Shaffer, SG, et al. Postnatal weight changes in low birth weight infants. *Pediatrics.* 1987;79:702.

Example A: A preterm AGA baby weighs 2,000 g at birth. As shown on the chart above, an X is placed on the chart each day, marking the baby's weight for that day. As long as the Xs stay close to the curve that starts at 2,000 g, the baby's weight change is normal. The Xs show this baby's weight follows a normal curve.

---

*Growth curves may also be found at https://neonatal.rti.org/birth_curves/dsp_BirthCurves.cfm. This Web site allows you to enter the birth weight, birth length, and birth head circumference of a 501- to 1,500-g infant and construct individualized, expected growth curves based on the National Institute of Child Health and Human Development Neonatal Research Network Growth Observational Study (Ehrenkranz, et al. *Pediatrics.* 1999;104:280–289). Charts for babies with birth weights greater than 1,500 g may be found at www.biomedcentral.com/1471-2431/3/13 and other Web sites.

Growth curves differ slightly from each other, but each may be used to plot a newborn's growth. Whichever curve you select to use to plot a specific baby's growth, you should use it consistently over time for that baby. Do not switch between different curves for the same baby.

Example B: Using Figure 8.2, plot the weights below for a baby weighing 2,500 g at birth.

Day 1 2,450 g	Day 3 2,350 g	Day 5 2,250 g
Day 2 2,400 g	Day 4 2,300 g	Day 6 2,200 g
		Day 7 2,200 g

Is this baby's weight change normal? ___ Yes ___ No

(Check your answer with the list that follows the Recommended Routines.)

9. Does a Low Birth Weight Baby Need Multivitamin Supplementation?

A. Low Birth Weight Babies (<1,800 g or <4 lb)

Vitamins are substances that occur in many foods in small amounts and are necessary for normal metabolic functions. The formulas designed for preterm babies and breast milk supplements, both described earlier in this unit, provide vitamins in the amounts necessary for adequate growth of preterm babies.

Preterm infants need pediatric multivitamin supplementation only when discharged to home on

- Standard 20 kcal/oz formula

- Unfortified breast milk

B. Vitamin Supplements (if needed)

Vitamins and some drugs have high osmolarity. To make them less hyperosmolar, *vitamins* are administered in the following way:

- Dose of 1 mL/day of an infant multivitamin preparation

- After the baby is tolerating feedings well

- Mixed in the entire volume in one feeding or divided and mixed in several feedings

 Dilute medications or multivitamins given orally or by tube feeding to decrease their osmolarity. This is especially important for preterm babies.

Note: Always try to give *medications* intravenously or intramuscularly. If these routes of administration are not possible or appropriate, dilute medications for oral or tube feeding administration in the full volume of milk for a feeding.

10. Does a Low Birth Weight Baby Need Iron Supplementation?

Preterm infants should receive iron supplementation (2 mg/kg elemental iron per day) at approximately 6 to 8 weeks after delivery or when the baby begins to grow rapidly.

- *Non-breastfeeding babies:* This supplement may be given as formula containing iron, or as an additional medication. Formulas described earlier that are designed for preterm babies (Enfamil Premature Formula, Similac Special Care Formula, Similac NeoSure, Enfamil EnfaCare) contain iron sufficient to provide 2 mg/kg elemental iron per day for babies receiving full feeds.

- *Breastfeeding babies:* Preterm babies receiving either breast milk with fortifier or plain breast milk should be given 2 mg/kg per day of liquid ferrous sulfate daily, starting at approximately 6 to 8 weeks of age and continuing through the first 12 months of age.

When iron is given as an additional medication, make certain a baby is tolerating feedings well before beginning supplementation.

Self-Test

Now answer these questions to test yourself on the information in the last section. Refer to the graphs or charts in the unit, as necessary, to answer these questions.

B1. **True** **False** Vitamins given orally or through a feeding tube should be diluted with the volume of a full feeding or split over several feedings.

B2. A baby weighing 2,250 g (4 lb, 15 1/2 oz) will not take more than 30 mL (1 oz) of formula every 4 hours on the third day after birth. What should be done for this baby?

_____

B3. A preterm baby born weighing 1,800 g (4 lb) weighs this much on the following days:

1,700 g–5 days old
1,750 g–10 days old
1,900 g–15 days old
2,050 g–20 days old

Is this baby following the expected growth pattern?   ___ Yes   ___ No

B4. Vitamins for low birth weight babies

Yes **No**

___ ___ Are unnecessary if a baby is receiving breast milk
___ ___ Should be mixed in a baby's feedings
___ ___ Should be given separate from a feeding
___ ___ May be started when a baby is tolerating feedings well

Check your answers with the list that follows the Recommended Routines. Correct any incorrect answers and review the appropriate section in the unit.

Tube Feeding

Objectives

In Part 2 of this unit you will learn

A. To recognize the dangers of tube feedings

B. When tube feedings should be used

C. When tube feedings should not be used

D. How to determine the volume of milk a baby should receive with each feeding

E. How to feed a baby safely using a feeding tube

1. What Is Tube Feeding?

Tube feeding is a method of feeding babies who are too sick or too preterm to be fed by nipple (bottle or breast). A feeding tube is inserted into either the baby's nose or mouth, down the esophagus, and into the baby's stomach. Milk (formula or breast milk) is given through this tube.

2. When Are Tube Feedings Required?

A. Preterm Babies (<32–34 weeks' gestation)

To be able to be fed successfully by nipple, the baby must be able to coordinate the following:

- Sucking
- Swallowing
- Breathing

Also, the baby must have developed a

- Gag reflex

Preterm babies may be able to do all of these things separately. However, babies younger than 32 to 34 weeks' gestation usually *cannot coordinate* these activities. If these activities—sucking, swallowing, breathing—are uncoordinated or if the gag reflex is not yet present, a baby may aspirate milk while trying to feed.

 Every baby younger than 32 to 34 weeks' gestation should be fed with a nasogastric or orogastric tube, even if the baby has a strong suck reflex.

B. Certain Sick Babies (>34 weeks' gestation)

Certain conditions in babies older than 34 weeks' gestation will prevent them from being fed safely by nipple.

- *Severe neurologic problems* may be associated with an absent gag reflex. Any infant with an absent gag reflex should *not* be fed by nipple.

- *Severe medical problems* such as sepsis may make an infant so lethargic that he or she is unable to eat by nipple. Septic babies may also develop an ileus and may need to be made NPO and given intravenous (IV) fluids until they are stable and bowel sounds are heard.

C. At-Risk Babies Requiring Continuing Care

Babies who were sick and have recovered from their acute illness, but are not yet well, may need tube feedings. These may include infants who have a gag reflex and are able to coordinate sucking, swallowing, and breathing, but tire easily from the exertion of nipple feeding. Tube feedings may be needed to supplement nipple feedings in order for a baby to receive adequate nutrition.

D. Babies With Respiratory Distress

Any baby, regardless of gestational age, who either

- Has a respiratory rate greater than approximately 60 breaths/minute

or

- Requires oxygen

should *not* be fed by nipple. These babies should be kept NPO and receive only IV fluids for the first several days after birth.

If a baby requires long-term intensive care and is still in *mild* respiratory distress at several days of age, *cautious* tube feedings may be appropriate. If respiratory distress is severe or prolonged, parenteral nutrition should be provided in a newborn intensive care unit.

3. How Do You Decide Whether to Use a Nasogastric Tube or an Orogastric Tube?

The decision to use nasogastric (NG) or orogastric (OG) tubes is often based on simple personal preference. However, the following factors should be considered:

- Nasogastric tubes can usually be taped in place more securely.

- Because of the relatively large oral cavity, babies tend to push orogastric tubes out of their mouths with their tongues. Therefore, orogastric tubes may be more likely to become dislodged during a feeding, thus increasing the chance of aspiration.

- Babies weighing less than 2,000 g, who depend on nasal patency for breathing, move significantly less air when one nostril is partially blocked with an NG tube. OG tubes may, therefore, be preferable for small babies who are experiencing respiratory distress or apnea spells.

4. How Are Tube Feedings Given?

A feeding tube is inserted through the baby's nose or mouth, down the throat and esophagus, and into the stomach. The upper end of the tube is taped to the baby's lip or cheek to hold the tube in place, and the lower end of the tube lies in the baby's stomach.

A syringe barrel, with plunger removed, is connected to the tube. At each feeding, a calculated volume of milk is placed in the syringe barrel and drips by gravity into a baby's stomach.

The syringe should be changed with each feeding, but the same feeding tube may be used for several feedings. Tube placement should be checked before *every* feeding.

 Do not leave a baby unattended while a tube feeding is being given.

Whenever an x-ray is obtained of a baby with a feeding tube in place, check to be sure the tube tip is 1.5 to 2.0 cm below the lower esophageal sphincter. This location will ensure that the milk flows into the baby's stomach.

Details of all of these steps are given in the following skill unit.

Self-Test

Now answer these questions to test yourself on the information in the last section.

C1. Which of the following babies should have tube instead of nipple feedings?

Yes	No	
___	___	31-week, large for gestational age baby without respiratory distress
___	___	40-week active baby who requires treatment for hypoglycemia
___	___	35-week appropriate for gestational age baby with tachypnea, grunting, retractions, and requiring 60% oxygen

C2. List the 3 activities that the baby must be able to coordinate to take nipple feedings successfully.

_____

_____

_____

C3. What reflex must be well developed for the baby to take nipple feedings safely?

_____

Check your answers with the list that follows the Recommended Routines. Correct any incorrect answers and review the appropriate section in the unit.

5. How Are Tube Feedings Managed?

- Use the information in Part 1 of this unit to determine the volume of each feeding.

- Before *every* feeding, aspirate from the tube to check if any residual milk has remained in the stomach from the previous feeding.

- Reinsert the residual milk and stomach fluid into the feeding syringe. This fluid contains electrolytes and other necessary body chemicals. It is important to replace these stomach contents.

  Note: When *first* inserting a gastric tube, there may be a large volume of fluid in the stomach, particularly if a baby is only a few hours old. This residual amniotic fluid may be discarded.

- Subtract the amount of residual milk (if any was found when the tube was aspirated) from the total volume of the milk to be given at that feeding. The number obtained is the number of milliliters of "new" milk to be given. Record the amount of residual fluid and "new" milk on the baby's chart.

- Pour the amount of milk for a feeding into the syringe barrel and allow it to drip by gravity into the baby's stomach.

  Example: Baby Frances was fed at 10:00 am. At 1:00 pm the next feeding was prepared. When the tube was checked, 5 mL of "old" milk and stomach juices were withdrawn, and then refed to the baby through the feeding tube.

  The total volume to be fed at 1:00 pm is 40 mL.
  The amount withdrawn and refed is 5 mL.
  The amount of "new" milk to be fed is 35 mL.

- Recalculate the volume of milk a baby needs as the baby grows and gains weight. When tube feedings are used, a baby has no control over how much milk is taken with each feeding.

6. When Are Tube Feedings Stopped?

A. When They Are No Longer Needed

All of the following should be documented before tube feedings are stopped and nipple feedings started for a baby:

- Who attained 32 to 34 weeks' gestational age
- Who developed a gag reflex and can coordinate sucking, swallowing, and breathing
- With no respiratory problems
- With normal vital signs, color, and activity

B. When They Are Not Tolerated

When significant residual volume is found consistently before each feeding, or if bile appears in the residual, this indicates that the baby is so sick the intestines are not actively moving the milk from the stomach.

Tube feedings should be stopped, the baby's hydration maintained with IV fluids, and the cause of the baby's ileus or obstruction investigated.

 Consistent residual volumes, or even one large residual, in a baby who previously had no residuals may indicate a serious intestinal problem— necrotizing enterocolitis.

These babies must be carefully evaluated for abdominal distention and other signs of illness.

7. Are Any Other Techniques Used to Feed Preterm Babies?

Spoon feeding, finger feeding, and/ or cup feeding are used by some centers in feeding preterm infants. The value and safety of these techniques for preterm babies are undergoing evaluation and, therefore, will not be discussed here.

Recommended Routines

All of the routines listed below are based on the principles of perinatal care presented in the unit you have just finished. They are recommended as part of routine perinatal care.

Read each routine carefully and decide whether it is standard operating procedure in your hospital. Check the appropriate blank next to each routine.

Procedure Standard in My Hospital	Needs Discussion by Our Staff	
_____	_____	1. Establish a policy of withholding feedings and administering intravenous fluids to all babies who
_____	_____	• Have a history of maternal hydramnios, until a diagnosis is established
_____	_____	• Have excessive mucus, until a diagnosis is established
_____	_____	• Have depressed, rapid, or labored respirations
_____	_____	• Are vomiting, have distended abdomens, and/or have not stooled by 48 hours of age
_____	_____	• Required prolonged resuscitation
_____	_____	• Are acutely unstable for any other reason
_____	_____	2. Establish a policy of withholding nipple feedings (breast or bottle) and using tube feedings for all babies younger than 32 to 34 weeks' gestation.
_____	_____	3. Establish a policy for preterm babies of using only breast milk (from a baby's own mother) or isosmolar formulas designed specifically for preterm infants.
_____	_____	4. Establish a routine for determining the amount and frequency of feedings for babies, according to their gestational age and weight, or expected weight for small for gestational age babies.
_____	_____	5. Establish a policy of weighing every baby daily and plotting the weight on a growth curve.
_____	_____	6. Establish a policy of providing vitamin and iron supplementation to preterm babies, either through use of a formula designed specifically for preterm babies or with supplements added to formula or breast milk.

These are the answers to the self-test questions. Please check them with the answers you gave and review the information in the unit wherever necessary.

A1. The baby may aspirate the milk.

A2. C. Insert an orogastric or nasogastric tube, and evaluate for obstruction before feeding.

A3. False   Formulas, medications, or vitamins with high osmolarity are more likely to damage the gastrointestinal tract of a newborn, particularly a preterm baby, than are isosmolar substances (same osmolarity as breast milk). Formulas designed specifically for preterm babies contain extra calories, vitamins, and minerals in an isosmolar concentration.

A4. Every 3 hours

A5. A.   Every 3 to 4 hours

B.   Small for gestational age

C.   60 mL every 3 hours or 80 mL every 4 hours (Expected weight at 10th percentile = 2,600 g) or more if baby appears hungry and tolerates feedings well.

A6. A.   Intravenous fluids only

Answer for Example B: No. Initially the baby's weight loss seems to follow the expected curve, but by day 6 and 7 clearly becomes abnormal.

B1. True

B2. Peripheral intravenous line started to supplement baby's fluid intake; check blood glucose screening tests

B3. Yes

B4. Yes   No

Yes	No	
___	_x_	Are unnecessary if a baby is receiving breast milk
_x_	___	Should be mixed in a baby's feedings
___	_x_	Should be given separate from a feeding
_x_	___	May be started when a baby is tolerating feedings well

C1. Yes. Tube feedings should be used.

No.   Tube feedings are not necessarily indicated. As long as the blood glucose has been brought to normal and the infant is alert, the baby may feed by bottle or breast in addition to the intravenous glucose therapy used to treat the baby's hypoglycemia.

No.   Tube feedings should not be given. This baby should be kept NPO and receive only intravenous fluids for the first several days after birth.

C2. Sucking
Swallowing
Breathing

C3. Gag reflex

Unit 8 Posttest

Without referring back to the information in the unit, please answer the following questions. Select the **one best** answer to each question (unless otherwise instructed). Record your answers on the answer sheet that is the last page in this book *and* on the test.

1. A 4-hour-old, term, appropriate for gestational age baby is fussy, with a distended abdomen. What should you do?
    - **A.** Feed the baby 60 mL (2 oz) glucose water (5% dextrose).
    - **B.** Obtain a serum sodium.
    - **C.** Feed the baby 60 mL (2 oz) formula.
    - **D.** Insert a nasogastric or orogastric tube.

2. Which of the following conditions is *most* suggestive that a baby may have difficulty with the first feeding?
    - **A.** Baby with excessive mucus
    - **B.** Twins with estimated gestational age of 36 weeks
    - **C.** Large for gestational age baby
    - **D.** Cesarean section baby

3. When calculating the volume of milk a small for gestational age baby needs, it is important to consider the baby's gestational age and
    - **A.** Actual weight
    - **B.** Length
    - **C.** Expected weight
    - **D.** History of the pregnancy

4. **True**   **False**   A baby whose estimated gestational age is 30 weeks may develop pneumonia if fed with a nipple.

5. **True**   **False**   As a general rule, preterm infants should not be fed until they are 48 hours old.

6. **True**   **False**   A 2-month-old preterm baby receiving full feedings with breast milk does not need iron supplementation.

7. **True**   **False**   Isosmolar formulas are preferred for preterm infants.

8. Which of the following babies requires tube instead of nipple feedings?
    - **A.** 31-week, appropriate for gestational age baby with a strong suck reflex
    - **B.** 38-week, small for gestational age baby with myelomeningocele
    - **C.** 39-week baby with hyperbilirubinemia requiring phototherapy
    - **D.** 40-week baby with a strong suck reflex receiving intravenous fluids for hypoglycemia

9. **True**   **False**   It is important to aspirate and discard the stomach contents before each new tube feeding.

10. **True**   **False**   A baby requiring oxygen may be fed safely by nipple as long as the environmental oxygen concentration is maintained.

11. **True**   **False**   Tube feedings are used only for preterm infants.

12. **True**   **False**   Once a feeding tube is inserted, checked, and taped in position, placement does not need to be checked again until a new tube is inserted.

13. A baby requires tube feedings of 40 mL of milk every 3 hours. While preparing the baby for the next feeding, you find that the baby has 5 mL of residual milk left in the stomach from the previous feeding. The baby's abdomen is not distended; vital signs, color, and activity are normal. What should you do?
    - **A.** Refeed the residual milk and feed the baby 40 mL of new milk.
    - **B.** Discard the residual milk and skip this feeding.
    - **C.** Refeed the residual milk and feed the baby 35 mL of new milk.
    - **D.** Discard the residual milk and feed the baby 40 mL of new milk.

For each question, please make sure you have marked your answer on the test and on the answer sheet (last page in book). The test is for you; the answer sheet will need to be turned in for continuing education credit.

Skill Unit   Nasogastric Tube Feedings

This skill unit will teach you how to insert a nasogastric (NG) tube and how to feed a baby using an NG tube. The techniques for inserting an orogastric (OG) tube and using it to feed a baby are very similar to those for an NG tube. The differences between NG tubes and OG tubes are indicated at the appropriate steps.

Study this skill unit and attend a skill session to practice and demonstrate this skill. Then arrange with your coordinator(s) to insert a feeding tube the next time a baby in your hospital needs one.

To master the skill, you will need to demonstrate correctly each of the following steps:

1. Collect and prepare equipment.

2. Measure the tube.

3. Insert the tube.

4. Check the placement of the tube.

5. Tape the tube in place.

6. Position the baby for a tube feeding.

7. Feed the baby.

Actions	**Remarks**

Deciding if Tube Feeding Is Appropriate

1. Should enteral feeding be used for this baby?

   - Does the baby have acute respiratory distress or other acute illness, particularly during the first few days after birth?

   Yes: Enteral feedings, given by any method, may *not* be appropriate.

   No: Does the baby have any of these conditions?
   - Gestational age below 32 to 34 weeks?
   - Lacks a gag reflex or cannot coordinate sucking, swallowing, or breathing?
   - Too weak to feed well by nipple?
   - Is recovering from acute respiratory disease, and is several days of age or older but is still requiring supplemental oxygen and/or has an increased respiratory rate?

   Yes to any of these questions: Consider tube feedings or maintain intravenous nutrition.

Preparing to Insert a Nasogastric Tube

2. Collect the following items:

• 5 F feeding tube	
• Clean syringes	
– One 3, 5, or 6 mL	To check tube placement
– One 12 or 20 mL	To hold milk for feeding
• Stethoscope	To check tube placement
• 1/2-inch adhesive tape	
– One 1-inch piece	To mark length of tube
– One 3-inch piece	To hold tube to baby's lip
• 1 piece of masking tape 10 inches long	To hold barrel of syringe with milk to top of incubator or to caregiver's or parent's clothing, if baby will be held during the feeding
• Clear adhesive dressing film (several commercial brands are available)	To protect baby's lip from adhesive tape

Actions	**Remarks**

Inserting a Nasogastric Tube

3. Measure length of feeding tube needed for the particular baby.

   - Turn baby's head to one side.
   - Hold the tube as you measure
     1. From a point midway between the umbilicus and the tip of the sternum
     2. To earlobe
     3. To nose

Note: When inserting an OG tube, measure to the baby's mouth rather than the nose.

4. If the tube has markers on it, note the one that is closest to the baby's nose. Record it on the baby's chart. As the baby grows, be sure to remeasure often and note new insertion length.

   If the tube is unmarked, wrap the small piece of adhesive tape around it to mark the point where the tube touches the end of the baby's nose.

Note: For very low birth weight babies, minimal insertion lengths have been identified.

Daily Weight (not birth weight) in **Grams**

	<750	750–999	1,000–1,249	1,250–1,499
Insertion Length	13 cm	15 cm	16 cm	17 cm

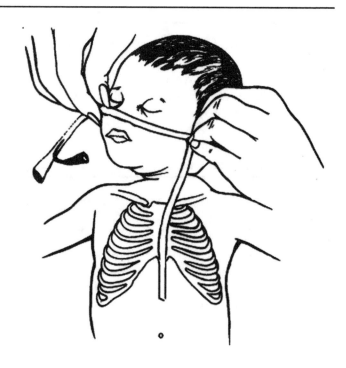

Only a few hospitals care for babies this size. For those that do, these minimal insertion lengths should be used *only as a guide*. Each baby should be measured and tube placement checked whenever a feeding tube is inserted.

5. Cut a piece of clear adhesive dressing (3 in. x 1/2 in.). Place this across the baby's upper lip (not shown).

   This is used to protect the baby's skin from the adhesive tape. The adhesive tape is placed on top of the clear adhesive dressing.

6. Prepare adhesive tape that will hold the NG tube to the baby's lip.

   - Use 3-inch length of tape.
   - Cut tape in Y shape as shown.
   - Put base of Y and 1/2 of split section on baby's lip.
   - Leave 1/2 of split tape loose to wrap around the tube later.

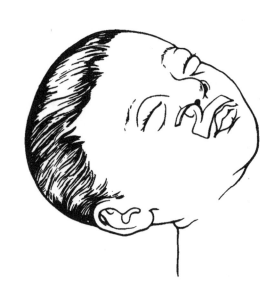

Actions	**Remarks**

Inserting a Nasogastric Tube (continued)

7. Restrain baby's arms.

8. Flex the baby's head forward and hold it so it will not move.

9. Insert NG tube into baby's nose. Continue pushing tube gently and quickly into nose and down the throat.

    Stop when the tape marker or measured marker is at baby's nose.

    If the tube comes out the baby's mouth instead of going down the baby's throat, or if the baby continues to gag, remove the tube and start again.

    Remarks: Some babies gag when the tube touches the back of their throat. This is normal. Continue inserting the tube.

    If the baby turns blue, remove the tube immediately. An uncommon complication of this procedure has occurred. The tube has entered the trachea rather than the esophagus.

10. Wrap the tube once with the loose end of the tape. This will hold the tube temporarily.

Checking the Placement of a Feeding Tube

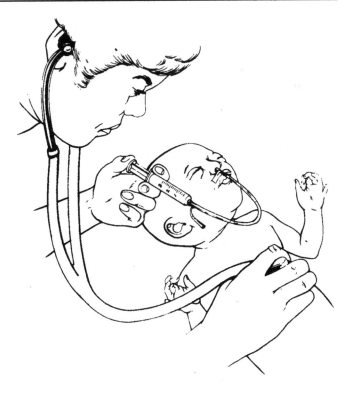

11. Draw 1 to 2 mL of air into the small syringe.

12. Attach the syringe to the open end of the tube.

13. Put a stethoscope over the baby's stomach (upper left quadrant of abdomen).

343

Actions	**Remarks**

Checking the Placement of a Feeding Tube (continued)

14. While listening with the stethoscope over the baby's stomach, quickly push in 1 to 2 mL of air with the syringe. Listen for the sound of the air entering the baby's stomach.

Rumbling heard in the stomach when air is pushed through the tube suggests it is in the stomach and not the lungs. However, air may sometimes be heard in the stomach when the tube tip is in the esophagus.

You hear the air in the stomach ⟶

Go to step 16.

You do *NOT* hear the air in the stomach ⟶

Remove the tube, remeasure it, and insert it again.

15. Withdraw the air from the baby's stomach.

16. Wrap the remainder of the loose end of adhesive tape in a spiral around the tube to hold it in place.

Note: An OG tube may be taped to a baby's cheek, using the same method described for taping an NG tube to a baby's lip.

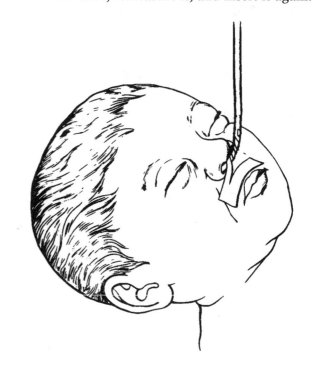

First Feeding Through the Tube

17. Position baby for feeding: Incline incubator so the baby's head is raised.

Consider positioning the baby on the right side because this position aids emptying of the stomach.

18. Remove plunger from larger syringe (12- or 20-mL syringe).

19. Attach barrel of syringe to the tube.

20. Attach masking tape to barrel of syringe so that half of the tape hangs free. This half will be used to attach the barrel to the top of the incubator or to the caregiver's clothing.

If the baby will be held throughout the feeding, the syringe barrel may be taped to the clothing of the caregiver or parent so the bottom of the barrel hangs a few inches above the baby.

Actions	**Remarks**

First Feeding Through the Tube (continued)

21. Pour measured amount of milk into the barrel of the syringe.

22. Start gravity flow of milk.

    • Insert plunger loosely in syringe.

    • Push plunger a little to start milk.

    • Tilt plunger to side to release vacuum in barrel.

    • Remove plunger.

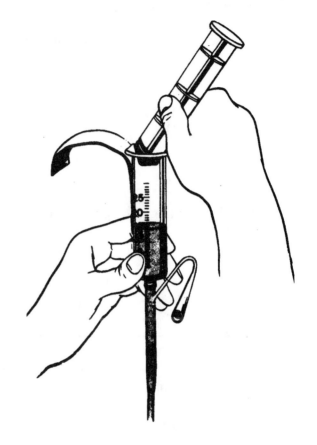

Do not push plunger in very far. You must be able to remove the plunger without withdrawing milk from the tube.

23. Tape the barrel to the top of the incubator or caregiver's clothing with the masking tape.

It is recommended that the baby suck on a pacifier during the feeding. This may be soothing to the baby, facilitate later nipple feeding, and has been shown to aid gastric motility.

24. Feed the baby for 10 to 20 minutes.

    If milk runs in too fast, a baby may have rapid gastric distention, making it more likely the baby will regurgitate some of the feeding or develop diarrhea.

    Use a 5 F rather than an 8 F feeding tube. The larger 8 F tube allows the milk to run in too quickly.

Never leave a baby unattended during a tube feeding. If the tube slips out of position, a baby can easily aspirate a large amount of milk.

Actions	Remarks

First Feeding Through the Tube (continued)

25. When all milk has run into tube

- Remove the barrel of the syringe from the tube.

Depending on the volume of milk a baby should receive, you may need to fill the barrel of the 12- or 20-mL syringe more than once during a feeding.

- Leave the tube open.

This allows a "vent" for the baby's stomach and minimizes the chance a baby will aspirate milk or stomach juices. The "vent" makes it less likely a baby will burp or vomit between feedings.

- Keep the baby in the head up position for 30 minutes.

Some people prefer to remove the tube after the feeding and insert a new tube before each feeding. Be sure there is no milk left in the syringe or visible in the feeding tube. Then pinch the tube tightly and withdraw it quickly.

Later Feedings With the Tube

26. Position baby for feeding.

- Incline the incubator so the baby's head is raised.

- Consider positioning the baby on his or her right side with blanket roll behind the baby for support.

  The baby may also be in a blanket nest (not shown). Usual monitoring equipment is also not shown.

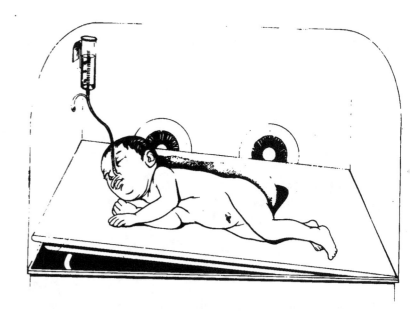

27. Check the position of the tube by listening over the stomach while pushing a small amount of air down the tube, as described previously.

ALWAYS check the position of the tube, before EVERY feeding. Even a correctly placed tube can slip out of the stomach between feedings.

Actions	Remarks

Measuring Milk Left in Stomach From Previous Feeding

28. Attach 3-, 5-, or 6-mL syringe to the tube and *gently* pull back the plunger until you feel increased pressure. Withdraw liquid from the stomach until no more fluid can be aspirated.

You are withdrawing the residual food and digestive juices left in the stomach from the previous feeding.

29. Observe how much liquid from the previous feeding is in the syringe.

30. Record the amount of liquid from the previous feeding on the patient record.

31. This liquid is generally too thick to drip by gravity. Therefore, gently push the liquid back into the tube with the syringe. Push *slowly* so the liquid goes in at a rate of 1 to 2 mL per minute.

If you push the liquid back quickly, the baby may vomit.

Generally you do not want to throw away the liquid from the baby's stomach. It contains electrolytes the baby needs to maintain stable body chemistries. However, excessive thick mucus or meconium in the stomach may be discarded before the first feeding.

32. Compute the amount of milk needed to complete the feeding. Subtract the amount of residual stomach liquid from the total amount of milk scheduled for feeding.

Large or repeated aspirates may indicate a baby has an ileus or is otherwise sick.

Example
Regular feeding	= 15 mL
Residual from stomach	= 5 mL
Feed this much new milk	= 10 mL

What Can Go Wrong?

1. The tube may be inserted into the airway instead of the stomach or the tube may not have been inserted far enough and thus may still be in the esophagus.

The most dangerous consequence of tube feedings is that milk may go into a baby's lungs.

This can happen because the tube is

- Positioned in the esophagus rather than the stomach. The milk may fill the esophagus and overflow into the trachea and lungs.
- Inserted into the trachea rather than down the esophagus, and milk is instilled directly into the lungs.

You must check the placement of a tube before EVERY feeding.

Actions	Remarks

What Can Go Wrong? *(continued)*

Actions	Remarks
2. You may overfeed or underfeed the baby.	Calculate volumes carefully and be sure to check for residual milk before each feeding. When tube feedings are used, the baby has very little control over how much milk is taken with each feeding.
3. The tube may perforate the stomach or esophagus.	This is a *rare* complication that may happen during insertion of the tube. Do not force the tube during insertion.
4. You leave a baby unattended.	The feeding tube may slip or be pulled loose by the baby. If this happens, milk may flow into the baby's lungs. — OR — The milk may stop flowing, causing a delay in the baby receiving the feeding.
5. You fail to check the tube position when an x-ray is taken.	Whenever an x-ray is taken of a baby with a feeding tube in place, the position of the tube tip should be noted. Be sure the end and side holes are in the stomach. The tube tip and 1.5 to 2.0 cm above the tip should be below the lower esophageal sphincter. This sphincter is at the level of the diaphragm, which is approximately at the level of the 9th thoracic vertebra.
6. You use the minimal insertion length for a very low birth weight baby, but do not increase the insertion length as the baby grows.	You should use the minimal insertion length for a baby's *current* weight. The insertion length will change as a baby grows. In addition, the minimal insertion lengths given in step 4 are guidelines only, and only for very small babies. Similar guidelines for larger babies have not been established. Each baby should be measured, and the placement of the tube always checked.

Unit 9

Hyperbilirubinemia

349

Objectives

In this unit you will learn

A. The causes of hyperbilirubinemia and factors affecting its severity

B. To recognize infants at risk for hyperbilirubinemia

C. To determine appropriate treatment(s) for hyperbilirubinemia

D. To operate phototherapy lights for maximum effectiveness

E. To assess a baby's risk for severe hyperbilirubinemia

 Recommendations in this unit incorporate guidelines given in the American Academy of Pediatrics Subcommittee on Hyperbilirubinemia. Management of hyperbilirubinemia in the newborn infant 35 or more weeks of gestation. Pediatrics. 2004;114:297–316.

Unit 9 Pretest

Before reading the unit, please answer the following questions. Select the *one best* answer to each question (unless otherwise instructed). Record your answers on the answer sheet that is the last page in this book *and* on the test.

1. Which of the following would concern you the *most*?

    A. Bilirubin of 12 at 30 hours of age in a full-term baby
    B. Bilirubin of 8 at 2 weeks of age in a breastfeeding baby
    C. Bilirubin of 9 at 10 hours of age in a full-term baby
    D. Bilirubin of 17 in a 3-day-old breastfeeding baby

2. For which of the following babies would you expect the binding capacity of serum protein for bilirubin to be *un*affected?

    A. A baby receiving ceftriaxone
    B. A baby who had a 5-minute Apgar score of 3
    C. A baby with an infection
    D. A baby with hypertension

3. When a baby is jaundiced, which of the following is the *first* action you should take?

    A. Begin phototherapy.
    B. Obtain blood samples for laboratory tests.
    C. Restrict feedings.
    D. Perform exchange transfusion.

4. Jaundice appearing within 24 hours of birth is usually

    A. Physiologic
    B. Due to breast milk
    C. Abnormal

5. Newborns are *more* likely than adults to have hyperbilirubinemia because

    A. They have decreased removal of bilirubin by the liver.
    B. Their diet consists only of formula or breast milk.
    C. They have fewer red blood cells.
    D. They have decreased reabsorption of bilirubin in the intestines.

6. The bilirubin of babies with very low Apgar scores may be dangerous at _____ bilirubin level than for a baby with high Apgar scores.

    A. A lower
    B. The same
    C. A higher

7. All of the following are possible complications of phototherapy *except*

    A. Increased number of stools
    B. Anemia
    C. Obstructed nasal breathing
    D. Hyperthermia

8. All of the following laboratory tests are routine in the investigation of hyperbilirubinemia, *except*

    A. Platelet count
    B. Coombs test
    C. Hematocrit
    D. Blood smear

9. When treating a girl baby with phototherapy lights, you would

    Yes No
    ___ ___ Cover the baby's eyes only for the first 8 hours of phototherapy.
    ___ ___ Discontinue phototherapy immediately if a rash appears.
    ___ ___ Completely undress the baby.
    ___ ___ Restrict the baby's fluid intake.
    ___ ___ Restrict the baby's feedings.

10. True   **False**   All jaundiced babies should receive phototherapy.

11. True   **False**   Jaundice associated with breastfeeding is seen only during the first 3 days after birth.

12. True   **False**   Sepsis increases the risk from hyperbilirubinemia.

For each question, please make sure you have marked your answer on the test and on the answer sheet (last page in book). The test is for you; the answer sheet will need to be turned in for continuing education credit.

1. What Is Bilirubin?

Bilirubin is formed from hemoglobin as a by-product of red blood cell breakdown. It is a waste product that must be eliminated from the body. In high concentrations, bilirubin is toxic to the brain and most tissues of the body.

 Excess bilirubin can cause brain damage.

Bilirubin toxicity is preventable in nearly all cases.

If toxicity occurs, *acute bilirubin encephalopathy* is used to describe the clinical findings during the first weeks after birth; *kernicterus* is used for the chronic and permanent clinical findings of bilirubin toxicity.

Bilirubin can be present in the blood in 2 forms.

- Direct or conjugated form

- Indirect or unconjugated form

2. How Is Bilirubin Removed From the Body?

Elimination of bilirubin occurs in several steps.

A. Bound to Serum Albumin

Unconjugated bilirubin in the blood is bound to serum albumin and then transported to the liver.

B. Processed by the Liver

In the liver, bilirubin becomes conjugated so that it can be excreted.

C. Excreted in the Stool

Conjugated bilirubin is carried in the bile into the intestine where it is further processed and then excreted in the stool. In newborns, as in fetuses, the conjugated bilirubin in the gut can be deconjugated and reabsorbed into the serum as unconjugated bilirubin.

3. How Is Bilirubin Measured?

Laboratories report bilirubin levels as conjugated (also called "direct") bilirubin, unconjugated (also called "indirect") bilirubin, and "total" bilirubin, which is the sum of the conjugated and unconjugated levels. Most of the bilirubin elevations seen in newborns result from elevated unconjugated bilirubin. In babies, therefore, the unconjugated and total bilirubin values are nearly equal to each other. Unless stated otherwise, bilirubin levels given in this unit are total serum bilirubin (TSB) values.

Bilirubin is expressed as milligrams per 100 mL of blood (eg, 5 mg/100 mL). This value may be noted as 5 mg/dL.

Transcutaneous bilirubin (TcB) may also be measured with any one of several commercially available noninvasive devices. Transcutaneous bilirubin measurement devices can be used as screening tools. They provide valid estimates when the TSB level is less than 15 mg/dL, although some experts use 12 mg/dL as the cutoff for accurate correlation between TcB and TSB.

4. What Is Hyperbilirubinemia?

Hyperbilirubinemia is an elevated level of bilirubin in the blood, which causes jaundice. Jaundice is characterized by a yellowish appearance of the skin and, as it progresses, a yellowish coloring of the whites of the eyes.

For reasons that are not entirely clear, babies with increasing bilirubin levels show a progression of jaundice from head to toe. If a baby is yellow all over, the bilirubin level is probably higher than if jaundice is visible only in the face.

In dark-skinned babies, the yellow skin coloring may be seen more easily by pressing your finger on the baby's skin, as if testing capillary refill time. Observe the color of the skin in the blanched area before capillary refill occurs.

Jaundice occurs in most newborns and, in most cases, is benign. Because bilirubin is potentially toxic, however, it should be monitored. Assess jaundice whenever you check a newborn's vital signs. Visual estimation of the *degree* of jaundice is unreliable. If jaundice is present, the only way to know the bilirubin level is to obtain a TcB or TSB measurement.

Phototherapy bleaches the skin, making TcB measurements unreliable when phototherapy is being used. Phototherapy also makes it more difficult to recognize jaundice with visual inspection. TSB measurements should be used.

5. What Causes Hyperbilirubinemia?

Bilirubin is higher in the blood of newborns because there is

- *Faster breakdown* of a larger number of red blood cells (overproduction of bilirubin)

- *Less efficient removal* of bilirubin by the liver

- *Increased reabsorption* from the intestines of bilirubin that has been secreted by the liver

Although there are many causes of hyperbilirubinemia (see Appendix), the most common are

A. Physiologic

Because of the 3 factors noted previously, approximately 65% of all newborns and 80% of all preterm newborns develop sufficient elevation of bilirubin to result in jaundice during the first few days after birth.

B. Hemolytic Disease (such as Rh or ABO incompatibility, or G6PD deficiency)

Hemolysis, the rapid destruction of red blood cells, may result from a variety of conditions. With blood group incompatibility, an antibody from the mother causes hemolysis of the baby's red blood cells. With glucose-6-phosphate dehydrogenase (G6PD) enzyme deficiency, or other inherited red blood cell abnormalities, hemolysis results from inherent fragility of the red blood cell membrane.

C. Various Neonatal Conditions

Any condition that tends to worsen any of the 3 factors noted previously will increase the severity of hyperbilirubinemia. For example,

- Polycythemia, a cephalohematoma, or widespread bruising will intensify overproduction.
- Prematurity is associated with decreased conjugation by the liver.
- Deconjugation and reabsorption will increase with intestinal obstruction or ileus.

6. When Is Bilirubin Dangerous to the Brain?

Bilirubin is dangerous when it leaves the blood and enters the brain. In the normal state, nearly all bilirubin is bound to serum protein (primarily albumin). The capacity of serum protein to attract and hold bilirubin is called the binding capacity. When there is an excess amount of bilirubin or an insufficient amount of serum protein, there is not enough binding space, and free bilirubin will result. Free bilirubin enters the brain very easily. Under certain circumstances involving severe stress, the blood-brain barrier is disturbed and even bilirubin bound to protein may enter the brain and cause damage.

Therefore, bilirubin is most likely to cause brain damage when

- There is too much bilirubin for the serum protein.

- Serum protein (albumin) levels are low.

- The binding capacity of serum protein is decreased.

- The baby has been severely stressed.

7. What Factors Influence Hyperbilirubinemia?

Some factors increase the likelihood that hyperbilirubinemia will develop. Other factors increase the risk of damage occurring as a result of hyperbilirubinemia. Still other factors are likely to influence the risk *of* hyperbilirubinemia and the risk *from* hyperbilirubinemia.

A. Increase Likelihood That Hyperbilirubinemia Will Develop

1. *Hemolysis:* Rapid breakdown of red blood cells may be caused by

   - Blood group incompatibility between mother and baby

   - G6PD deficiency (inherited enzyme deficiency), which is more common in populations originally from Mediterranean regions,

Middle East, Arabian peninsula, Southeast Asia, and Africa, but immigration and intermarriage have resulted in G6PD becoming widespread. G6PD deficiency occurs in 11% to 13% of African Americans and should be considered if severe hyperbilirubinemia develops, because African American infants generally have much lower TSB levels than white or Asian infants.

- Variety of neonatal illnesses, such as sepsis.

B. Increase Risk of Damage From Hyperbilirubinemia

1. *Perinatal compromise*

2. *Serum albumin less than 3.0 g/dL*

3. *Sick baby,* with any of the following:
   - Significant lethargy
   - Temperature instability
   - Acidosis

4. *Certain drugs**
   Some medications decrease serum albumin binding capacity by competing for binding sites. Examples of medications with high binding ratios include
   - Salicylates
   - Sulfonamides
   - Some cephalosporin antibiotics, such as ceftriaxone

C. Both Increase the Likelihood of Hyperbilirubinemia and the Risks Associated With It

1. *Prematurity*

   Preterm infants have immature livers with decreased ability to process bilirubin. Preterm babies are also more likely to be stressed and, therefore, are at risk for an impaired blood-brain barrier. Further, preterm babies often have low serum protein and thus have fewer bilirubin binding sites with a resultant increased likelihood of free bilirubin.

2. *Sepsis* (blood infection)

   Hemolysis, hepatocellular damage, ileus, and/or acidosis may occur as a result of sepsis. As noted previously, these factors may increase bilirubin production (hemolysis), decrease bilirubin removal (liver cell damage), increase reabsorption of bilirubin (ileus), and/or increase the risk of hyperbilirubinemia (acidosis).

 Prematurity, perinatal compromise, and infection are 3 important factors that increase the risks associated with hyperbilirubinemia.

---

*Additional information may be found in Robertson A, Carp W, Broderson R. Bilirubin displace effect of drugs used in neonatology. *Acta Paediatr Scand.* 1991;80:1119–1127.

Self-Test

Now answer these questions to test yourself on the information in the last section.

A1. What problem can result from hyperbilirubinemia? _____

A2. What are 3 reasons newborns have higher bilirubin levels than adults?

_____

_____

_____

A3. What does the binding capacity of serum protein mean?
   A. It is the cohesive property of blood that aids in clotting.
   B. It is the capacity of protein to bind bilirubin to hemoglobin.
   C. It is the capacity of serum protein to attract and hold bilirubin.

A4. **True False**   Under certain conditions, bilirubin bound to protein can enter the brain.

A5. **True False**   Careful visual inspection of a baby's jaundice provides reliable estimation of the serum bilirubin level.

A6. **True False**   Transcutaneous bilirubin measurements are as reliable as serum bilirubin measurements at every level of bilirubin.

A7. When is bilirubin dangerous to the brain?

_____

A8. Name at least 2 conditions that make hyperbilirubinemia more dangerous.

_____

_____

Check your answers with the list that follows the Recommended Routines. Correct any incorrect answers and review the appropriate section in the unit.

8. What Should Be Done When an Infant Becomes Jaundiced?

If an infant becomes jaundiced during the first 24 hours after birth, or is significantly jaundiced at any time, the bilirubin level should be measured. The infant should be examined and laboratory and other data obtained to determine the cause of the hyperbilirubinemia. A common mistake is to assume too quickly that jaundice is simply the result of physiologic hyperbilirubinemia. There are many causes for elevated bilirubin. Jaundice should be considered a possible sign of other conditions affecting the infant.

In general, jaundice should NOT be considered physiologic if
- *It appears in the first 24 hours after birth.*
- *Bilirubin levels rise faster than 0.5 mg/dL per hour.*
- *There is evidence of hemolysis.*
- *Physical examination is abnormal.*
- *Direct serum bilirubin exceeds 20% of total bilirubin.*
- *Jaundice persists for more than 3 weeks.*

There are 3 kinds of information that should be collected to determine the cause and appropriate treatment for hyperbilirubinemia.

A. History

- Review prenatal, labor, and delivery histories.

- Review notes for infant's feeding pattern and changes in activity.

- Interview family for history of significant hemolytic disease.

- Determine baby's ethnicity because enzyme abnormalities, such as G6PD deficiency, and other causes of hyperbilirubinemia are more common in individuals from Mediterranean, Middle Eastern, Arabian peninsula, African, or Asian origin.

B. Physical Examination

- Look for signs of infection, either acute or congenital. (See the next unit, Infections).

- Look for areas of accumulated blood (bruising, cephalohematoma).

- Check size of liver and spleen (enlargement suggests presence of hemolysis).

C. Laboratory Tests

- Serum bilirubin (total and direct reacting bilirubin)

- Mother's blood group and type and baby's blood group and type

- Coombs test

- Hematocrit/hemoglobin

- Blood smear and reticulocyte count

- Other tests as indicated

A more detailed description of how to determine the causes of jaundice and appropriate treatment is given in the Appendix.

9. Does Breastfeeding Cause Jaundice?

There is an association between breastfeeding and hyperbilirubinemia in newborns. Two syndromes are discussed. Most experts believe there is considerable overlap between the two.

A. Breastfeeding Jaundice: Early Onset

Breastfed babies typically have higher levels of bilirubin than bottle-fed babies in the first several days after birth. The cause of this is not well understood, but is likely related to decreased caloric intake and/or relative dehydration, and increased rate of bilirubin reabsorption from the intestines in breastfed babies.

If a breast-fed baby develops significant jaundice during the *first* week after birth

- Evaluate as described previously to rule out other causes of hyperbilirubinemia.

- Encourage and support frequent breastfeeding (at least 8–12 times per 24 hours).

- If the bilirubin exceeds approximately 15 mg/dL, consider temporarily interrupting breastfeeding, substituting formula, and possibly using phototherapy for 48 to 72 hours to allow the bilirubin to decline. Breastfeeding may then be resumed. While formula is used, the mother can maintain her milk supply with hand expression or use of a breast pump.

Note: Unless dehydration can be documented, supplementation with water or glucose water has been shown to be of no value in healthy, term, or near-term infants.

B. Breastfeeding Jaundice: Late Onset

As many as 20% to 30% of breastfed babies develop prolonged hyperbilirubinemia associated with breastfeeding. The bilirubin level increases progressively after the fourth day of age and reaches a maximum by 10 to 15 days of age. Once again, the cause is not clear but is probably related to increased rate of bilirubin reabsorption from the intestines in some breastfed babies.

If a breastfed baby develops significant jaundice during the *second* or *third* week

- If not already done, consider instituting the measures outlined in section 9A.

- If hyperbilirubinemia persists for more than 3 weeks, consider consultation with regional center experts.

10. How Is Hyperbilirubinemia Treated?

Babies with hyperbilirubinemia should be well hydrated. If there are no contraindications to feeding, infants should also be fed to promote the excretion of bilirubin in the stool.

A. Phototherapy

Certain types of fluorescent, tungsten-halogen, and fiberoptic lights are effective in lowering bilirubin levels in the blood by changing the shape of the bilirubin molecule so it can be excreted more readily. Phototherapy is useful for term and preterm infants with physiologic jaundice and is commonly used to lower TSB levels.

Phototherapy equipment and lights vary widely, but all can be effective in lowering bilirubin. Effectiveness relates to the dose of phototherapy received by the infant. Commercially available devices, or radiometers, are available to measure the irradiance emitted by the lights.

B. Exchange Transfusion

Another way to treat hyperbilirubinemia is to exchange the infant's blood with that of an adult donor with a normal bilirubin level. Although exchange transfusions are more effective than phototherapy in lowering bilirubin levels rapidly, they also carry considerably greater risks and are not performed unless intensive phototherapy fails to lower the bilirubin level.

Self-Test

Now answer these questions to test yourself on the information in the last section.

B1. True   False   Phototherapy needs to be started whenever jaundice is detected in a baby.

B2. True   False   Breastfed babies are likely to have higher bilirubin levels than formula-fed babies.

B3.   To establish the cause of hyperbilirubinemia, which of the following types of information should always be reviewed?

Yes	No	
___	___	Laboratory tests
___	___	Chest x-ray
___	___	Oxygen saturation
___	___	History
___	___	Physical examination

B4.   When is hyperbilirubinemia not physiologic? Give at least 2 situations.

_____

_____

B5. True   False   A healthy-appearing baby girl is noted to be jaundiced on the first day after birth. She is active and eating well. This is physiologic jaundice.

B6. True   False   Exchange transfusion is more effective than phototherapy in rapidly lowering bilirubin levels.

B7. True   False   The increased incidence of hyperbilirubinemia in breastfed babies may be due to increased bilirubin reabsorption from the intestines.

B8.   Which laboratory tests are obtained initially for the evaluation of hyperbilirubinemia?

Yes	No	
___	___	Blood smear
___	___	Hematocrit/hemoglobin
___	___	Coombs test
___	___	Mother's and baby's blood group

Check your answers with the list that follows the Recommended Routines. Correct any incorrect answers and review the appropriate section in the unit.

11. When Are Babies Treated With Phototherapy for Hyperbilirubinemia?

A. Healthy Babies Born at 35 or More Weeks of Gestation

Bilirubin levels should be interpreted according to an infant's age in hours. For the guidelines in the graph below, use *intensive* phototherapy when a baby's TSB exceeds the line indicated for the baby's risk category and age.

Bilirubin levels can be lowered by using phototherapy lights that provide radiant flux or irradiance of 4 μW/cm^2/nm (microwatts per square centimeter per nanometer), or higher. *Intensive phototherapy* refers to an irradiance of at least 30 μW/cm^2/nm, measured at the infant's skin, directly below the center of the phototherapy lights, and delivered to as much of the baby's skin as possible.

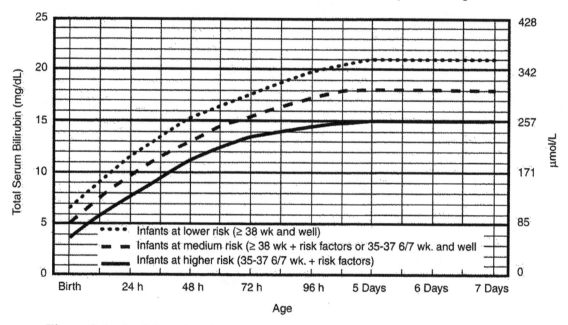

Figure 9.1. Guidelines for Phototherapy for Infants 35 or More Weeks' Gestation*

- Use TSB. Do not subtract direct reacting or conjugated bilirubin.

- **Risk factors**
  - Isoimmune hemolytic disease
  - G6PD deficiency
  - Perinatal compromise
  - Significant lethargy
  - Temperature instability
  - Sepsis
  - Acidosis
  - Albumin (if measured) less than 3.0 gm/dL

- Consider intervening at lower TSB levels for babies closer to 35 weeks and at higher TSB levels for those closer to 37 6/7 weeks.

- If the TSB continues to rise or does not decrease in a newborn receiving intensive phototherapy, consider that hemolysis may be present.

*Graph and legend adapted from American Academy of Pediatrics Subcommittee on Hyperbilirubinemia. Management of hyperbilirubinemia in the newborn infant 35 or more weeks of gestation. *Pediatrics* 2004;114:304.

- Consider conventional phototherapy in hospital or at home at TSB levels 2 to 3 mg/dL below those shown, but home phototherapy should not be used for any infant with risk factors.

Examples: You would follow the middle dashed line in the graph to determine that

- Phototherapy *is not indicated* for a well baby born at 36 weeks' gestation with TSB of 4 mg/dL at 24 hours.
- *Intensive* phototherapy *is indicated* for a well baby born at 36 weeks' gestation with TSB of 11 mg/dL at 24 hours.

B. Preterm Babies

Management of preterm babies differs from the guidelines noted previously for healthy, term, or near-term infants. Management decisions are based on the cause of the jaundice, the degree of illness of the baby, risk factors, and the rate of rise of the bilirubin. Some experts recommend the following general guidelines for starting phototherapy in preterm infants.

Guidelines for Initiating Phototherapy in Preterm Neonates

Birth Weight	Total Serum Billrubin Level (mg/dL)	
	Healthy	Sick
2,001–2,500 g	12–15	10–12
1,500–2,000 g	10–12	8–10
1,001–1,500 g	7–10	6–8
<1,000 g	5–7	4

Adapted from Table 46-2 in Halamek LP, Stevenson DK. Neonatal jaundice and liver disease. In: Fanaroff AA, Martin RJ, eds. *Neonatal-Perinatal Medicine, Diseases of the Fetus and Infant.* 7th ed. St Louis, MO: Mosby; 2002:1335.

For all babies, if intensive phototherapy is unsuccessful at preventing the bilirubin level from rising significantly, an exchange transfusion should be preformed. It should be emphasized, however, that when phototherapy is used appropriately, exchange transfusion is *rarely* required for the treatment of hyperbilirubinemia.

12. What Are the Techniques of Phototherapy?

Cover the baby's eyes completely. The strong lights may cause eye damage if the eyes are not covered.

Keep the baby as undressed as possible. Because the lights affect the bilirubin that has collected in the skin, as much of a baby's skin as possible must be exposed for maximum effectiveness.

Preserve temperature control. It is often helpful to keep a baby in an incubator or under a servocontrolled radiant warmer during phototherapy. Phototherapy lights may overheat a baby, especially if cared for in an incubator. Therefore, it is important to check a baby's temperature periodically during phototherapy. Even if an incubator is not needed to supply heat, it can be useful to minimize convective heat loss from an unclothed baby.

Increase fluid intake and check body weight frequently. Phototherapy lights can more than double a baby's stool and evaporative water losses.

363

Provide output (radiant flux or irradiance) at a minimum of 4 μW/cm²/nm. There is a direct relationship between irradiance and the effectiveness of phototherapy in reducing bilirubin levels. The radiant flux should be measured with a radiometer sensor held at the level of the infant's skin, directly below the center of the phototherapy lights. Irradiance measured below the center of the light source will be much higher than that measured at the light periphery. A minimum of 30 μW/cm²/nm, measured at the center of the light source, should be used for babies who require *intensive* phototherapy.

Replace bulbs as recommended by the manufacturer or when measurements show inadequate irradiance. After being used for a number of hours, phototherapy bulbs may lose effectiveness. Perform periodic checks to be sure the phototherapy lights provide adequate irradiance.

Position phototherapy lights an appropriate distance from the baby. Effectiveness decreases as the distance between the light source and the skin increases. However, problems with temperature control (overheating) and lack of clear visibility of the baby may be caused by phototherapy lights placed too close to a baby. A distance of approximately 45 cm from the baby for fluorescent lights has been recommended. Halogen spotlights need to be positioned according to the manufacturers' recommendations because burns can result if the lamps are too close to a baby.

Keep the shield that covers the bulbs in place. This helps to screen the light and reduces the baby's exposure to ultraviolet rays. In addition, a bulb will sometimes burst. The shield prevents glass fragments from falling onto the baby.

Use multiple lights and a fiberoptic phototherapy blanket to provide intensive phototherapy. In cases of very high or rapidly rising bilirubin, double or triple lights directed from different angles onto a baby's skin, to expose as much of the skin as possible to phototherapy, are more effective than a single set of lights. Large, term babies may need 2 lights to start to provide effective therapy over their entire surface area. A fiberoptic phototherapy blanket placed under a baby with a conventional phototherapy light(s) over the baby also increases the surface area of the baby exposed to phototherapy and the total radiant flux of the phototherapy.

In summary, the points to consider when providing phototherapy are

- Cover baby's eyes (see possible complications in next section).
- Keep baby naked.
- Monitor baby's temperature and thermal environment.
- Increase fluid intake to compensate for water loss through evaporation and more frequent stools.
- Monitor stools for excess fluid loss.
- Measure irradiance (radiant flux) of phototherapy light(s).
- Provide irradiance of *at least* 4 μw/cm²/nm.
- Provide irradiance of 30 μw/cm²/nm or more if *intensive* phototherapy is needed.

- Position lights to avoid overheating and to allow clear visibility of baby.
- Keep manufacturer's bulb shield in place.
- Use double or triple lights, and consider adding a phototherapy blanket, for babies with high or rapidly rising bilirubin.

In most cases, *brief* interruption of phototherapy during feeding or a portion of parental visiting time will not interfere with phototherapy treatment. It is essential, however, that any interruption be as brief as possible. Treatment can only be effective when the baby is under phototherapy lights.

13. What Are the Complications of Phototherapy?

Possible phototherapy complications include

- Eye damage, if baby's eyes are not covered (eye patches should be used)
- Obstructed nasal breathing, if eye patches slip and cover the nose (deaths have occurred; consider electronic cardiorespiratory monitoring for all babies receiving phototherapy)
- Skin rash (reasons are unknown; continue therapy)
- Increase in stools (increase fluid intake)
- Increased water loss through evaporation (increase fluid intake)
- Hyperthermia (monitor temperature frequently)

Other complications, such as bronze infant syndrome due to cholestasis (stoppage of bile flow) and severe skin blistering due to congenital photosensitivity are possible, but *rare*.

14. When Is an Exchange Transfusion Needed?

If the TSB reaches levels at which brain damage has been reported, despite *intensive* phototherapy, an exchange transfusion should be considered. Significant morbidity, in the form of apnea, bradycardia, cyanosis, vasospasm, necrotizing enterocolitis, thrombosis, as well as complications of blood transfusions, can occur. Deaths have occurred. Because exchange transfusions are rarely performed now, the risks are difficult to quantify, but are likely higher than when exchange transfusions were more common and more perinatal health care providers were skilled in doing them.

Figure 9.2 will help you identify if a term or near-term baby in your care has a bilirubin level approaching the need for an exchange transfusion, and regional center consultation should be considered. The American Academy of Pediatrics recommends an exchange transfusion be performed only by trained personnel in a neonatal intensive care unit with full monitoring and resuscitation capabilities.*

---

*American Academy of Pediatrics Subcommittee on Hyperbilirubinemia. Management of hyperbilirubinemia in the newborn infant 35 or more weeks of gestation. *Pediatrics* 2004;114:302.

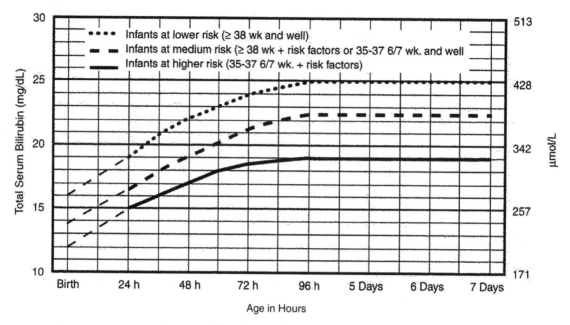

Figure 9.2. Guidelines for Exchange Transfusion in Infants 35 or More Weeks' Gestation*

- Use TSB. Do not subtract direct reacting or conjugated bilirubin.

- If exchange transfusion is being considered, obtain a serum albumin level and calculate the bilirubin/albumin ratio.

- **Risk factors**
  - Isoimmune hemolytic disease
  - G6PD deficiency
  - Perinatal compromise
  - Sepsis
  - Acidosis
  - Temperature instability
  - Significant lethargy
  - Low albumin

- *Immediate* exchange transfusion is recommended if the infant shows signs of acute bilirubin encephalopathy (hypertonia, arching, retrocollis, opisthotonos, fever, high-pitched cry) or if TSB is ≥5 mg/dL above the lines.

- Dashed lines for first 24 hours indicate uncertainty due to wide range of clinical circumstances and responses to phototherapy.

15. When Can Phototherapy Be Stopped?

Skin color is not a reliable index of the degree of hyperbilirubinemia, particularly if a baby is receiving phototherapy. Just because a baby is no longer jaundiced, does not necessarily mean the bilirubin in the blood has fallen sufficiently to stop treatment.

After starting phototherapy, serum bilirubin should be measured at least every 4 to 6 hours in babies with rapidly rising bilirubin, in preterm babies, or in sick babies. For otherwise healthy, term infants, who do not have rapidly rising bilirubin levels, serum bilirubin may be checked less frequently. Continue to check serum bilirubin until levels begin to decline.

*Graph and legend adapted from the American Academy of Pediatrics Subcommittee on Hyperbilirubinemia. Management of hyperbilirubinemia in the newborn infant 35 or more weeks of gestation. *Pediatrics.* 2004;114:305.

It is important to use only TSB rather than TcB measurements when babies are receiving phototherapy. This is because of skin bleaching and reliability of TcB measurements only for levels below 15 mg/dL, as noted earlier.

Discontinuation of phototherapy is a clinical decision based on

- Risk factors (such as history of perinatal compromise, acidosis, illness, etc)
- Serum bilirubin level
- Age of baby (gestational age at birth and postnatal age)
- Assessment of the baby's risk of severe hyperbilirubinemia

In most cases, if serum bilirubin levels are clearly decreasing, and are less than 13 to 14 mg/dL, phototherapy may be discontinued. However, a rebound increase of serum bilirubin may occur. Therefore, bilirubin levels should be checked for at least 12 hours after phototherapy has been stopped. If a significant rebound increase in bilirubin occurs, phototherapy may need to be restarted.

16. When Is it Safe to Discharge a Baby With Hyperbilirubinemia?

Babies who are preterm, have evidence of hemolysis, or have received phototherapy require individual consideration regarding appropriate timing of discharge and follow-up.

Figure 9.3 is for well newborns born at 36 or more weeks' gestation with birth weight of 2,000 g or more or babies 35 or more weeks' gestation with birth weight 2,500 g or more. The babies used to construct the figure had no identifiable risk factors. It can be used to estimate the likelihood that a baby with a given bilirubin value will reach a level of severe hyperbilirubinemia on a subsequent value. "Severe" was defined as a level of bilirubin that is greater than that achieved by 95% of well babies at the specified age. For the babies used to generate the figure, the results were as follows:

Risk Zone	Chance of Having Severe Hyperbilirubinemia on a Subsequent Value
High	40%
High intermediate	13%
Low intermediate	2%
Low	0%

To use Figure 9.3, note the baby's exact age in hours when the bilirubin sample was taken and mark it on the graph. The zone in which the value falls predicts the likelihood of a subsequent bilirubin level reaching a severe level. This assessment is particularly important for babies discharged before 72 hours of age.

Examples

- A 3,000-g baby born at 36 weeks' gestation had a TSB level of 13 mg/dL at 36 hours of age. The value falls in the high-risk zone, which indicates the baby has a significant risk of having another TSB falling in the severe range. This risk for severe hyperbilirubinemia is increased further as the number of risk factors increase.

- A 2,500-g baby born at 37 weeks' gestation had a TSB level of 8 mg/dL at 36 hours of age. The value falls in the low-intermediate risk zone, which indicates the baby has a relatively low likelihood of having a subsequent TSB value fall in the severe range. This risk for severe hyperbilirubinemia is increased further as the number of risk factors increase.

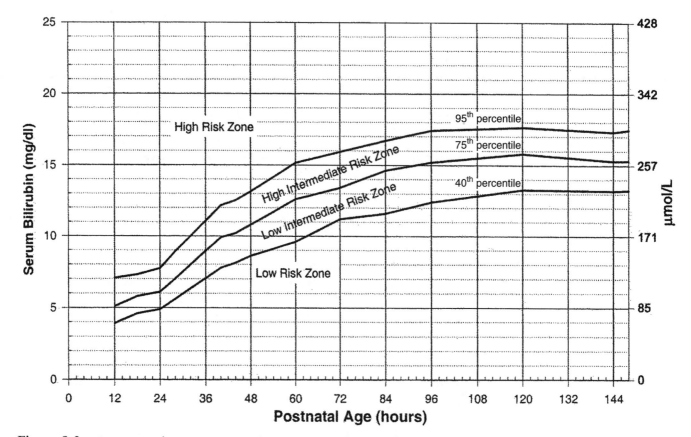

Figure 9.3. Nomogram for Designation of Risk for Severe Hyperbilirubinemia in Term and Near Term Well Newborns*

All newborns discharged 48 hours or less after birth should be evaluated by a health care professional within 48 hours after discharge. Use the identified risk zone as well as a baby's risk factors, plus clinical judgments, to determine when and how often the bilirubin level should be checked after discharge. The baby's weight, feeding, urine, and stool output should also be assessed.

At the time of discharge, all parents should have written and verbal explanations of jaundice, the need for further monitoring, and an identified plan for additional monitoring.

*Graph printed with permission from Bhutani VK, Johnson L, Sivieri EM. Predictive ability of a predischarge hour-specific serum bilirubin for subsequent significant hyperbilirubinemia in healthy term and near-term newborns. *Pediatrics.* 1999;103:6–14.

Self-Test

Now answer these questions to test yourself on the information in the last section.

C1. Use the graphs in the previous sections to help you answer these questions. For each of the following examples, decide if you should

- **A.** Consider phototherapy.
- **B.** Begin phototherapy.
- **C.** Begin intensive phototherapy.
- **D.** Consider an exchange transfusion.
- **E.** No other action needed at this time.

a. ____ A vigorous infant of 38 weeks' gestation with no risk factors who is jaundiced at 30 hours of age with a bilirubin of 10 mg/dL

b. ____ A 1,900-g baby of 33 weeks' gestation with respiratory distress and a bilirubin of 10 mg/dL at 36 hours of age

c. ____ A 3,000-g (6 lb, 10 oz) term baby with hemolytic disease from ABO incompatibility and a bilirubin of 20 mg/dL at 36 hours of age, while undergoing intensive phototherapy since 8 hours of age

d. ____ A formula-fed baby of 40 weeks' gestation with no complications who has a serum bilirubin of 15 mg/dL at 36 hours of age

e. ____ A baby of 36 weeks' gestation with a serum bilirubin of 8 mg/dL at 30 hours of age

f. ____ A baby of 39 weeks' gestation with a 1-minute Apgar score of 2 who required prolonged resuscitation, became jaundiced by 12 hours of age, and has a serum bilirubin of 10 mg/dL

C2. Name 3 common problems that can develop as a result of phototherapy.

_____

_____

_____

C3. **True False** The best way to know when to stop phototherapy is when the baby is no longer jaundiced.

C4. **True False** Phototherapy light irradiance should be at least 30 $\mu W/cm^2/nm$ for intensive phototherapy.

C5. Name the 4 pieces of information that must be considered when deciding when to discontinue phototherapy.

_____

_____

_____

_____

Check your answers with the list that follows the Recommended Routines. Correct any incorrect answers and review the appropriate section in the unit.

17. Is Home Phototherapy Useful?

For selected babies, phototherapy given in the home may be appropriate. Keep in mind that most babies requiring treatment for hyperbilirubinemia will warrant continued hospitalization. If discharged home, some infants may need rehospitalization for treatment of hyperbilirubinemia. The following are guidelines* for home phototherapy.

Infants should meet the following criteria:
- Term or near term, otherwise healthy, infants, who are at least 48 hours of age
- Serum bilirubin level below the curve for low-risk infants in Figure 9.1.
- No elevation in direct-reacting (conjugated) bilirubin concentration
- Physiologic hyperbilirubinemia, as determined by perinatal history, physical examination, and laboratory tests
- All other requirements for discharge are met

The rate of rise of the bilirubin should be estimated by obtaining at least 2 bilirubin levels, at least 4 hours apart. If the bilirubin is rising rapidly (more than 1 mg/dL in 3–4 hours), or if the initial bilirubin level obtained, before 48 hours of age, is in the high-risk zone in Figure 9.3 home phototherapy is not recommended. If there is no increase in bilirubin concentration over 4 hours or the baby's risk assessment is in the low-risk zone, and phototherapy is not being used in the hospital, there is no reason to initiate phototherapy in the home. Individual consideration of a baby's condition and risk factors needs to be given when the initial bilirubin value falls in the low-intermediate or high-intermediate zones in Figure 9.3.

If home phototherapy is appropriate, it is accomplished with a fiberoptic phototherapy blanket under the baby. The risk of nasal occlusion from a slipped eye patch is too great to allow recommendation for home use of overhead phototherapy lights that require eye patches for the baby.

Arrangements for home care should include the following:
- Parent(s) willing and able to provide home phototherapy
- Daily communication between parent(s) and physician or nurse practitioner
- Serum bilirubin measured every 12 to 24 hours, depending on previous level, rate of rise, and predischarge assessment of the risk for severe hyperbilirubinemia
- Verbal and written instructions for the parents regarding
  - Risks and benefits of phototherapy

---

*Adapted from American Academy of Pediatrics Committee on Fetus and Newborn. Home phototherapy. *Pediatrics*. 1985;76:136 and American Academy of Pediatrics Subcommittee on Hyperbilirubinemia. Management of hyperbilirubinemia in the newborn infant 35 or more weeks of gestation. *Pediatrics*. 2004;114:297–316.

- Use of phototherapy equipment

- Adequate hydration for the baby

- Need to report problems promptly

- Removal of baby from phototherapy during feedings, baths, and diaper changes, and when the parent(s) is asleep

- Possible need for rehospitalization if the baby becomes ill or the bilirubin rises sufficiently to enter the high-risk zone (see Figure 9.3)

Home phototherapy should be stopped when the bilirubin concentration drops below 13 to 14 mg/dL. To determine if a rebound in the bilirubin concentration occurs, levels should be rechecked 12 to 24 hours after phototherapy is discontinued.

Recommended Routines

All of the routines listed below are based on the principles of perinatal care presented in the unit you have just finished. They are recommended as part of routine perinatal care.

Read each routine carefully and decide whether it is standard operating procedure in your hospital. Check the appropriate blank next to each routine.

Procedure Standard in My Hospital	Needs Discussion by Our Staff	
_____	_____	1. Establish a policy of defining each case of jaundice as either physiologic or non-physiologic.
_____	_____	2. Establish a policy of always investigating the cause of hyperbilirubinemia whenever phototherapy is started.
_____	_____	3. Establish a policy that allows nurses to obtain a transcutaneous bilirubin (TcB) level or to order a total serum bilirubin (TSB) measurement any time jaundice is noted in a term or preterm newborn or to obtain follow-up levels at defined intervals.
_____	_____	4. For all babies receiving phototherapy, establish a policy of • Covering the eyes • Checking vital signs frequently • Monitoring intake and output and assessing hydration
_____	_____	5. Establish a policy of obtaining a TcB or TSB level within 48 hours after birth for term and near-term babies and of using Figure 9.3 to predict the course of bilirubin and likelihood of a subsequent value being in the high-risk zone.
_____	_____	6. Establish a protocol so all newborns discharged 48 hours or less after birth are evaluated by a health care professional within 48 hours after discharge.

These are the answers to the self-test questions. Please check them with the answers you gave and review the information in the unit wherever necessary.

A1. Brain damage

A2. Increased production of bilirubin due to breakdown of more red blood cells, at a faster rate.
Less efficient removal of bilirubin by the liver.
Increased reabsorption of bilirubin from the intestines.

A3. C. The capacity of the serum protein to attract and hold bilirubin.

A4. True

A5. False   A baby's serum bilirubin level cannot be reliably estimated from visual assessment of jaundice.

A6. False   Transcutaneous bilirubin and total serum bilirubin correlate closely when the bilirubin level is 15 mg/dL or lower. Some experts use 12 mg/dL as the cutoff for accurate correlation. In addition, transcutaneous bilirubin should not be used for babies under phototherapy lights because the lights bleach the skin, making transcutaneous bilirubin measurements unreliable.

A7. When it leaves the blood and enters the brain.

A8. Any 2 of the following:
- Prematurity
- Sepsis
- Perinatal compromise
- Acidosis
- Illness (lethargy, temperature instability)
- Low serum albumin (<3.0 g/dL)
- Certain medications

B1. False   Many babies will not require any treatment. The baby's physical examination, age, weight, risk factors, bilirubin level, and other tests, as indicated, need to be evaluated to determine the appropriate treatment.

B2. True

B3.

Yes	No	
x	___	Laboratory tests
___	x	Chest x-ray
___	x	Oxygen saturation
x	___	History
x	___	Physical examination

B4. Hyperbilirubinemia is not physiologic when
- It appears in the first 24 hours after birth.
- Bilirubin levels rise faster than 0.5 mg/dL per hour.
- There is evidence of hemolysis.
- Physical examination is abnormal.
- Direct bilirubin exceeds 20% of total bilirubin.
- Jaundice persists for more than 3 weeks

B5. False   Jaundice is not considered physiologic if it appears within 24 hours after birth, even if the baby appears well.

B6. True

B7. True

B8.

Yes	No	
x	___	Blood smear
x	___	Hematocrit/hemoglobin
x	___	Coombs test
x	___	Mother's and baby's blood group

C1. a. E. No other action needed at this time.
   b. B. Begin phototherapy.
   c. D. Consider an exchange transfusion.
   d. C. Begin intensive phototherapy.
   e. A. Consider phototherapy.
   f. C. Begin intensive phototherapy.

C2. Any 3 of the following:
   • Eye damage (if eyes not covered)
   • Skin rash
   • Nasal obstruction (from slipped eye patch)
   • Increase in stools
   • Increase in evaporative water loss
   • Hyperthermia

C3. False   Skin color is not a reliable indicator of the degree of hyperbilirubinemia, especially for babies receiving phototherapy. The baby may no longer appear jaundiced but may still have a high serum bilirubin level. Total serum bilirubin (not transcutaneous bilirubin) measurement should be taken to determine baby's bilirubin level.

C4. True

C5. Risk factors in the baby's history
   Serum bilirubin level
   Age of baby (gestational age at birth and postnatal age)
   Assessment of the baby's risk of severe hyperbilirubinemia

Appendix: Identification and Treatment of Jaundice During the First Week After Birth*

	Physical Examination	Laboratory Findings	Cause	Treatment (in addition to management given in unit)
1.	Jaundice; normal appearing infant, may be preterm	• Negative Coombs • Normal: Hct†, reticulocytes, and smear	Immature liver; decreased conjugation of bilirubin	Maintain hydration.
2.	Jaundice; normal appearing infant with perhaps some paleness and/or evidence of tachypnea or mild congestive heart failure	• Direct Coombs: positive in Rh incompatibility, may be positive in ABO incompatibility • In both Rh and ABO incompatibility: decreased Hct, increased reticulocyte count, and polychromasia seen on smear	Hemolysis secondary to Rh, ABO, or a minor blood group incompatibility	Monitor for anemia in hospital and post-discharge, as antibodies may continue to cause hemolysis for weeks or months.
3.	Jaundice; hepatosplenomegaly; lethargy; hypothermia; poor feeding	• Increased direct and indirect bilirubin • Perhaps some evidence of hemolysis with decreased Hct, increased reticulocyte count • Negative Coombs	Sepsis	Obtain cultures, give antibiotics.
4.	Jaundice; ruddy color; frequently SGA or baby of a multifetal pregnancy	• Negative Coombs • Increased hematocrit • Normal: reticulocytes, smear	Polycythemia with increased bilirubin load from excess red blood cells	Consider treatment of high hematocrit (see Book III, Tests and Results).
5.	Jaundice; abnormalities on exam: • Hepatosplenomegaly • Possible: congenital heart disease, microcephaly, cataracts, hydrocephaly	• Increased direct bilirubin • Positive viral cultures or antibody rise and/or serology positive for syphilis • Negative Coombs	Congenital viral infection	Provide medical treatment of herpes, toxoplasmosis, or syphilis. (See Book II: Neonatal Care, Infections.)
6.	Jaundice; normal appearance with the exception of abdominal distension, history of vomiting and delayed or absent stooling	• Increased indirect bilirubin • Negative Coombs • Normal: smear, reticulocytes	Bowel obstruction	Provide supportive treatment • IV hydration, keep NPO • NG suction • Abdominal x-ray • Surgical consult
7.	Jaundice; normal appearing infant with multiple bruises from difficult labor and delivery	• Negative Coombs • Normal: smear, reticulocytes	Hemorrhaging under skin leads to increased breakdown of red blood cells	
8.	Jaundice; normal appearing infant; possible hepatosplenomegaly; may become acutely ill with hypoglycemia, vomiting, diarrhea, seizures, and clinical signs similar to sepsis	• Increased indirect and direct bilirubin • Urine positive for reducing substances if fed human milk or formula • Obtain blood sample for measurement of enzyme level	Galactosemia	Remove galactose from diet—change to formula that contains no galactose or lactose.
9.	Jaundice; normal appearing infant of Mediterranean, Middle East, Southeast Asia, or African American heritage	• Decreased Hct, increased reticulocyte count, and polychromasia seen on smear • Sudden increase in bilirubin can occur	G6PD deficiency	• Test for G6PD G6PD-deficient infants require intervention at lower TSB levels.

*Table is for detecting causes of jaundice only during the first few days of after birth. If jaundice persists or is late appearing, evaluate further for more rare conditions.

†Hct, hematocrit; ABO, major blood group isohemaglutanins; SGA, small for gestational age; IV, intravenous; NPO, nothing by mouth; NG, nasogastric; G6PD, glucose-6-phosphate dehydrogenase; TSB, total serum bilirubin.

Unit 9 Posttest

Without referring back to the information in the unit, please answer the following questions. Select the *one best* answer to each question (unless otherwise instructed). Record your answers on the answer sheet that is the last page in this book *and* on the test.

1. A baby has an infection. You would anticipate this baby's bilirubin level to be

   A. Lower than normal
   B. Normal
   C. Higher than normal

2. For which of the following babies is the binding capacity of serum protein *least* likely to be affected?

   A. Preterm baby
   B. Baby receiving sulfonamides
   C. Baby who had a 1-minute Apgar score of 2
   D. Baby who has hypocalcemia

3. When a baby is jaundiced, which of the following is the *first* action you should take?

   A. Start antibiotics.
   B. Obtain blood samples for laboratory tests.
   C. Restrict the baby's fluids.
   D. Perform an exchange transfusion.

4. All of the following conditions are possible complications of phototherapy *except*

   A. Alkalosis
   B. Dehydration
   C. Skin rash
   D. Eye damage

5. All of the following conditions are added risk factors for a baby with hyperbilirubinemia *except*

   A. Prematurity
   B. Infection
   C. Acidosis
   D. High blood pH

6. All of the following laboratory tests are recommended for the investigation of hyperbilirubinemia *except*

   A. Blood glucose
   B. Hematocrit/hemoglobin
   C. Blood smear
   D. Mother's blood type

7. When you are treating a baby with phototherapy, you

   Yes No
   ___ ___   Cover the baby's eyes.
   ___ ___   Dress the baby in special clothing.
   ___ ___   May have to restrict the baby's fluid intake.
   ___ ___   Take the baby's temperature more frequently.

8. Newborns are *more* likely than adults to have hyperbilirubinemia because

   A. They have increased removal of bilirubin by the liver.
   B. Their diet consists only of formula or breast milk.
   C. They have fewer red blood cells.
   D. They have increased reabsorption of bilirubin in the intestines.

9. **True   False**   Some babies with mild hyperbilirubinemia do not need phototherapy.

10. **True   False**   A sick term baby will require treatment for hyperbilirubinemia at a lower bilirubin level than a healthy term baby.

11. True   False   Brain damage can result from excess bilirubin.

12. True   False   Breastfed babies should receive water supplementation to help prevent the development of hyperbilirubinemia.

For each question, please make sure you have marked your answer on the test and on the answer sheet (last page in book). The test is for you; the answer sheet will need to be turned in for continuing education credit.

Unit 10   Infections

Objectives

In this unit you will learn

A. Why newborn babies can easily become infected

B. Which babies are at risk for infection

C. The types of neonatal infections

D. The clinical signs and laboratory findings suggestive of infection

E. What to do when infection is suspected

F. The importance of the appropriate use of antibiotics

G. How to control spread of infections in the nursery

Note: Certain recommendations, guidelines, and charts in this unit are adapted from material published by The American College of Obstetricians and Gynecologists and the American Academy of Pediatrics in the sources listed below. For more detailed discussion of specific perinatal infections and their management, consult

- *Guidelines for Perinatal Care.* 5th ed. American Academy of Pediatrics and American College of Obstetricians and Gynecologists, 2002

- *Red Book: 2006 Report of the Committee on Infectious Diseases.* 27th ed. American Academy of Pediatrics, 2006

For a detailed description of infection control procedures to prevent the transmission of bloodborne and nosocomial pathogens, see the recommendations of the Centers for Disease Control and Prevention.

- Garner JS. Guideline for isolation precautions in hospitals. Available at: www.cdc.gov/ncidod/dhqp/gl_isolation.html.

Unit 10 Pretest

Before reading the unit, please answer the following questions. Select the *one best* answer to each question (unless otherwise instructed). Record your answers on the answer sheet that is the last page in this book *and* on the test.

1. Which of the following is the *most* common clinical sign indicating a newborn baby has a systemic infection?
   A. A low body temperature
   B. An elevated body temperature
   C. Persistent cough
   D. Skin rash

2. Which of the following statements is true?
   A. Medication is available to cure infants with congenital rubella.
   B. An infected baby will always have an abnormal white blood cell count.
   C. An infected baby may develop metabolic acidosis.
   D. Gentamicin should be given by rapid intravenous push to obtain therapeutic blood levels.

3. Of the procedures listed below, what is the *first* thing that should be done for an infant suspected of having a systemic infection?
   A. Begin antibiotic therapy.
   B. Wash the baby with diluted hexachlorophene (Phisohex).
   C. Obtain blood cultures.
   D. Give intravenous gamma globulin.

4. Which of the following procedures is *most* effective in controlling the spread of infection in the nursery?
   A. Have everyone wear hospital scrub clothes.
   B. Require handwashing between handling babies.
   C. Put all babies in incubators.
   D. Have everyone wear masks.

5. What is one reason infants become infected more often than adults?
   A. The level of complement in the blood is excessively high.
   B. They are exposed to more virulent organisms.
   C. They have fewer white blood cells.
   D. Their immune system is immature.

6. **True   False**   Babies with mild localized staphylococcal infections require only mild soap and water washes of the affected area and application of an antibiotic ointment.

7. **True   False**   An umbilical arterial catheter increases a baby's risk for infection.

8. **True   False**   Neonatal group B beta hemolytic streptococcus sepsis is rarely a life-threatening infection.

9. **True   False**   Even if a baby shows no sign of infection, congenital syphilis should be treated with intravenous antibiotics for 10 to 14 days.

10. **True   False**   Hepatitis B virus vaccine is recommended only for babies with mothers positive for hepatitis B surface antigen.

11. **True   False**   Antiretroviral treatment of HIV-positive women during pregnancy and labor can dramatically reduce the number of babies who become infected with the virus.

12. **True   False**   Gonococcal conjunctivitis is a localized infection that requires systemic antibiotic treatment.

13. For each of the following conditions, determine if they place the infant at risk for developing an infection.

    Yes   No
    ___   ___   Rupture of membranes 24 hours prior to delivery
    ___   ___   Active labor for 24 hours
    ___   ___   Father's skin colonized with staphylococcal epidermidis

381

14. A pregnant woman's membranes ruptured 36 hours before delivery. Twenty-four hours after birth the baby has a reduced temperature and low activity level.

Yes	No	
___	___	The baby was at risk for infection at the time of birth.
___	___	Reduced temperature is a clinical sign of infection in babies.
___	___	This baby probably has a localized infection.
___	___	The first actions to take are to begin supportive care and obtain cultures from this baby.
___	___	You should obtain blood cultures and promptly begin antibiotics.
___	___	Ampicillin alone is an appropriate treatment for this baby.

For each question, please make sure you have marked your answer on the test and on the answer sheet (last page in book). The test is for you; the answer sheet will need to be turned in for continuing education credit.

A newborn infant with systemic infection (sepsis) has a very high probability of either dying or being permanently damaged if the infection is not suspected and treated quickly.

1. Why Do Babies Become Infected?

A. Defense Mechanisms Are Immature

Babies are less capable of handling infections than are older children and adults because babies' immune systems are immature.

B. Antibodies Against Specific Microorganisms Have Not Developed

Normally, while in utero a fetus is not exposed to any microorganisms and therefore does not have the opportunity to develop resistance to specific infectious agents.

C. IgG Antibody Levels May Be Low (if Baby Is Preterm)

Some of the woman's antibodies (IgG type) are normally transferred across the placenta to the fetus during the third trimester. If a baby is significantly preterm, there will be a decreased amount of maternally acquired antibodies.

D. All Babies Have Low Amounts of IgM Antibody

One type of maternal antibody (IgM) is too large to be transferred across the placenta. Therefore, all newborns, term and preterm, are deficient in IgM antibodies.

2. How Are Types of Infections Grouped?

A. Acute Life-Threatening Infection of the Blood (Sepsis)

There is a very high mortality rate for babies with these infections. Also, infections of the blood in newborns can become an infection of the spinal fluid (meningitis). The most common causative organisms are bacterial.

- Gram-positive bacteria (eg, group B, beta hemolytic streptococcus [GBS])

- Gram-negative bacteria (eg, *E coli* and *Klebsiella*)

Viral infections (eg, herpes simplex or cytomegalovirus) can also cause severe blood infections in the newborn, but are less common.

B. Localized Infections

Infections in this category are confined to a specific area or part of the infant. These infections are usually not life-threatening, but may become so if not treated properly. The most common conditions are

- Staphylococcal pustulosis

- Abscess

- Omphalitis (infection of the umbilical stump)

- Conjunctivitis
- Wound infections

C. Congenital Infections

These infections are associated with an infection of the woman during pregnancy. The fetus acquires the infection in utero. If infected early in pregnancy, the fetus may develop cataracts, congenital heart disease, or other abnormalities. If infected late in pregnancy or around the time of delivery, a baby may be born with symptoms of an acute systemic infection. The common intrauterine infections are often referred to as TORCHS infections.

T   Toxoplasmosis
O   Other (varicella, coxsackie B, HIV, etc)
R   Rubella
C   Cytomegalovirus
H   Herpes simplex
S   Syphilis

In addition to these infections, it is also known that many infants born to women who tested positive for hepatitis B surface antigen will become infected with hepatitis B virus, unless treatment is started soon after birth.

Although TORCHS infections may be diagnosed on the basis of the effect they have already had on the infant prior to birth, identification of the infecting agent is important because appropriate therapy may alter the outcome.

D. Hospital-Acquired Infections

Hospital-acquired infections (also called nosocomial infections) often result in systemic, life-threatening illness in newborns. Babies who require continued hospitalization are at risk for nosocomial infections. There are several reasons for this.

- Likelihood of needing a greater number of invasive procedures.

- Longer time period to be exposed to a greater number of health care workers, who may have also cared for other babies and for patients in other hospital areas.

- Inadequate use of infection control measures, such as standard precautions and proper handwashing.

- Overuse and/or misuse of some antibiotics, which then allows resistant strains of bacteria to develop. *Nationwide, infections with drug-resistant organisms are a serious and increasing problem.*

Self-Test

Now answer these questions to test yourself on the information in the last section.

A1. Inadequate handwashing by hospital staff may result in a newborn developing a _____ infection.

A2. Why do infants become infected? (Choose as many as appropriate.)

    A. Their immune systems are immature.
    B. They cannot receive antibiotics routinely used in adults.
    C. They have not built up antibodies against specific organisms.
    D. If preterm, their maternally acquired antibody levels will be low.

A3. For each of the following infections, determine the general type or category.

    A. Acute, systemic (blood) infection
    B. Localized infection
    C. Congenital intrauterine infection

      _____ *E coli* infection
      _____ Staphylococcal pustulosis
      _____ Conjunctivitis
      _____ Group B beta hemolytic streptococcus infection
      _____ Cytomegalovirus

A4. **True False** Sepsis (blood infection) is rarely life-threatening in babies.

A5. **True False** Overuse of antibiotics is one reason drug-resistant forms of bacteria develop.

A6. **True False** Prolonged hospitalization increases a baby's risk for infection.

Check your answers with the list that follows the Recommended Routines. Correct any incorrect answers and review the appropriate section in the unit.

3. Which Infants Are At Risk for Infection?

To be at risk for infection means having been exposed to certain conditions or circumstances that predispose a baby to developing an infection.

A. Life-Threatening Systemic Infections

The following conditions place an infant at risk for developing a systemic infection:

- Rupture of amniotic membranes longer than 18 hours
  Note: Although uncommon, it is also possible for a fetus to become infected through intact membranes (ascending infection).

- Labor longer than 20 hours

- Maternal fever (38°C [100.4°F] or higher) during labor

- Maternal illness (varicella, gastroenteritis, urinary tract infection, etc)

- Preterm delivery

- Woman with genital herpes simplex lesions at the time amniotic membranes rupture

- Birth canal or maternal rectum colonized with GBS, history of a previous infant with GBS infection, or maternal GBS bacteriuria at any time during this pregnancy

- Invasive procedure or any foreign body, such as an umbilical catheter

- Prolonged hospitalization (more than several days)

B. Localized Infections

Infants are at risk for developing localized infections if subjected to any of the following conditions:

- High staphylococcal colonization rates in other newborns in the nursery

- Any puncture site, such as from an intravenous (IV) or fetal monitoring scalp electrode

- Staphylococcal, gonococcal, or chlamydial infections predisposing the infant to conjunctivitis (eye infection)

C. Congenital Intrauterine Infections

The following conditions place an infant at risk for becoming infected in utero:

- Pregnant woman contracts rubella (German measles) during pregnancy

- Pregnant woman has syphilis (or converts her serology) during pregnancy

- Pregnant woman is exposed to cat litter during pregnancy (cats are frequently carriers of toxoplasmosis)

- Pregnant woman has active genital herpes

- Pregnant woman contracts cytomegalovirus during pregnancy

- Pregnant woman contracts varicella during pregnancy

- Pregnant woman is positive for hepatitis B surface antigen (HBsAg)

- Pregnant woman is positive for HIV antibody

4. How Do You Know a Baby Is Infected?

It is very difficult to diagnose infections in babies because the signs and symptoms usually seen with infections in older children and adults are frequently absent, or opposite of what you would expect. The single best clue is if the baby is known to be at risk for infection.

Clinical signs must also be used to suspect infection. The most frequent clinical signs seen in an infected baby are changes in the vital signs, color, feeding pattern, or general activity.

Certain laboratory studies can also help to indicate whether the baby is infected. In addition, cultures should be obtained at the first suspicion of sepsis. Although results will not be available for several days, if the cultures are positive it will provide strong evidence that the baby is infected and guide you in adjustment of therapy to provide the most appropriate antibiotics.

A. Life-Threatening Systemic Infections (Sepsis)

1. *Risk Factors*

   Newborns are at risk for developing systemic infection if subjected to any of the conditions listed in section 3A.

2. *Clinical Signs*

   The signs and symptoms of systemic infection may be subtle and easily missed. Any change in vital signs should suggest the possibility of sepsis.

   - Respiratory difficulty (grunting, nasal flaring, retracting, tachypnea, or an apnea spell)

   - Marked increase or decrease in heart rate

   - Unexplained hypotension

   - Reduced body temperature (or, less commonly, an elevated body temperature)

   - Pale, gray, or mottled color; poor capillary refill

   - Poor feeding

   - Change in activity, either reduced activity levels (lethargy or decreased tone) or irritability

- Abdominal distension, vomiting, jaundice

- Seizure activity

3. *Laboratory Findings*

An infected baby may or may not have abnormal laboratory findings. Even if the laboratory findings are normal, suspect sepsis if the baby appears sick on examination. The laboratory studies most strongly associated with sepsis include

- White blood cell count with the number of total neutrophils falling outside (either above or below) the shaded area in Figure 10.1

- Ratio of immature to total polymorphonuclear white blood cells of greater than 0.2 (20%)

- Low blood pH or serum bicarbonate level (An infected baby may develop a gray color from poor perfusion; low blood pH or low serum bicarbonate level may result from this poor perfusion.)

- Abnormal coagulation values and low platelet count

- Unexplained hypoglycemia or hyperglycemia

Many of these findings are also seen in sick but noninfected neonates. Because timing is so important in identification and initiation of drug therapy for systemic infections, *you cannot wait for culture results to differentiate between infectious and noninfectious conditions.* You must rely on your knowledge of risk factors and observation of clinical signs to suspect neonatal systemic infection.

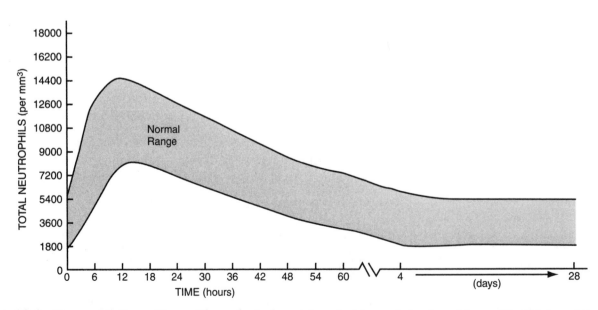

Figure 10.1. Neutrophil Count Versus Chronologic Age. Adapted with permission from Manroe BL, Weinberg AG, Rosenfeld CR, Browne R. The neonatal blood count in health and disease. I. Reference values for neutrophilic cells. *J Pediatr.* 1979;95:91–92.

Example of abnormal white blood cell count: An 18-hour-old baby develops respiratory distress and is suspected of having pneumonia. His laboratory results are

- White blood count: 5,000

- Polymorphonuclear cells
  (polys or polymorphs) = 33%

- Bands —————— = 15% ⎱ Total immature cells
- Juveniles —————— = 4% ⎰ = 19% of 5,000

  Total neutrophils = 52% of 5,000

- Lymphocytes —————— = 48%

This baby's total neutrophil count is less than 7,200, which is below the normal range for a baby 18 hours old, as shown in Figure 10.1. The ratio of immature to total polymorphonuclear cells for this baby is 19% to 52% or a ratio of 0.37 (37%), which is greater than 0.2 (20%). Both of these findings suggest the baby has a high likelihood of being infected.

Note: A baby who has had severe perinatal compromise or who has been recently stressed (eg, following circumcision) may have laboratory findings suggestive of sepsis without actually being infected.

B. Localized Infection

Localized infections in the neonate are easier to diagnose than systemic infections.

1. *Risk Factors*

   Newborns will be at risk for localized infection if subjected to any of the conditions listed earlier (section 3B).

2. *Observational Factors*

   The clinical signs and symptoms of localized infections are easily recognizable.

   - Swelling at the infected site

   - Warmth of the infected area

   - Erythema (redness) of the infected site

   - Pustules

   - Conjunctivitis (red, swollen, watery, or pus-filled eye[s])

   Localized infections must be promptly detected and treated. If not properly managed, a localized infection may quickly develop into a systemic, life-threatening infection.

C. Congenital Intrauterine Infections

   Babies with congenital intrauterine infections may seem extremely ill but more commonly will have subtle findings.

1. *Risk Factors*

   Newborns will be at risk for congenital intrauterine infections if their mothers had any of the conditions listed in section 3C. Refer to the list in section 3C, as well as Book II: Maternal and Fetal Care, Perinatal Infections, for additional information regarding maternal and neonatal management. *Most infants with congenital infections, however, have no maternal history indicating an infection.*

2. *Observational Factors*

   A newborn with congenital infection may have any or all of the signs of a baby with sepsis. Other findings may include

   - Spots of bleeding within the skin (petechiae or purpura)

   - Blisters on skin (vesicles)

   - Jaundice lasting more than several days (both direct and indirect forms of bilirubin may be elevated, see the previous unit, Hyperbilirubinemia)

   - Enlarged liver or spleen

   - Rapidly enlarging head or a particularly small head

   - Cataracts or abnormal retinas

   - Poor response to sound

   - Rash

   - Pneumonia

   - Anemia

   - Thrombocytopenia (low platelet count)

   - Lymphadenopathy (enlarged lymph nodes)

3. *Laboratory Findings*

   The laboratory findings for many congenital intrauterine infections take several weeks to become positive. Most of the tests involve measuring the level of antibody in the baby's blood and the mother's blood at the time of the illness and again during the first few weeks after birth. Consult your state infectious disease laboratory for the proper technique and timing for obtaining these samples.

D. Hospital-Acquired Infections

   1. *Risk Factors*

      The babies at highest risk for nosocomial infection are babies who

      - Are hospitalized for more than several days

      - Require invasive procedures

2. *Clinical Signs*

Hospital-acquired infections are usually systemic infections. Babies with nosocomial infections, therefore, exhibit the same clinical signs as those listed earlier in section 4A.2.

3. *Laboratory Findings*

These findings will be the same as those listed in section 4A.3 for systemic infections. Hospital-acquired infections, however, are more likely to be due to drug-resistant organisms.

Drug-resistant bacteria grown from a baby's cultures will show resistance to the usual antibiotics. Check culture results and antibiotic sensitivities carefully. Consider consultation with infectious disease experts regarding appropriate antibiotics.

Now answer these questions to test yourself on the information in the last section.

B1. What does "at risk for infection" mean?

    A. There are certain predisposing conditions that make it likely the infant will become infected.

    B. The infant will give infections to other people.

    C. The infant will definitely become sick because of being exposed to other infected infants.

B2. Name at least 3 conditions that put a newborn at risk for sepsis.

_____

_____

_____

B3. Name 2 conditions that would put an infant at risk for localized infections.

_____ and _____

B4. What is (are) the best clinical sign(s) that an infant may have a systemic infection?

    A. Change in heart rate

    B. Reduced temperature

    C. Reduced activity

    D. All of the above

B5. What are the common clinical signs of localized infections?

_____

_____

_____

_____

_____

B6. Name at least 2 conditions occurring during pregnancy that put the infant at risk for a congenital infection.

_____

_____

B7. **True** **False** Results of white blood cell count and differential reliably indicate whether a baby has bacterial sepsis.

Check your answers with the list that follows the Recommended Routines. Correct any incorrect answers and review the appropriate section in the unit.

5. What Should Be Done if an Infant Is Suspected of Being Infected?

From the time the first clinical sign(s) appears or you become suspicious that a baby may have sepsis, you have a very short time to obtain cultures and initiate drug therapy.

As soon as you suspect an infant is septic, immediately begin supportive care, obtain blood cultures, and then begin antibiotic therapy.

Drug therapy must be initiated as quickly as possible after obtaining cultures. Do not wait for culture results before starting drug therapy.

When the culture results are known (in 2–3 days), antibiotic therapy can be stopped or adjusted, according to the culture results, antibiotic sensitivities, and baby's clinical condition.

A. Systemic Life-Threatening Infections

If a baby is suspected of having a life-threatening infection, take these actions in this order.

1. Provide supportive care–*quickly.*

2. Obtain cultures and laboratory tests–*quickly.*

3. Administer antibiotics–*quickly.*

4. Adjust antibiotics according to culture results.

5. Monitor antibiotic levels.

Supportive Care

As soon as an infant is suspected of having a systemic infection, the following should be done immediately:

- Connect the baby to a heart rate monitor.

- Establish an IV line for
  - Fluids (Unstable babies suspected of sepsis should be placed NPO until their vital signs are stable.)
  - Antibiotics and possible emergency medications

- Check all vital signs frequently (heart rate, respirations, temperature, blood pressure).

- Obtain frequent blood glucose screening tests to check for hypoglycemia and hyperglycemia.

Culture and Laboratory Tests

Once supportive care has been started, appropriate laboratory studies and cultures should be obtained. Essential studies for all babies suspected of sepsis include

- Blood cultures

- White blood count with differential

- Chest x-ray, if the baby has signs of respiratory distress

- Platelet count

It may also be helpful to check blood pH and serum bicarbonate levels.

Additional studies for babies sufficiently stable to tolerate the procedure(s) include

- Lumbar puncture (for spinal fluid glucose, protein, microscopic examination, and culture)

- Blood glucose (obtained at same time as lumbar puncture for comparison with spinal fluid glucose)

Note: Many experts advise delaying a lumbar puncture until a baby is stable because early therapy will not be changed by the results and the procedure can be very stressful for a baby.

Antibiotic Therapy

 If an infant is suspected of having a systemic infection, obtain blood cultures, then, immediately begin antibiotics. Do not wait for laboratory and culture reports before starting antibiotics.

Antibiotics should be selected to be effective against gram-positive and gram-negative organisms. A general suggestion for choice of antibiotics is

| **Ampicillin** (gram-positive organisms) | ⟵ PLUS ⟶ | **Gentamicin** (gram-negative organisms) |

Table 10.1. Antibiotic Therapy

Antibiotic	Gestational Age	Chronologic Age	Dosage*	Route	Interval[||]
Ampicillin*	All babies	0–7 days	100 mg/kg/dose	IV[†] or IM	q 12 hr
	All babies	>7 days	100 mg/kg/dose	IV or IM	q 6–8 hr
Gentamicin[‡]	34 weeks or less	0–7 days	2.5 mg/kg/dose	IV[§] over 30 min	q 24 hr
	35 weeks and older	0–7 days	2.5 mg/kg/dose	IV[§] over 30 min	q 12 hr
	29 weeks or less	>7 days	2.5 mg/kg/dose	IV[§] over 30 min	q 24 hr
	30–34 weeks	>7 days	2.5 mg/kg/dose	IV[§] over 30 min	q 12 hr
	35 weeks and older	>7 days	2.5 mg/kg/dose	IV[§] over 30 min	q 8 hr

*This is the initial dosing for babies suspected of sepsis or meningitis. Lower doses may be indicated for other infections.
[†]IV, intravenously; IM, intramuscularly; q, every.
[‡]Monitoring serum levels is essential if gentamicin is administered for longer than 48 hours. The optimal **peak** serum level is 4 to 10 mcg/mL, 1 hour after the infusion of an intravenous dose has been completed. Serum **trough** level should be 0.5 to 2 mcg/mL immediately preceding a dose. The dose should be reduced and/or the interval between doses increased when renal function is impaired.
[§]Gentamicin may be given by intramuscular injection, although absorption is variable in small babies.
[||]Follow a different schedule involving longer intervals for extremely preterm babies and other babies with significant perinatal compromise.

Gentamicin given intravenously should be infused over 30 minutes. Avoid bolus infusion of gentamicin to minimize the drug's ototoxic and nephrotoxic complications. Ampicillin may be given by slow IV push or by intramuscular injection.

The infection control service in each hospital should monitor prevalent organisms and, if resistant organisms appear, the choice of first-line antibiotics should be adjusted. For example, cephalosporins are used in some hospitals. Vancomycin is often instituted in infants who develop infections later during their hospitalization.

If the infant is infected with a known organism (the infecting organism has been identified and confirmed), then antibiotics specific for that organism should be started. Also, when culture results reveal a specific organism is resistant to a specific antibiotic, then antibiotic therapy should be changed accordingly.

Note: In addition to ruling out infection by a drug-resistant organism, the use of acyclovir for treatment of possible herpes simplex infection should be considered for babies who become more ill while receiving antibiotic therapy or who develop signs of sepsis, including an elevated temperature, at several days of age. Consult regional center staff.

Use only antibiotics that culture and sensitivity results indicate are effective against the particular infecting organism.

If culture results demonstrate the infecting organism is resistant to a particular antibiotic, do not use that drug or discontinue use of it.

If infection is proven, or strongly suspected from clinical and laboratory findings, IV antibiotic therapy is usually given for 7 to 10 days.

If blood cultures show no growth and the baby appears well at 48 to 72 hours, you might elect to stop antibiotic therapy at that time.

B. Localized Infection

The **general principles** of treating localized infections in adults also apply to babies.

- Incision and drainage of abscesses (Material from abscess should be cultured and a gram stain prepared.)

- Debridement of wound infections

- Culture, gram stain, and topical treatment of conjunctivitis, except gonococcal and chlamydial infections that require systemic therapy

Because an abscess may sometimes form at the site where a scalp electrode was placed for fetal monitoring during labor, some experts advise a scrub with antimicrobial soap to the electrode site for all babies who received internal fetal heart rate monitoring. This is not a treatment measure but is used to help prevent the development of a scalp abscess.

 In infants, localized infections are much more likely to develop into systemic life-threatening infections than are such infections in adults, and therefore must be treated promptly and thoroughly.

Chlamydia Infections (conjunctivitis, pneumonia)

Topical prophylaxis with silver nitrate, erythromycin, or tetracycline routinely used to prevent gonococcal ophthalmia, will *not* reliably prevent chlamydial conjunctivitis. Chlamydial conjunctivitis is treated with systemic erythromycin, given orally. Babies born to women with untreated or incompletely treated *Chlamydia* infection should be monitored for development of disease. Prophylactic antibiotics, however, are not recommended; neither is cesarean delivery.

If chlamydial conjunctivitis develops, treat it with
• Erythromycin 12.5 mg/kg given orally, every 6 hours for 14 days

Erythromycin therapy, however, is only about 80% effective so a second course of treatment may be necessary. Erythromycin may be poorly tolerated in some infants, in which case oral sulfonamides may be used after the neonatal period.

Chlamydial pneumonia can develop from infection acquired at the time of delivery. Onset of symptoms, however, is usually between 2 and 19 weeks after birth. Treatment is with oral erythromycin or sulfonamides.

Gonococcal Infections (conjunctivitis, scalp abscess)

Topical antibiotic treatment is not adequate when localized gonococcal infection is present. Systemic antibiotic therapy should be used. Because of the high frequency of penicillin-resistant *Neisseria gonorrhoeae*, ceftriaxone is the preferred antibiotic treatment. Treat the baby with

• Ceftriaxone 25 to 50 mg/kg (not to exceed 125 mg), one dose, given intramuscularly or intravenously

Ceftriaxone should be given cautiously to infants with hyperbilirubinemia, especially preterm infants. Cefotaxime is recommended for babies with hyperbilirubinemia who are being treated for gonococcal infections.

• Cefotaxime 100 mg/kg, one dose, given intramuscularly or intravenously

Because topical treatment is inadequate by itself, and unnecessary when systemic antibiotic therapy is used, there is no need to use ophthalmic antibiotic ointment for babies with gonococcal conjunctivitis. Instead, those babies should have their eyes irrigated frequently with sterile saline, until the discharge is eliminated.

Staphylococcal Pustulosis Infections

- *Mild:* Thoroughly wash the affected area with mild soap. Follow this cleansing with application of a topical antibiotic ointment such as mupirocin or bacitracin.

  Note: Epidemic *Staphylococcus aureus* outbreaks in newborn nurseries require special measures, such as possible use of hexachlorophene (Phisohex) baths. Consult with regional center staff.

- *Moderate or Severe:* Provide therapy for mild localized infection, *plus* obtain blood cultures and administer oral, intramuscular, or IV antistaphylococcal antibiotics (eg, nafcillin, cephalothin, or vancomycin). Be certain to check culture sensitivities because drug-resistant organisms are becoming more common.

Self-Test

Now answer these questions to test yourself on the information in the last section.

C1. **True** **False** It is necessary to know the bacterial culture results before beginning antibiotic therapy for a baby suspected of being septic.

C2. What are the 4 *supportive procedures* that must be initiated if an infant is suspected of having a systemic infection?

_____

_____

_____

_____

C3. What are the 4 essential *tests or studies* that should be obtained for all infants suspected of having a life-threatening infection?

_____

_____

_____

_____

C4. What *other tests* may be helpful in evaluating an infant with severe life-threatening infection?

_____

_____

C5. In selecting antibiotics to administer when an infection is suspected, what 2 general types of organisms need to be considered?

_____ and _____

C6. Which of the following statements best describes the treatment of localized infections?

    A. Follow the same procedure as for adults.

    B. Make sure the infection does not spread by washing the baby often with undiluted hexachlorophene (Phisohex).

    C. The same procedures used on adults apply, but special care must be taken to keep the infection from developing into a systemic life-threatening infection.

C7. What is a first-line drug to use against gram-negative organisms? _____

C8. **True** **False** Chlamydial conjunctivitis can be treated effectively with an ophthalmic preparation of erythromycin.

C9. **True** **False** If gonococcal conjunctivitis develops, treatment with systemic ceftriaxone or cefotaxime is recommended.

C10. **True** **False** Mild staphylococcal pustulosis infections require treatment with systemic antibiotics.

Check your answers with the list that follows the Recommended Routines. Correct any incorrect answers and review the appropriate section in the unit.

C. Congenital Infections

Babies with congenital rubella and certain other infections require special isolation precautions. Women with varicella-zoster virus (chickenpox) infection near the time of delivery, as well as their babies, might require special precautions depending on the timing of the infection. Many congenital intrauterine infections and some acquired during the birth process (perinatal acquisition) require particular isolation precautions and cannot be treated with specific drug therapy. For these and other infectious diseases not discussed below, consult the resources listed on page 2 and/or your regional center staff.

Cytomegalovirus (CMV)

- *Transmission and risk:* Congenital infection can cause varying degrees of illness in the baby, with primary (first time) maternal infection, especially early in pregnancy, carrying the highest risk of damage to the fetus. Most infants, however, are not symptomatic at birth, but some of those will go on to demonstrate hearing loss and/or learning disability in childhood.

  Infection can also occur as a result of passage through an infected birth canal, by ingestion of CMV-positive breast milk, or by transfusion of CMV-positive blood. Most infants infected during or shortly after birth do not develop signs of infection. Premature infants are at greater risk for illness than are term infants.

- *Clinical findings:* Babies with symptomatic CMV infection may present with intrauterine growth retardation, jaundice (especially direct hyperbilirubinemia), thrombocytopenia, purpura, "blueberry muffin" spots, hepatosplenomegaly, microcephaly, cerebral calcifications, chorioretinitis, and/or cataracts.

- *Diagnosis and treatment:* Viral culture of urine or saliva is used to confirm CMV infection. Neonatal treatment may be appropriate for some situations. Consult regional perinatal center staff.

- *Precautions:* Standard precautions for blood and body fluids are indicated. Meticulous handwashing is particularly important for pregnant women caring for patients with known CMV infection. Keep in mind, however, that about 1% of all live-born babies are infected in utero and excrete CMV at birth, but only a small fraction of those babies are recognized as having CMV disease.

- *Follow-up:* Regardless of their initial clinical presentation, infants with congenital CMV infection, as well as babies with infection acquired soon after birth, should have long-term follow-up, with assessment of hearing, vision, psychomotor development, and learning abilities.

Hepatitis B Virus (HBV)

- *Transmission and risk:* Infected persons carry HBV in all body fluids. The virus is transmitted primarily by intimate (usually sexual) contact and less often by transfusion of contaminated blood (rare in the

United States) or sharing of needles by drug users. More than one third of adults positive for HBsAg have no easily identified risk factor.

Routine testing at the first prenatal visit is recommended for *all* women. Vaccination during pregnancy should be offered to HBsAg-negative women. Women who were not screened during pregnancy should be tested when admitted for delivery.

Transplacental transmission from the pregnant woman to her fetus occurs but is uncommon. Neonatal infection seems to result mainly through direct contact with the mother's blood at the time of delivery. The rate of transmission to the newborn is not affected by whether the woman is a chronic carrier or has an acute infection at the time of delivery or by the route of delivery (cesarean or vaginal). If a baby was not infected at delivery, postnatal transmission through close personal contact between mother and child is likely during early childhood.

If untreated, more than half the babies born to women with hepatitis B infection will become infected, and up to 25% of those babies will develop fatal liver disease (chronic active hepatitis, cirrhosis, or hepatocellular carcinoma) during early childhood.

- *Precautions:* For babies of HBsAg-positive women, the baby should be cleansed promptly of maternal blood following delivery. Standard precautions should be used by health care providers.

- *Treatment:* Transmission of HBV infection can be prevented for approximately 95% of infants born to HBsAg-positive women by administration of HBV vaccine and hepatitis B immune globulin (HBIG), with the first dose given within 12 hours of birth.

The HBV vaccine alone is also highly effective in preventing infection, and is recommended for *all* newborns regardless of whether the mother is HbsAg positive or negative. In either case, a series of 3 doses is required.

 All newborns should receive hepatitis B vaccine*. Babies born to HBsAg-positive women should also receive HBIG.

Herpes Simplex Virus (HSV)

- *Transmission and risk:* Congenital HSV infection is rare. Transmission to the baby most often occurs during passage through a

---

**Guidelines for Perinatal Care.* 5th ed. American Academy of Pediatrics and American College of Obstetricians and Gynecologists; 2002:288.

Table 10.2. Hepatitis B Immunoprophylaxis by Infant Birth Weight*

Maternal Status	Infant ≥2,000 g	Infant <2,000 g
HBsAg positive	Hepatitis B vaccine + HBIG (within 12 h of birth)	Hepatitis B vaccine + HBIG (within 12 h of birth)
	Continue vaccine series beginning at 1–2 mo of age according to recommended schedule for infants born to HBsAg-positive mothers (see Table 10.3)	Continue vaccine series beginning at 1–2 mo of age according to recommended schedule for infants born to HBsAg-positive mothers (see Table 10.3)
		Immunize with 4 vaccine doses; do not count birth dose as part of vaccine series
	Check anti-HBs and HBsAg after completion of vaccine series†	Check anti-HBs and HBsAg after completion of vaccine series†
	HBsAg-negative infants with anti-HBs levels ≥10 mIU/mL are protected and need no further medical management	HBsAg-negative infants with anti-HBs levels ≥10 mIU/mL are protected and need no further medical management
	HBsAg-negative infants with anti-HBs levels <10 mIU/mL should be reimmunized with 3 doses at 2-mo intervals and retested	HBsAg-negative infants with anti-HBs levels <10 mIU/mL should be reimmunized with 3 doses at 2-mo intervals and retested
	Infants who are HBsAg positive should receive appropriate followup, including medical evaluation for chronic liver disease	Infants who are HBsAg positive should receive appropriate follow-up, including medical evaluation for chronic liver disease
HBsAg status unknown	Test mother for HBsAg immediately after admission for delivery	Test mother for HBsAg immediately after admission for delivery
	Hepatitis B vaccine (by 12 h)	Hepatitis B vaccine (by 12 h)
	Administer HBIG (within 7 days) if mother tests HBsAg positive	Administer HBIG if mother tests HBsAg positive or if mother's HBsAg result is not available within 12 h of birth
	Continue vaccine series beginning at 1–2 mo of age according to recommended schedule based on mother's HBsAg result (see Table 10.3)	Continue vaccine series beginning at 1–2 mo of age according to recommended schedule based on mother's HBsAg result (see Table 10.3)
		Immunize with 4 vaccine doses; do not count birth dose as part of vaccine series
HBsAg negative	Hepatitis B vaccine at birth‡	Hepatitis B vaccine dose 1–30 days of chronologic age if medically stable, or at hospital discharge if before 30 days of chronologic age
	Continue vaccine series beginning at 1–2 mo of age (see Table 10.3)	Continue vaccine series beginning at 1–2 mo of age (see Table 10.3)
	Follow-up anti-HBs and HBsAg testing not needed	Follow-up anti-HBs and HBsAg testing not needed

Reprinted with permission from *Red Book: 2006 Report of the Committee on Infectious Diseases*. 27th ed. Elk Grove Village, IL: American Academy of Pediatrics; 2006:327

HBsAg indicates hepatitis B surface antigen; HBIG, hepatitis B Immune Globulin; anti-HBs, antibody to hepatitis B surface antigen.

*Extremes of gestational age and birth weight no longer are a consideration for timing of hepatitis B vaccine doses.

†Test at 9 to 18 months of age, generally at the next well-child visit after completion of the primary series. Use testing method that allows determination of a protective concentration of anti-HBs (≥10 mIU/mL).

‡The first dose may be delayed until after hospital discharge for an infant who weighs ≥2,000 g and whose mother is HBsAg negative, but only if a physician's order to withhold the birth dose and a copy of the mother's original HBsAg-negative laboratory report are documented in the infant's medical record.

Table 10.3. Hepatitis B Vaccine by Maternal Hepatitis B Surface Antigen (HBsAg) Status*[†]

Maternal HBsAg Status	Single-Antigen Vaccine		Single-Antigen + Combination	
	Dose	Age	Dose	Age
Positive	1[‡]	Birth (≤12 h)	1[‡]	Birth (≤12 h)
	HBIG[§]	Birth (≤12 h)	HBIG	Birth (≤12 h)
	2	1–2 mo	2	2 mo
	3[‖]	6 mo	3	4 mo
			4[‖]	6 mo (Pediarix) or 12–15 mo (Comvax)
Unknown[¶]	1[‡]	Birth (≤12 h)	1[‡]	Birth (≤12 h)
	2	1–2 mo	2	2 mo
	3[‖]	6 mo	3	4 mo
			4[‖]	6 mo (Pediarix) or 12–15 mo (Comvax)
Negative	1[‡,#]	Birth (before discharge)	1[‡,#]	Birth (before discharge)
	2	1–2 mo	2	2 mo
	3[‖]	6–18 mo	3	4 mo
			4[‖]	6 mo (Pediarix) or 12–15 mo (Comvax)

Reprinted with permission from *Red Book: 2006 Report of the Committee on Infectious Diseases.* 27th ed. Elk Grove Village, IL: American Academy of Pediatrics; 2006:348

*Centers for Disease Control and Prevention. A comprehensive immunization strategy to eliminate transmission of hepatitis B virus infection in the United States. Recommendations of the Advisory Committee on Immunization Practices (ACIP) part 1: immunization of infants, children, and adolescents. *MMWR Recomm Rep.* 2005;54(RR-16):1–23

[†]See Table 10.2 for vaccine schedules for preterm infants weighing <2,000 g.

[‡]Recombivax HB or Engerix-B should be used for the birth dose. Comvax and Pediarix cannot be administered at birth or before 6 weeks of age.

[§]Hepatitis B Immune Globulin (0.5 mL) administered intramuscularly in a separate site from vaccine.

[‖]The final dose in the vaccine series should not be administered before 24 weeks (164 days) of age.

[¶]Pregnant women should have blood drawn and tested for HBsAg as soon as possible after admission for delivery; if the woman is found to be HBsAg-positive, the infant should receive HBIG as soon as possible but no later than 7 days of age.

[#]On a case-by-case basis and only in rare circumstances, the first dose may be delayed until after hospital discharge for an infant who weighs ≥2,000 g and whose mother is HBsAg negative, but only if a physician's order to withhold the birth dose and a copy of the mother's original HBsAg-negative laboratory report are documented in the infant's medical record.

birth canal with active lesions present. There is a very low risk of infection to babies born

- Vaginally to women with a history of recurrent genital herpes but who have no symptoms at the time of delivery
- By cesarean delivery, before or within 4 to 6 hours of rupture of membranes, to women with symptoms at the time of delivery

Neonatal HSV infection is uncommon but, if it occurs, the risk of permanent neurological damage or death is high.

- *Clinical findings:* Neonatal HSV infection can present in different ways.

  - *Systemic disease* involves the liver, lungs, skin, and other organs, including the central nervous system (CNS). More than one third of these infants do not have the vesicular lesions characteristic of herpes. Herpes simplex virus infection should be considered if a baby who is several days of age, or who was born after prolonged rupture of membranes, develops respiratory distress, seizures, temperature instability, and other signs of sepsis.

  - *Infection localized to the CNS* presents with seizures, lethargy, irritability, poor feeding, temperature instability, and/or bulging fontanel.

  - *Disease localized to the skin, eyes, and/or mouth* may include conjunctivitis, keratitis, and/or chorioretinitis. Vesicles and/or ulcers can be seen on the skin or in the mouth.

  Symptoms may be present at birth, especially if rupture of membranes was prolonged, or occur as late as 4 to 6 weeks after birth. The onset of systemic disease is usually during the first 2 weeks after birth.

- *Diagnosis:* Viral cultures should be taken from skin lesions, mouth, eyes, blood, stool (or rectum), urine, and/or cerebral spinal fluid. Immunodiagnostic techniques using vesicle scrapings are available in some institutions. Serologic testing is of little value when an acute infection is suspected.

- *Treatment:* Whenever an infant appears ill at birth, if vaginal delivery occurs with active maternal disease, consult regional center experts. If treatment with IV acyclovir is recommended, it should be started promptly. In addition to cultures, other tests may be advisable. Recommendations to treat asymptomatic infants may be made on the basis of culture results. Consultation with infectious disease experts and often care at a regional perinatal center is generally recommended for these babies.

  Neonatal illness is treated with acyclovir 60 mg/kg per day in 3 divided doses given intravenously every 8 hours for 14 to 21 days, depending on whether disease is limited to skin, eyes, and/or mouth or is disseminated. Dosing interval should be increased if renal or hepatic function is impaired, and renal and hepatic function should be monitored, regardless of function at initiation of therapy.

- *Precautions:* Contact precautions should be used by health care providers.

  Newborns known to have been exposed to active HSV lesions, and their mothers, should be isolated from all other babies. Postnatal infection through direct contact with lesions (may be around an adult's mouth or mother's breasts) or through indirect contact from the hands of family or health care providers can occur.

A private room for the mother, with continuous rooming-in, may be used as long as the infant is not ill and the mother uses good handwashing technique. The mother should use a clean barrier whenever she handles her baby to be sure the infant does not come in contact with lesions or potentially infectious material. If the mother or another family member has "cold sores," a disposable surgical mask should be worn, until the lesions have crusted and dried, whenever the baby is touched or held. Even with a mask, nuzzling and kissing the infant should be avoided until the lesions have cleared. If there are no breast lesions, the mother may safely breastfeed.

- *Follow-up:* Parents and health care providers need to be alert to the possibility of the onset of HSV illness at several weeks of age in high-risk babies. Consideration should be given to delaying circumcision beyond 1 month of age because herpes infection is more likely to occur at the site of skin trauma.

Human Immunodeficiency Virus (HIV)

- *Transmission and testing:* An increasing number of women are infected with HIV. Women at particular risk are those with a history of substance use, multiple sexual partners, and/or sexually transmitted disease(s). Because of heterosexual transmission, even women with no apparent risk factors may be HIV-positive. Despite the recommendation for universal HIV testing of all pregnant women, infected babies continue to be born to undiagnosed infected women. Treatment of an HIV-positive pregnant woman can

  – Delay the onset of active disease for the woman.

  – Dramatically reduce the likelihood that the virus will be passed to the baby.

 Routine testing of ALL pregnant women for HIV infection is recommended.*

If a woman's HIV status during pregnancy or postpartum is unknown, HIV testing of the newborn is important for care of the baby.*

Nearly all babies born to HIV-positive women, even babies not actually infected with the virus, will test positive at birth because of antibodies acquired in utero from the mother.

Test infants born to HIV-positive women at 1 month and at 4 to 6 months of age. Nearly 100% of HIV-infected babies can be identified by 4 to 6 months of age. Early antiviral therapy is indicated for all babies exposed to HIV.

---

*For further information about HIV testing, see *Guidelines for Perinatal Care.* 5th ed. American Academy of Pediatrics and American College of Obstetricians and Gynecologists; 2002:298, 299.

- *Precautions:* After delivery, all blood should be removed from the infant's skin. There is no need to isolate either the mother or the baby, although standard precautions should be used. If desired, the baby may room-in with the mother. Breastfeeding should be discouraged, however, because the virus can be transmitted in breast milk.

- *Treatment:* Combination antiretroviral therapy or monotherapy with zidovudine given during pregnancy and labor has been shown to reduce mother-to-child transmission by two thirds.

  Cesarean delivery, performed before the onset of labor and before rupture of membranes, may be of particular benefit to babies whose mothers have a high viral-RNA load, of 1,000 copies/mL or greater, at the time of delivery.

  If antenatal and intrapartum zidovudine treatment was used, continue zidovudine therapy for the baby. Even if a woman did not receive antepartum or intrapartum zidovudine, recommended neonatal therapy is

  – 2 mg/kg of zidovudine syrup given orally every 6 hours

  – Beginning 8 to 12 hours after birth

  – Continuing for 6 weeks

  Arrange for comprehensive follow-up care for HIV-positive babies, their mothers, and their families.

 Evaluation, monitoring, and management of babies born to HIV-positive women can be complex. Information changes rapidly. Consultation with regional center experts is essential. In addition, refer to www.cdc.gov and www.aidsinfo.nih.gov.

Syphilis

- *Transmission:* Over the past several years, there has been a nationwide increase in congenital syphilis. Transmission to the fetus can occur at any stage in the woman's illness and at any time during pregnancy.

 No newborn should be discharged from a hospital without determination of the mother's serologic status for syphilis.*

- *Precautions:* **Contact precautions** should be used **until penicillin therapy has been given for at least 24 hours.** Parents, visitors, and health care providers should use gloves when handling the infant during this time.

**Guidelines for Perinatal Care.* 5th ed. American Academy of Pediatrics and American College of Obstetricians and Gynecologists; 2002:321 and *Red Book: 2006 Report of the Committee on Infectious Diseases.* 27th ed. American Academy of Pediatrics; 2006:634.

- *Evaluation*

  1. Who to evaluate? Any infant, if syphilis in the woman was
     - Untreated or inadequately treated
     - Treated with a non-penicillin regimen (such as erythromycin) or an inadequate penicillin dose
     - Treated appropriately with penicillin but the expected decrease in nontreponemal antibody titer did not occur
     - Treated less than 1 month before delivery
     - Treated, but treatment or penicillin dose is not documented, or
     - Treated, but with insufficient serologic follow-up to assess the response to treatment and current infection status

  2. What to include?
     - Physical examination: Clinical findings suggestive of congenital syphilis include unexplained jaundice, rash, hepatosplen-omegaly, pneumonia, anemia, lymphadenopathy, or thrombocytopenia. Most infected babies, however, will not have any of these findings.
     - Nontreponemal serologic test of the infant's blood (not cord blood because false-positive and false-negative results can occur)
     - Lumbar puncture with testing of cerebral spinal fluid for Venereal Disease Research Laboratory (VDRL) cells, and protein
     - X-rays of the long bones
     - Other tests as indicated, such as chest x-ray, complete blood count (CBC), liver function tests, ophthalmologic examinations, auditory brain stem response test

Infants can have congenital syphilis without displaying any clinical signs of infection.

If untreated, syphilis will cause irreversible damage to a baby's brain and other organs, although the damage may not become apparent until many years after birth.

- *Tests:* Two types of serologic tests, nontreponemal (VDRL, rapid plasma reagin, and automated reagin test) and treponemal (micro-hemagglutination assay–*Treponema pallidum* and florescent treponemal antibody absorption), are used to detect an infection, but neither type of test by itself is sufficient to make a diagnosis. (See Table 10.4.)

- *Treatment:* If a baby had risk factors that prompted evaluation for congenital syphilis, treatment should be given if
  - Infection is documented.
  - Tests results cannot rule out infection.
  - The infant cannot be fully evaluated.
  - Adequate follow-up cannot be ensured.

  Follow the treatment guidelines in Table 10.5.

- *Follow-up:* Newborns treated for congenital syphilis should have follow-up evaluations at 1, 2, 4, 6, and 12 months of age, with nontreponemal tests performed at 2 to 4, 6, and 12 months after

Table 10.4. Guide for Interpretation of Syphilis Serologic Test Results of Mothers and Their Infants

Nontreponemal Test Result (eg, VDRL, RPR, ART)		Treponemal Test Result (eg, TP-PA, FTA-ABS)		Interpretation*
Mother	Infant	Mother	Infant	
−	−	−	−	No syphilis or incubating syphilis in the mother or infant or prozone phenomenon
+	+	−	−	No syphilis in mother or infant (false-positive result of nontreponemal test with passive transfer to infant)
+	+ or −	+	+	Maternal syphilis with possible infant infection; mother treated for syphilis during pregnancy; or mother with latent syphilis and possible infant infection[†]
+	+	+	+	Recent or previous syphilis in the mother; possible infant infection
−	−	+	+	Mother successfully treated for syphilis before or early in pregnancy; or mother with Lyme disease (ie, false-positive serologic test result); infant syphilis unlikely

Reprinted with permission from *Red Book: 2006 Report of the Committee on Infectious Diseases.* 27th ed. Elk Grove Village, IL: American Academy of Pediatrics; 2006:636

VDRL, Venereal Disease Research Laboratory; RPR, rapid plasma reagin; ART, automated reagin test; TP-PA, *Treponema pallidum* particle agglutination test; FTA-ABS, fluorescent treponemal antibody absorption; +, reactive; −, nonreactive.

*Table presents a guide and not a definitive interpretation of serologic test results for syphilis in mothers and their newborn infants. Maternal history is the most important aspect for interpretation of test results. Factors that should be considered include timing of maternal infection, nature and timing of maternal treatment, quantitative maternal and infant titers, and serial determination of nontreponemal test titers in both mother and infant.

[†]Mothers with latent syphilis may have nonreactive nontreponemal test results.

treatment ended or until the tests become nonreactive or the titer has decreased 4-fold. Titers should decline by 3 months of age and become nonreactive by 6 months of age. Consider re-treatment if titers remain stable, including persistent low titers. Newborns who had abnormal CSF findings and neurosyphilis require more extensive and longer-term follow-up. Expert consultation is recommended for those babies.

Toxoplasmosis

- *Transmission and risk:* Toxoplasmosis infection is rarely recognized in a pregnant woman because the illness is self-limited, mild, with nonspecific symptoms often described as a "cold." Feces of infected cats and meat of infected sheep, pigs, and cattle harbor the organism, with human infection usually resulting from exposure to cat feces or ingestion of raw or under-cooked meat. Reinfection is uncommon and occurs only in immunosuppressed persons because the first infection normally confers life-long immunity. Infants born to women with HIV and toxoplasmosis infection are at significantly increased risk for becoming infected.

Maternal infection early in pregnancy is more likely to cause severe symptoms than is infection late in pregnancy. More than 70% of

Table 10.5. Recommended Treatment of Neonates (≤4 Weeks of Age) With Proven or Possible Congenital Syphilis

Clinical Status	Evaluation	Antimicrobial Therapy*
Proven or highly probable disease[†]	CSF analysis for VDRL, cell count, and protein CBC and platelet count Other tests as clinically indicated (eg, long-bone radiography, liver function tests, ophthalmologic examination)	Aqueous crystalline penicillin G, 100,000–150,000 U/kg per day, administered as 50,000 U/kg per dose, IV, every 12 h during the first 7 days of life and every 8 h thereafter for a total of 10 days OR Penicillin G procaine,[‡] 50,000 U/kg per day, IM, in a single dose for 10 days
Normal physical examination and serum quantitative nontreponemal titer the same or less than fourfold the maternal titer:		
(a) (i) Mother was not treated or inadequately treated or has no documented treatment; (ii) mother was treated with erythromycin or other nonpenicillin regimen; (iii) mother received treatment ≤4 weeks before delivery	CSF analysis for VDRL, cell count, and protein CBC and platelet count Long-bone radiography	Aqueous crystalline penicillin G, IV, for 10 days[§] OR Penicillin G procaine,[‡] 50,000 U/kg per day, IM, in a single dose for 10 days[§] OR Penicillin G benzathine,[‡] 50,000 U/kg, IM, in a single dose[§]
(b) (i) Adequate maternal therapy given >4 wk before delivery; (ii) mother has no evidence of reinfection or relapse	None	Clinical, serologic follow-up, and penicillin G benzathine, 50,000 U/kg, IM, in a single dose[∥]
(c) Adequate therapy before pregnancy and mother's nontreponemal serologic titer remained low and stable during pregnancy and at delivery	None	None[¶]

Reprinted with permission from *Red Book: 2006 Report of the Committee on Infectious Diseases*. 27th ed. Elk Grove Village, IL: American Academy of Pediatrics; 2006:638.

IV indicates intravenously; IM, intramuscularly; CSF, cerebrospinal fluid; and CBC, complete blood cell.

*If more than 1 day of therapy is missed, the entire course should be restarted.

[†]Abnormal physical examination, serum quantitative nontreponemal titer that is fourfold greater than the mother's titer, or positive result of darkfield or fluorescent antibody test of body fluid(s).

[‡]Penicillin G benzathine and penicillin G procaine are approved for IM administration *only*.

[§]A complete evaluation (CSF analysis, bone radiography, CBC) is not necessary if 10 days of parenteral therapy is administered but may be useful to support a diagnosis of congenital syphilis. If a single dose of penicillin G benzathine is used, then the infant must be evaluated fully, the full evaluation must be normal, and follow-up must be certain. If any part of the infant's evaluation is abnormal or not performed or if the CSF analysis is uninterpretable, the 10-day course of penicillin is required.

[∥]Some experts would not treat the infant but would provide close serologic follow-up.

[¶]Some experts would treat with penicillin G benzathine, 50,000 U/kg, as a single IM injection if follow-up is uncertain.

infants with congenital infection have no symptoms at birth, although visual impairment, learning disability, and/or mental retardation may become apparent months or years later.

- *Clinical findings:* Neonatal symptoms of congenital toxoplasmosis may include hepatosplenomegaly, jaundice, thrombocytopenia, anemia, seizures, microcephaly, hydrocephalus, intracranial calcifications, and/or lymphadenopathy.

- *Diagnosis and treatment:* Consult regional center neonatal and infectious disease experts. Serologic tests are the primary diagnostic methods. Availability and interpretation of sensitive and specific assays usually require specialized expertise. Treatment requires multiple drugs over a prolonged period. Investigational drugs may be appropriate in some circumstances.

- *Precautions:* Standard precautions are recommended.

D. Hospital-Acquired Infections

Care for babies with nosocomial infections is the same as for any baby with a systemic infection. Because hospital-acquired infections are more likely to be due to drug-resistant organisms, pay close attention to culture results and antibiotic sensitivities and adjust antibiotic therapy accordingly.

Self-Test

Now answer these questions to test yourself on the information in the last section.

D1. True   False   Results of testing for syphilis of every mother should be known before any baby is discharged from a hospital.

D2. True   False   Most babies with congenital syphilis show characteristic physical findings at birth.

D3. True   False   Onset of illness may be as late as 4 to 6 weeks after birth for babies who develop infection after being exposed to herpes simplex virus at birth.

D4. True   False   Babies treated for congenital syphilis should have follow-up examinations and testing for evidence of continued infection for 12 months or longer after birth.

D5. True   False   Risk of neonatal herpes infection is very high when a woman with a history of herpes infections delivers vaginally, even when there are no active lesions at the time of delivery.

D6. True   False   Intravenous therapy with acyclovir is used to treat neonatal herpes simplex virus infection and may be appropriate for some babies who show no evidence of illness but were exposed to active lesions at the time of delivery.

D7. True   False   Hepatitis B virus vaccine is recommended for *all* newborns.

D8. True   False   Newborns who appear well but are known to have been exposed to active herpes lesions at the time of delivery may room-in with the mother but should be separated from all other babies.

D9. True   False   Babies who develop hepatitis B infection are at risk for serious liver disease later in childhood.

Check your answers with the list that follows the Recommended Routines. Correct any incorrect answers and review the appropriate section in the unit.

6. How Do You Care for a Baby Whose Mother Received Antibiotics During Labor?

Women may receive antibiotics during labor for the prevention of early-onset GBS disease. See Book II: Maternal and Fetal Care, Perinatal Infections for a description and flow diagram of recommended intrapartum antibiotic therapy.

It has been shown that penicillin or ampicillin given during labor to women at risk for transmitting GBS disease decreases the number of babies who become infected. Neonatal GBS infection can cause life-threatening, systemic illness.

Although intrapartum antibiotics are given to help prevent neonatal GBS disease, a small number of babies will still become infected. However, routine administration of antibiotics to all newborns born to women who received intrapartum antibiotics for the prevention of GBS infection is not recommended.

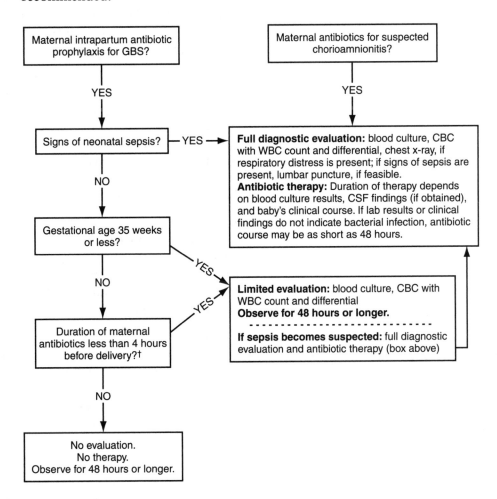

Figure 10.2. Management of a Newborn Whose Mother Received Intrapartum Antibiotics for Prevention of Neonatal GBS* Disease

Adapted from *Red Book: 2006 Report of the Committee on Infectious Diseases.* 27th ed. American Academy of Pediatrics; 2006:626.

*GBS, group B beta hemolytic streptococcal; CBC, complete blood count; WBC, white blood cell; CSF, cerebrospinal fluid.

†Applies only to recommended dosing regimens of penicillin, ampicillin, or cefazolin.

Figure 10.2 outlines one approach to management of babies whose mothers received intrapartum antibiotics; but it is not the only approach that may be used. Individual maternal and neonatal history and clinical condition need to be considered.

7. How Do You Provide for Infection Control in the Nursery?

GOOD HANDWASHING and use of waterless antiseptic agents are the most important techniques for preventing spread of infection.

A. Health Care Providers

Because screening of pregnant women for the presence of HIV or hepatitis infections is recommended but not mandatory, and because physical examination cannot identify either adults or newborns infected with these viruses, blood and body fluid precautions should be used for *all* patients. These precautions will also help protect patients and health care providers against the spread of other bacterial and viral pathogens

"Standard precautions" should be used at all times. Many hospital protocols specify that gloves should be worn for *every* contact, with patients or patient equipment that may involve
• Blood
• Any body fluid, secretion, or excretion *except sweat*, regardless of whether they contain visible blood
• Nonintact skin
• Mucous membranes

Gloves should be changed between babies. In addition, the use of gloves does not replace handwashing or use of waterless antiseptic agents. Gloves may be defective or may become torn with wear. Therefore, you should wash your hands with water and an antiseptic solution or rub your hands with a waterless antiseptic agent each time you change your gloves.

Protective gowns and eyewear, masks, or face shields are recommended when exposure to splashed blood or body fluids is likely, such as in the delivery room or during suctioning, and other such procedures.

Standard (blood and body fluid) precautions should be used consistently
• *For all patients*
• *By all health care providers*
• *At all times*

In addition to protecting themselves from infection, all health care workers need to be vigilant in preventing transmission of infection between babies and from personnel or other patients to babies. Hospital-acquired infections can and should be prevented. This is of increasing importance in light of the growing problem of drug-resistant organisms.

Certain illnesses require transmission-based precautions (airborne, droplet, and/or contact) in addition to standard precautions used for all patients. Consult with the sources listed on page 2 and/or infection control staff in your hospital.

The importance of GOOD HANDWASHING and use of waterless antiseptic agents cannot be overstated in preventing transmission of infections from

- *Infant to infant*
- *Personnel to infant*
- *Infant to personnel*

B. Babies

For infants with "closed space" infections (such as sepsis, meningitis, or urinary tract infections), good handwashing technique should suffice for prevention of the spread of these infections.

Certain infants are more likely to be shedding organisms and, ideally, should be isolated from other infants. These include infants with
- Diarrhea
- Bacterial or viral pneumonia
- Open infections such as wound infections
- Staphylococcal disease such as pustulosis, abscess, etc
- Congenital infections

It may be impractical to isolate such infants in a separate room, particularly if an infant is critically ill. Physical separation within the nursery is acceptable, although separate staffing is recommended. In general, pregnant women should not care for infants with congenital viral infections.

A small number of infections are transmitted by airborne droplets and should be isolated from the nursery altogether. These include infants with
- Chickenpox (varicella-zoster virus)
- Congenital tuberculosis

See Book II: Maternal and Fetal Care, Perinatal Infections for further discussion of maternal and neonatal management of tuberculosis and varicella-zoster.

Each hospital should have written protocols for control of infections in the obstetrical area and in the nursery. You should be familiar with these procedures.

C. Use of Antibiotics

Appropriate use of antibiotics will help curtail the development of drug-resistant organisms. Care should be taken to use first-line antibiotics first. For example, do not use vancomycin when ampicillin would be equally effective. Switch to other antibiotics only when culture sensitivities indicate the first choice is not effective against the specific infecting agent or a patient develops new signs of infection while receiving first-line antibiotics.

Promptly discontinue use of any antibiotic shown to be ineffective against a particular organism.

Self-Test

Now answer these questions to test yourself on the information in the last section.

E1. What is the single most important thing that can be done to prevent the spread of infection?

_____

E2. Blood and body fluid precautions should be used for

A. All infants

B. Infants with a known viral infection

C. Infants of HIV-positive mothers

D. Infants of all mothers with no prenatal care

E3. What should be done if a culture report indicates the gram-positive infecting bacteria are not sensitive to an antibiotic a baby is receiving?

A. Stop antibiotics and begin acyclovir.

B. Increase the dose of the antibiotic.

C. Continue use of the antibiotic and begin use of another antibiotic known to be effective against gram-positive organisms.

D. Stop the antibiotic and begin use of another antibiotic known to be effective against gram-positive organisms.

E4. True   False   The use of gloves eliminates the need for handwashing.

E5. Infection control means to

Yes	No	
___	___	Prevent transmission of organisms from an infected baby to other babies in the nursery.
___	___	Wash hands before and after caring for each baby.
___	___	Keep all babies with proven infections in isolation.
___	___	Prevent transmission of organisms between health care providers and patients.
___	___	Prevent transmission of organisms from an infected baby to health care providers.
___	___	Use broad-spectrum antibiotics for all at-risk patients.

Check your answers with the list that follows the Recommended Routines. Correct any incorrect answers and review the appropriate section in the unit.

Recommended Routines

All of the routines listed below are based on the principles of perinatal care presented in the unit you have just finished. They are recommended as part of routine perinatal care.

Read each routine carefully and decide whether it is standard operating procedure in your hospital. Check the appropriate blank next to each routine.

Procedure Standard in My Hospital	Needs Discussion by Our Staff	
_____	_____	1. Establish a system to review periodically the use of infection control measures and to ensure that good handwashing or a waterless antiseptic agent and standard precautions are used *at all times*.
_____	_____	2. Establish a mechanism to invoke additional transmission-based precautions, as appropriate, for individual patients.
_____	_____	3. Establish a system for ensuring that maternal risk factors for infection are reliably transferred to a baby's chart and that the baby's health care providers are notified.
_____	_____	4. Establish a policy of obtaining a blood culture before starting antibiotic therapy.
_____	_____	5. Establish a routine of withholding feedings, starting an intravenous line, and attaching an electronic heart rate monitor for all babies in whom sepsis is suspected.
_____	_____	6. Establish written protocols for management of infants and pregnant or postpartum women with suspected or proven contagious diseases.
_____	_____	7. Establish a system to provide hepatitis B immunization for *all* babies, according to the recommendations for baby's birth weight and maternal hepatitis B surface antigen status.
_____	_____	8. Consider establishing a policy to provide antimicrobial cleansing of scalp electrode site for all babies who received internal fetal heart rate monitoring.

These are the answers to the self-test questions. Please check them with the answers you gave and review the information in the unit wherever necessary.

A1. Hospital-acquired or nosocomial

A2. A, C, and D

A3. *E coli* infection—A
    Staphylococcal pustulosis—B
    Conjunctivitis—B
    Group B beta hemolytic streptococcus infection—A
    Cytomegalovirus—A and C

A4. False   There is a high mortality rate for babies with sepsis. Also, blood infections in babies may develop into meningitis, which may result in severe damage.

A5. True

A6. True

B1. A

B2. Any 3 of the following:
- Rupture of membranes longer than 18 hours (Although uncommon, it is also possible for a fetus to become infected through intact membranes [ascending infection].)
- Labor longer than 20 hours
- Maternal fever (38°C [100.4°F] or higher) during labor
- Maternal illness (varicella, gastroenteritis, urinary tract infection, etc)
- Preterm delivery
- Pregnant woman with genital herpes simplex lesions at the time membranes rupture
- Birth canal and/or rectum colonized with group B beta hemolytic streptococcus (GBS) or history of a previous infant with GBS infection or GBS bacteriuria at any time during this pregnancy
- Invasive procedure or any foreign body, such as an umbilical catheter
- Prolonged hospitalization (more than several days)

B3. Any 2 of the following:
- High staphylococcal colonization rates in other newborns in the nursery
- Puncture site
- Staphylococcal, gonococcal, or chlamydial infections predisposing an infant to conjunctivitis

B4. D

B5. Swelling at the infected site
    Warmth of the infected area
    Erythema of infected site
    Pustules
    Red, swollen, watery, or pus-filled eye(s), if conjunctivitis

B6. Any 2 of the following:
- Rubella (German measles), syphilis, varicella, or cytomegalovirus infection in the mother during pregnancy
- Maternal exposure to cat litter during pregnancy
- Mother with active genital herpes simplex at the time of delivery
- Mother positive for hepatitis B surface antigen
- Mother positive for HIV

B7. False   A baby with sepsis may have normal laboratory findings. In a baby with risk factors and/or clinical signs of sepsis, the white blood cell (WBC) count and differential findings, if abnormal, may provide further evidence of sepsis. However, a baby who experienced perinatal compromise or who was stressed may have an abnormal WBC count and differential without being infected.

C1. False   While blood cultures should be obtained before antibiotics are started, antibiotic therapy should not be delayed until the culture results are known. As soon as a baby suspected of being septic is stabilized, and cultures are drawn, antibiotics should be started. Many institutions believe this should be done immediately (within 1 hour of birth) or, if the baby becomes sick later, within 1 hour of when sepsis is first suspected. If necessary, the antibiotics used may be readjusted once culture and sensitivity results are known.

C2. Connect the baby to a cardiac monitor.
Establish an intravenous line; consider making NPO.
Check vital signs frequently.
Obtain blood glucose screening tests frequently.

C3. Blood culture
Chest x-ray, if signs of respiratory distress
White blood cell count and differential
Platelet count

C4. Blood pH and serum bicarbonate levels
Lumbar puncture (for stable babies able to tolerate procedure) with simultaneous blood glucose

C5. Gram-positive and gram-negative

C6. C. Gonococcal, chlamydial, and certain staphylococcal infections, however, also require systemic therapy.

C7. Gentamicin

C8. False   Chlamydial conjunctivitis requires treatment with systemic erythromycin or a sulfonamide antibiotic.

C9. True

C10. False   Mild staphylococcal pustulosis can be washed with mild soap and treated with a topical antibiotic. Moderate or severe infections require those measures, plus systemic treatment with suitable antibiotics.

D1. True

D2. False   Most babies with congenital syphilis show no signs or symptoms of the infection at birth. Only a few infected babies will have characteristic findings.

D3. True

D4. True

D5. False   Risk of neonatal herpes infection is very *low* when a woman with a history of herpes infections delivers vaginally and *no active lesions* are present at the time of delivery. The risk of neonatal herpes infection is much higher if active lesions are present
• When vaginal delivery occurs
• When membranes were ruptured for 6 hours or longer before cesarean delivery occurs

D6. True

D7. True

D8. True

D9. True

E1. Good handwashing before and after handling each infant

E2. A

E3. D

E4. False   Gloves may be defective or may become damaged. Hands should be washed each time gloves are changed.

E5.

Yes	No	
x	___	Prevent transmission of organisms from an infected baby to other babies in the nursery.
x	___	Wash hands before and after caring for each baby.
___	x	Keep all babies with proven infections in isolation.
x	___	Prevent transmission of organisms between health care providers and patients.
x	___	Prevent transmission of organisms from an infected baby to health care providers.
___	x	Use broad-spectrum antibiotics for all at-risk patients.

Without referring back to the information in the unit, please answer the following questions. Select the **one best** answer to each question (unless otherwise instructed). Record your answers on the answer sheet that is the last page in this book *and* on the test.

1. What is one reason preterm infants become infected more often than adults?

   A. Some antibodies do not cross the placenta.
   B. They are exposed to more virulent organisms.
   C. They have fewer white blood cells.
   D. The level of complement in the blood is excessively high.

2. Which of the following laboratory findings is *most* suggestive of a systemic infection?

   A. Hyponatremia
   B. Elevated spinal fluid pH
   C. Low blood pH
   D. A ratio of immature to total polymorphonuclear white blood cells of less than 0.2

3. Which of the following procedures is *most* effective in controlling the spread of infection in the nursery?

   A. Have everyone wear hospital scrub clothes.
   B. Require handwashing between handling babies.
   C. Have an air lock between nursery rooms.
   D. Put all babies in incubators.

4. What does it mean for an infant to be at risk for infections?

   A. The probability of an infant becoming sick is proportional to the amount of time the infant is exposed to an infecting organism.
   B. The infant will transfer his or her infection to other people.
   C. An infant is almost ensured of developing an infection.
   D. An infant has been exposed to certain conditions that increase his or her chances of becoming infected.

5. **True**   **False**   When maternal history and laboratory findings indicate a baby needs to be evaluated for congenital syphilis, that evaluation should include a lumbar puncture and testing of the cerebral spinal fluid for evidence of infection.

6. **True**   **False**   Congenital intrauterine cytomegalovirus infection causes severe damage in most fetuses.

7. **True**   **False**   A baby born to a woman with untreated syphilis needs treatment only if the baby is symptomatic or the spinal fluid is abnormal.

8. **True**   **False**   A baby with suspected or proven herpes infection should be isolated from all other babies.

9. **True**   **False**   Human immunodeficiency virus can be passed from an infected mother to her baby in breast milk.

10. **True**   **False**   A baby was born to a woman with membranes ruptured for 48 hours. If the baby has an elevation in the number of immature white blood cells, it is very *unlikely* that he has a blood infection.

11. **True**   **False**   When a baby is suspected of having an infection, starting antibiotics immediately is the only recommended management.

12. **True**   **False**   Once identified, congenital toxoplasmosis infection is easily treated.

13. For each of the following conditions, determine if they place the infant at risk for developing an infection.

    Yes   No
    ___   ___   Infant born preterm
    ___   ___   Mother's vagina colonized with group B beta hemolytic streptococcus
    ___   ___   Father's skin colonized with staphylococcal epidermidis

14. A woman had a normal pregnancy and delivery. The baby weighed 3,300 g (7 lb, 4 oz) and had a 5-minute Apgar score of 9. Thirty-six hours after birth the baby's heart rate increased and the baby began grunting.

Yes	No	
___	___	A change in heart rate is a sign of possible infection in the baby.
___	___	You should suspect that the baby has a systemic infection.
___	___	The first action to take is to begin antibiotic therapy.
___	___	Begin antibiotic therapy only after blood culture results are known.
___	___	Ampicillin and gentamicin would be appropriate drugs for this baby.

For each question, please make sure you have marked your answer on the test and on the answer sheet (last page in book). The test is for you; the answer sheet will need to be turned in for continuing education credit.

PCEP

Perinatal Continuing Education Program

Answer Key
Book II: Neonatal Care
Unit 1: Thermal Environment

Pretest

1. A	8. False
2. D	9. False
3. C	10. True
4. B	11. True
5. A	12. False
6. True	13. False
7. False	

Posttest

1. C	7. True
2. A	8. True
3a. C	9. True
3b. B	10. False
4. False	11. True
5. C	12. True
6. False	13. True

Unit 2: Oxygen Therapy

Pretest

1. B	8. False
2. B	9. True
3. C	10. False
4. A	11. False
5. D	12. True
6. D	13. True
7. True	

Posttest

1. A	8. True
2. D	9. False
3. B	10. False
4. A	11. D
5. True	12. C
6. True	13. C
7. True	

Unit 3: Respiratory Distress

Pretest

1. C	8. B
2. B	9. D
3. D	10. A
4. C	11. False
5. B	12. True
6. A	13. True
7. D	14. C
	15. A
	16. C
	17. B
	18. True

Posttest

1. Tachypnea	6. True
Grunting	7. False
Retracting	8. C
Nasal flaring	9. A
Cyanosis	10. A
2. B	11. D
3. A	12. B
4. D	13. C
5. D	14. C
	15. D
	16. A
	17. B
	18. True

Unit 4: Umbilical Catheters

Pretest

1. A
2. A
3. B
4. Yes   No

Yes	No	
x	___	Thrombosis
x	___	Blood infection
___	x	Brain damage
___	x	Kidney damage
___	x	Loss of toe from embolus

5. False
6. True
7. A
8. C

Posttest

1. B
2. A
3. B
4. D
5. False
6. True
7. False
8. Yes   No

Yes	No	
x	___	Thrombosis
x	___	Sepsis
___	x	Brain damage
x	___	Kidney Damage
x	___	Loss of toe from embolus

Unit 5: Blood Pressure

Pretest

1. D
2. C
3. B
4. A
5. C
6. D
7. E
8. False
9. B
10. C

Posttest

1. D
2. B
3. D
4. C
5. B
6. False
7. B
8. B
9. A
10. C

Unit 6: Hypoglycemia

Pretest

1. True
2. False
3. True
4. True
5. False
6. True
7. B
8. C
9. A
10. A
11. D

Posttest

1. False
2. False
3. False
4. True
5. True
6. True
7. D
8. C
9. A
10. B
11. B

424

Unit 7: Intravenous Therapy

Pretest

1. Yes No

  _x_   ___ 1,590-g vigorous baby on the first day after birth

  ___   _x_ 3,175-g baby with Apgar scores of 6 at 1 and 9 at 5 minutes

  _x_   ___ 3,620-g septic baby who has taken 120 mL of formula during the past 24 hours

  ___   _x_ 2,720-g vigorous baby, mother hospitalized with bacterial pneumonia at 20 weeks' gestation

2. B
3. D
4. C
5. False
6. A
7. B
8. C

Posttest

1. D
2. B
3. A
4. C
5. D
6. False
7. C
8. A

Unit 8: Feedings

Pretest

1. B
2. A
3. D
4. C
5. True
6. False
7. False
8. A
9. B
10. True
11. False
12. True
13. C

Posttest

1. D
2. A
3. C
4. True
5. False
6. False
7. True
8. A
9. False
10. False
11. False
12. False
13. C

Unit 9: Hyperbilirubinemia

Pretest

1. C
2. D
3. B
4. C
5. A
6. A
7. B
8. A
9. Yes   No
   ___   _x_ Cover baby's eyes for first 8 hours
   ___   _x_ Discontinue phototherapy if rash appears
   _x_   ___ Completely undress baby
   ___   _x_ Restrict baby's fluid intake
   ___   _x_ Restrict baby's feedings
10. False
11. False
12. True

Posttest

1. C
2. D
3. B
4. A
5. D
6. A
7. Yes   No
   _x_   ___ Cover baby's eyes
   ___   _x_ Dress baby in special clothing
   ___   _x_ May have to restrict baby's fluid intake
   _x_   ___ Take baby's temperature frequently
8. D
9. True
10. True
11. True
12. False

Unit 10: Infections

Pretest

1. A
2. C
3. C
4. B
5. D
6. True
7. True
8. False
9. True
10. False
11. True
12. True

13. Yes   No
    _x_   ___ Rupture of membranes 24 hours before delivery
    _x_   ___ Active labor for 24 hours
    ___   _x_ father's skin colonized with staphylococcal epidermidis
14. Yes   No
    _x_   ___ Baby at-risk for infection at birth
    _x_   ___ Reduced temperature
    ___   _x_ Localized infection
    _x_   ___ First, begin supportive care and obtain cultures
    _x_   ___ Obtain blood cultures and begin antibiotics
    ___   _x_ Ampicillin alone

Posttest

1. A
2. C
3. B
4. D
5. True
6. False
7. False
8. True
9. True
10. False
11. False
12. False

13. Yes   No
    _x_   ___ Infant born preterm
    _x_   ___ Mother's vagina colonized with Group B beta hemolytic streptococcus
    ___   _x_ Father's skin colonized with staphylococcal epidermidis
14. Yes   No
    _x_   ___ Change in heart rate
    _x_   ___ Suspect baby has systemic infection
    ___   _x_ First, begin antibiotic therapy
    ___   _x_ Begin antibiotic therapy after blood culture results are known
    _x_   ___ Ampicillin and gentamicin

Index

A

ABG. *See* Arterial blood gas (ABG)
Abscess, 383
Acidosis, 10, 114, 121, 136, 244
Acute bilirubin encephalopathy,
    353
Anemia, 114, 390
Antibiotic therapy, 394–395
Antibodies, 383
Apnea, 125
    anticipation and detection, 126
    monitoring to be discontinued,
        129
    recurrent and/or severe, 129
Arterial blood gas (ABG), 95, 119,
    134–135
Arterial blood oxygen (PaO$_2$), 50,
    56–57, 120, 135
    recommended responses to, 61
Arterial carbon dioxide (PaCO$_2$)
    concentration, 120, 135
Arterial spasm, 97
Aspiration syndrome, 114, 133
Automated reagin test, 406

B

Babies
    with additional blood glucose
        monitoring, 269–270
    with apneic spell, 128–129
    at risk for a pneumothorax, 133
    at risk for apnea, 125–126
    at risk for developing feeding
        problems, 317
    at risk for infection, 386–387
    born at term or near term, 318
    breastfeeding, 319, 326
    with certain digestive problems,
        319
    chilled or cold-stressed, 10
    difficulty controlling their own
        temperature, 11

extremely preterm, 290–291,
    291–292
fasted, 265
feeding guidelines for
    appropriate for gestational
        age, 320
following resuscitation, 291
growing satisfactorily, 324–325
guidelines for increasing feedings
    for preterm, 321
with hepatitis B
    immunoprophylaxis, 401
with hyperbilirubinemia,
    367–368
hypotensive, 246
in incubators, 43–44
infected with jaundice, 358–359
infection of, 383
inspired oxygen concentration
    measurement, 79
IV solutions for, 290–291
large for gestational age (LGA),
    264
likely to develop hypoglycemia,
    264
losing fluids, 290
losing heat, 4
low birth weight, 325
with low blood pressure, 244
with low blood glucose, 291
with low blood volume, 245–246
with low body temperature,
    22–23
milk appropriate for gestational
    age, 319–321
milk appropriate for small
    for gestational age,
    321–322
monitoring with oximetry, 93
neutral thermal environment,
    13–15
non-breastfeeding, 319, 325–326

Evaluation Form
Book II: Neonatal Care

Note: Completion of this form, as well as the unit pretests and posttests, is required for continuing education credit.

Date: _____

Your Name: _____   Your Hospital: _____

Work Area: Maternal/Fetal Care ____   Maternal/Fetal and Newborn Care ____
           Maternal/Newborn Care ____   Newborn Care ____   Neonatal Intensive Care ____

Discipline: Physician ___   RN ___   LPN ___   AIDE ___   CNM ___   NP ___   RRT ___   Other ____

For each scale, place an X on the line at the point which best describes how you feel.

1. Were the objectives listed on page 2 of each unit met? Please consider each unit separately when answering questions A through J.

   A. **Thermal Environment** ....
      all met   half met   none met

   B. **Oxygen** ....
      all met   half met   none met

   C. **Respiratory Distress** ....
      all met   half met   none met

   D. **Umbilical Catheters** ....
      all met   half met   none met

   E. **Low Blood Pressure** ....
      all met   half met   none met

   F. **Hypoglycemia** ....
      all met   half met   none met

   G. **Intravenous Therapy** ....
      all met   half met   none met

   H. **Feeding** ....
      all met   half met   none met

   I. **Hyperbilirubinemia** ....
      all met   half met   none met

   J. **Infections** ....
      all met   half met   none met

2. How useful is the material in this book to your work?

   very useful   not at all useful

3. How effectively was the material in this book conveyed?

   very effectively   not at all effectively

4. How confident do you feel that you know the material in this book?

   very confident   not at all confident

5. What is your overall impression of this book?

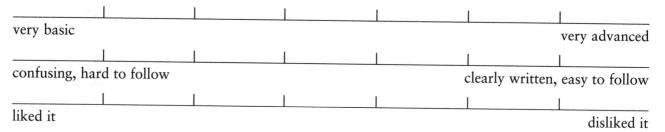

very basic   very advanced

confusing, hard to follow   clearly written, easy to follow

liked it   disliked it

Complete this form, cut it out, and submit it with your test answer sheet. It is required for *AMA PRA Category 1 Credit(s)™* or contact hours. If you are participating in the Perinatal Continuing Education Program through a regional outreach program, a copy may also be needed by the outreach center. See the first page in this book for further information or visit www.pcep.org/cec.html.

PCEP

Perinatal Continuing Education Program

Answer Sheet
Book II: Neonatal Care

Unit 1: Thermal Environment

Pretest

1. A B C
2. A B C D
3. A B C D
4. A B C D
5. A B C D
6. True False
7. True False
8. True False
9. True False
10. True False
11. True False
12. True False
13. True False

Posttest

1. A B C D
2. A B C D
3a. A B C D
3b. A B C D
4. True False
5. A B C D
6. True False
7. True False
8. True False
9. True False
10. True False
11. True False
13. True False

Unit 2: Oxygen

Pretest

1. A B C D
2. A B C D
3. A B C D
4. A B C D
5. A B C D
6. A B C D
7. True False
8. True False
9. True False
10. True False
11. True False
12. True False
13. True False

Posttest

1. A B C D
2. A B C D
3. A B C D
4. A B C D
5. True False
6. True False
7. True False
8. True False
9. True False
10. True False
11. A B C D
12. A B C D
13. A B C D

Unit 3: Respiratory Distress

Pretest

1. A   B   C   D
2. A   B   C   D
3. A   B   C   D
4. A   B   C   D
5. A   B   C   D
6. A   B
7. A   B   C   D
8. A   B
9. A   B   C   D
10. A   B   C
11. True   False
12. True   False
13. True   False
14. A   B   C   D
15. A   B   C   D
16. A   B   C   D
17. A   B   C   D
18. True   False

Posttest

1. _____
   _____
   _____
   _____
   _____
2. A   B   C   D
3. A   B   C   D
4. A   B   C   D
5. A   B   C   D
6. True   False
7. True   False
8. A   B   C   D
9. A   B   C   D
10. A   B   C   D
11. A   B   C   D
12. A   B   C   D
13. A   B   C   D
14. A   B   C   D
15. A   B   C   D
16. A   B   C   D
17. A   B   C   D
18. True   False

Unit 4: Umbilical Catheters

Pretest

1. A   B
2. A   B
3. A   B
4. Yes   No
   ___ ___ Thrombosis
   ___ ___ Blood infection
   ___ ___ Brain damage
   ___ ___ Kidney damage
   ___ ___ Loss of toe from embolus
5. True   False
6. True   False
7. A   B   C   D
8. A   B   C   D

Posttest

1. A   B
2. A   B
3. A   B   C   D
4. A   B   C   D
5. True   False
6. True   False
7. True   False
8. Yes   No
   ___ ___ Thrombosis
   ___ ___ Sepsis
   ___ ___ Brain damage
   ___ ___ Kidney Damage
   ___ ___ Loss of toe from embolus

Unit 5: Low Blood Pressure

Pretest

1. A B C D
2. A B C D
3. A B C D
4. A B C D
5. A B C D
6. A B C D
7. A B C D E
8. True   False
9. A B C D
10. A B C

Posttest

1. A B C D E
2. A B C D
3. A B C D
4. A B C D
5. A B C D
6. True   False
7. A B C D
8. A B C D
9. A B C D
10. A B C

Unit 6: Hypoglycemia

Pretest

1. True   False
2. True   False
3. True   False
4. True   False
5. True   False
6. True   False
7. A B C D
8. A B C D
9. A B C D
10. A B C D
11. A B C D

Posttest

1. True   False
2. True   False
3. True   False
4. True   False
5. True   False
6. True   False
7. A B C D
8. A B C D
9. A B C D
10. A B C D
11. A B C D

Unit 7: Intravenous Therapy

Pretest

1. Yes   No
   __   __   1,590 g vigorous baby on the first day after birth
   __   __   3,175 g baby with Apgar scores of 6 at 1 and 9 at 5 minutes
   __   __   3,620 g septic baby who has taken 120 mL of formula during the past 24 hours
   __   __   2,720 g vigorous baby, mother hospitalized with bacterial pneumonia at 20 weeks gestation
2. A B C D
3. A B C D
4. A B C D
5. True   False
6. A B C D
7. A B C D
8. A B C D

Posttest

1. A B C D
2. A B C D
3. A B C D
4. A B C D
5. A B C D
6. True   False
7. A B C D
8. A B C D

Unit 8: Feeding

Pretest

1. A B C D
2. A B C D
3. A B C D
4. A B C D
5. True   False
6. True   False
7. True   False
8. A B C D
9. A B
10. True   False
11. True   False
12. True   False
13. A B C D

Posttest

1. A B C D
2. A B C D
3. A B C D
4. True   False
5. True   False
6. True   False
7. True   False
8. A B C D
9. True   False
10. True   False
11. True   False
12. True   False
13. A B C D

Unit 9: Hyperbilirubinemia

Pretest

1. A B C D
2. A B C D
3. A B C D
4. A B C
5. A B C D
6. A B C
7. A B C D
8. A B C D
9. Yes   No

___ ___ Cover baby's eyes for first 8 hours
___ ___ Discontinue phototherapy if rash appears
___ ___ Completely undress baby
___ ___ Restrict baby's fluid intake
___ ___ Restrict baby's feedings

10. True   False
11. True   False
12. True   False

Posttest

1. A B C
2. A B C D
3. A B C D
4. A B C D
5. A B C D
6. A B C D
7. Yes   No

___ ___ Cover baby's eyes
___ ___ Dress baby in special clothing
___ ___ May have to restrict baby's fluid intake
___ ___ Take baby's temperature frequently

8. A B C D
9. True   False
10. True   False
11. True   False
12. True   False

Posttest

1. A B C D
2. A B C D
3. A B C D
4. A B C D
5. A B C D
6. True   False
7. True   False
8. True   False
9. True   False
10. True   False
11. True   False
12. True   False
13. Yes   No

___ ___ Rupture of membranes 24 hours before delivery

___ ___ Active labor for 24 hours

___ ___ Father's skin colonized with staphylococcal epidermidis

14. Yes   No

___ ___ Baby at-risk for infection at birth

___ ___ Reduced temperature

___ ___ Localized infection

___ ___ First, begin supportive care and obtain cultures

___ ___ Obtain blood cultures and begin antibiotics

___ ___ Ampicillin alone

Pretest

1. A B C D
2. A B C D
3. A B C D
4. A B C D
5. True   False
6. True   False
7. True   False
8. True   False
9. True   False
10. True   False
11. True   False
12. True   False
13. Yes   No

___ ___ Infant born preterm

___ ___ Mother's vagina colonized with Group B beta hemolytic streptococcus

___ ___ Father's skin colonized with staphylococcal epidermidis

14. Yes   No

___ ___ Change in heart rate

___ ___ Suspect baby has systemic infection

___ ___ First, begin antibiotic therapy

___ ___ Begin antibiotic therapy after blood culture results are known

___ ___ ampicillin and gentamicin